D1538643

Depression

Medical Psychiatry

Series Editor Emeritus

William A. Frosch, M.D.
*Weill Medical College of Cornell University
New York, New York, U.S.A.*

Advisory Board

Jonathan E. Alpert, M.D., Ph.D.
*Massachusetts General Hospital and Harvard
University School of Medicine
Boston, Massachusetts, U.S.A.*

Bennett Leventhal, M.D.
*University of Chicago School of Medicine
Chicago, Illinois, U.S.A.*

Siegfried Kasper, M.D.
*Medical University of Vienna
Vienna, Austria*

Mark H. Rapaport, M.D.
*Cedars-Sinai Medical Center
Los Angeles, California, U.S.A.*

1. Handbook of Depression and Anxiety: A Biological Approach, *edited by Johan A. den Boer and J. M. Ad Sitsen*
2. Anticonvulsants in Mood Disorders, *edited by Russell T. Joffe and Joseph R. Calabrese*
3. Serotonin in Antipsychotic Treatment: Mechanisms and Clinical Practice, *edited by John M. Kane, H.-J. Möller, and Frans Awouters*
4. Handbook of Functional Gastrointestinal Disorders, *edited by Kevin W. Olden*
5. Clinical Management of Anxiety, *edited by Johan A. den Boer*
6. Obsessive-Compulsive Disorders: Diagnosis • Etiology • Treatment, *edited by Eric Hollander and Dan J. Stein*
7. Bipolar Disorder: Biological Models and Their Clinical Application, *edited by L. Trevor Young and Russell T. Joffe*
8. Dual Diagnosis and Treatment: Substance Abuse and Comorbid Medical and Psychiatric Disorders, *edited by Henry R. Kranzler and Bruce J. Rounsaville*
9. Geriatric Psychopharmacology, *edited by J. Craig Nelson*
10. Panic Disorder and Its Treatment, *edited by Jerrold F. Rosenbaum and Mark H. Pollack*
11. Comorbidity in Affective Disorders, *edited by Mauricio Tohen*

Depression
Treatment Strategies and Management

edited by

Thomas L. Schwartz
SUNY Upstate Medical University
Syracuse, New York, U.S.A.

Timothy J. Petersen
Massachussetts General Hospital
Harvard Medical School
Boston, Massachusetts, U.S.A.

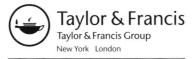

Taylor & Francis
Taylor & Francis Group
New York   London

Taylor & Francis is an imprint of the
Taylor & Francis Group, an informa business

Published in 2006 by
Taylor & Francis Group
270 Madison Avenue
New York, NY 10016

© 2006 by Taylor & Francis Group, LLC

No claim to original U.S. Government works
Printed in the United States of America on acid-free paper
10 9 8 7 6 5 4 3 2

International Standard Book Number-10: 0-8493-4027-6 (Hardcover)
International Standard Book Number-13: 978-0-8493-4027-7 (Hardcover)
Library of Congress Card Number 2005056856

Library of Congress Cataloging-in-Publication Data

Depression : treatment strategies and management / edited by Thomas L. Schwartz, Timothy J. Petersen.
    p. ; cm. -- (Medical psychiatry ; 34)
    Includes bibliographical references and index.
    ISBN-13: 978-0-8493-4027-7 (alk. paper)
    ISBN-10: 0-8493-4027-6 (alk. paper)
    1. Depression, Mental. I. Schwartz, Thomas L. II. Petersen, Timothy J. III. Series.
    [DNLM: 1. Depressive Disorder--therapy. WM 171 D4241997 2006]

RC537.D4462 2006
616.85'27--dc22
                           2005056856

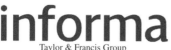

Taylor & Francis Group
is the Academic Division of Informa plc.

**Visit the Taylor & Francis Web site at
http://www.taylorandfrancis.com**

Dr. Schwartz would like to thank his family: Beth, Connor, Sarah, Christopher, Rose, Lauren, Marjorie, and Brian for their love and support. He would like to further acknowledge the excellent training he received under the guidance of the faculty at SUNY Upstate Medical University.

Dr. Petersen dedicates this book to his supportive family, his wonderful colleagues at the Depression Clinical and Research Program, and in particular his mentor, Dr. Maurizio Fava.

Finally, the editors would like to acknowledge the hard and dedicated work of Mark Chilton in the editing and compilation of chapters in this book.

Foreword

Drs. Schwartz and Petersen have put together a state-of-the-art book on depression that should be of great interest to psychiatrists and, indeed, to all mental health practitioners. The book is a collection of current issues in the treatment of depression, including the "hot topics" in this area and has been synthesized from contributions by some of the world's leading experts. Scholarly, highly referenced with many recently published citations, it covers the waterfront from clinical descriptions of depression, to the biological basis of depression, to the plethora of available treatments for depression, and beyond.

Beginning with an excellent description of the syndrome, this text then explores a very comprehensive analysis of the pathophysiology of depression, beyond the monoamine hypothesis, to include contemporary ideas that incorporate other neurotransmitters, neuroendocrine links, signal transduction theories, and genetic links—a topic that is expanded later in the text in a dedicated chapter. Another chapter covers recent advances in the burgeoning field of neuroimaging as well as neurophysiology of depression.

Perhaps one of the most unique aspects of this text is how it deals with therapeutics in depression. Rather than recount a litany of drugs, with an emphasis mostly on the new agents as is typical for many texts, here there is a major effort over several chapters, to deal with therapeutics in a balanced manner that is very relevant to clinical practice, namely, old drugs and therapies as well as new ones, how to combine therapies, how to maintain therapies, and how to get the best outcomes. If the data do not yield clear answers, these chapters deal with the best theories and hypotheses in regards to best treatment practices. Specifically, the therapeutics section of this book speaks in detail about combining drugs with psychotherapies, assessing the randomized clinical trials of a wide range of psychotherapies alone or in combination with antidepressants, combining drugs, not only to get better efficacy for lack of remission or treatment resistance, but also to improve tolerability. There is a balanced and refreshing approach to using and combining new as well as old, psychopharmacology as well as psychotherapy, that will be of immediate practical use to the clinician. The theme is pragmatic and outcomes oriented, not theoretically lopsided toward either biological/psychopharmacologic or psychological approaches to treatment. There is even a modern chapter on various somatic treatments including electroconvulsive therapy (ECT) and its related new therapeutics transcranial magnetic stimulation (TMS), vagal nerve stimulation (VNS), deep brain stimulation (DBS), and magnetic seizure therapy (MST).

In sum, the reader will enjoy a useful, comprehensive approach to depression and its treatment and will emerge well informed from a scholarly yet practical approach.

Stephen Stahl, M.D.
Professor of Psychiatry
University of California
San Diego School of Medicine
San Diego, California, U.S.A.

Preface

Major depressive disorder (MDD) is one of the most prevalent mental illnesses and may be one of the most dangerous considering resultant suicide rates. Bona fide treatment options date back to the 1800s. Research and clinical experience have offered us several effective forms of psychotherapy and multiple effective medications. There are also newer medications and somatic treatments in the pipeline that may offer additional treatment options in the future. Despite treatment, it is rare to bring a depressed patient to a full, sustained remission. Therefore, polypharmacy, psychotherapy, and multi-modal treatments are the norm.

The book provides an authoritative and up-to-date review of current knowledge regarding the treatment of MDD. We briefly cover symptomatology, diagnosis, epidemiology, and etiological theories as a review, followed by a more in-depth look at the pharmacodynamic history of FDA antidepressant approval and the purported mechanism of action by which these drugs treat depression. This gives a clear review of the antidepressants with links to the etiological theories. At the close of every pharmacologic chapter, the parallels for psychotherapy are considered. A final chapter describes newer treatment options and research endeavors currently in development.

The major clinical segments of this book discuss research data and clinical experience regarding acute outcomes, long-term outcomes, and combination treatment outcomes to improve effectiveness and tolerability. Rational polypharmacy and combination with psychotherapy are discussed, and future treatments that may be used in combination strategy are discussed as well.

The closing segment evaluates the possible future of treating major depression. We attempt to evaluate the pharmacotherapy and psychotherapy pipeline of treatments soon to be available or currently being studied.

We discuss, as well, genetics and neuro-imaging as cutting-edge techniques that will eventually improve our ability to treat major depressive disorder.

This book was written by key authors and provides a state-of-the-art review and clinical compendium about treating depression with multiple therapies. The fundamental focus was a book tailored to the multiple needs of those who prescribe psychotropics and/or perform psychotherapy, serving as a reference, practical review, journal watch, and clinical guideline in one convenient form. Psychiatrists, residents in training, nurse practitioners, psychologists, social workers, and even primary care physicians who do the majority of antidepressant prescribing should find this book a useful tool.

Thomas L. Schwartz
Timothy J. Petersen

Contents

Contributors

Jeremy Barowski Department of Psychiatry, SUNY Upstate Medical University, Syracuse, New York, U.S.A.

Boadie W. Dunlop Department of Psychiatry and Behavioral Sciences, Emory University School of Medicine, Atlanta, Georgia, U.S.A.

Giovanni A. Fava Department of Psychology, University of Bologna, Bologna, Italy and Department of Psychiatry, State University of New York at Buffalo, Buffalo, New York, U.S.A.

Holly Garriock Interdisciplinary Program in Genetics and Psychiatry, University of Arizona, Tucson, Arizona, U.S.A.

Mark Goldman Brown University, Providence, Rhode Island, U.S.A.

Corey Goldstein Department of Psychiatry, Rush University Medical Center, Chicago, Illinois, U.S.A.

Geoffrey Hopkins Department of Psychiatry, SUNY Upstate Medical University, Syracuse, New York, U.S.A.

Dan V. Iosifescu Depression Clinical and Research Program, Massachusetts General Hospital, Harvard Medical School, Boston, Massachusetts, U.S.A.

Arun Kunwar   Department of Psychiatry, SUNY Upstate Medical University, Syracuse, New York, U.S.A.

Antonio Mantovani   Department of Neuroscience, Division of Brain Stimulation and Neuromodulation, Columbia University, New York, New York, U.S.A. and Department of Neuroscience, Postgraduate School in Applied Neurological Sciences, Siena University, Siena, Italy

James L. Megna   Department of Psychiatry, SUNY Upstate Medical University, Syracuse, New York, U.S.A.

Francisco Moreno   Department of Psychiatry, College of Medicine, The University of Arizona Health Sciences Center, Tucson, Arizona, U.S.A.

Nikhil Nihalani   Department of Psychiatry, University of Rochester School of Medicine, Rochester, New York, U.S.A.

George I. Papakostas   Massachusetts General Hospital/Harvard Medical School, Boston, Massachusetts, U.S.A.

Timothy J. Petersen   Massachusetts General Hospital/Harvard Medical School, Boston, Massachusetts, U.S.A.

Chiara Ruini   Department of Psychology, University of Bologna, Bologna, Italy and Department of Psychiatry, State University of New York at Buffalo, Buffalo, New York, U.S.A.

Thomas L. Schwartz   Department of Psychiatry, SUNY Upstate Medical University, Syracuse, New York, U.S.A.

Richard C. Shelton   Department of Psychiatry, Vanderbilt University School of Medicine, Nashville, Tennessee, U.S.A.

Mihai Simionescu   Department of Psychiatry, SUNY Upstate Medical University, Syracuse, New York, U.S.A.

Lynn Stormon   Department of Psychiatry, SUNY Upstate Medical University, Syracuse, New York, U.S.A.

Michael E. Thase   University of Pittsburgh Medical Center, Western Psychiatric Institute and Clinic, Pittsburgh, Pennsylvania, U.S.A.

John M. Zajecka   Department of Psychiatry, Rush University Medical Center, Chicago, Illinois, U.S.A.

1

Epidemiology, Symptomatology, and Diagnosis

James L. Megna and Mihai Simionescu

Department of Psychiatry, SUNY Upstate Medical University, Syracuse, New York, U.S.A.

INTRODUCTION

The core elements of what we now call major depressive disorder (MDD) are as old as the history of mankind. Nevertheless, the ways in which we choose to approach these elements reflect the unfolding of human knowledge in this expanding area of clinical care and research. Hippocrates of Cos (460–377 B.C.) talked about melancholia, a condition that was essentially described very similarly to today's MDD specifier (1) including prolonged despondency, blue moods, detachment, anhedonia, irritability, restlessness, sleeplessness, aversion to food, diurnal variation, and suicidal impulses. An essential element in the identification of melancholia was the groundless character of the despondency. It was thus recognized that human beings have a potential for experiencing intense states of sadness often in response to adversity. Mourning and grief were viewed in a normalizing perspective and only the presence of excessive, psychotic, or unmotivated sadness was construed as "disordered." This distinction was maintained for many years in the definition of "depressive neurosis" as described in the Diagnostic and Statistical Manual of Mental Disorders (DSM)-II (2). Starting with DSM-III (3), however, any theoretical underpinnings regarding the causes of illnesses, including depression, were removed. Mental illnesses were now conceptualized as symptom-based, categorical diseases (4).

This nonetiological and atheoretical classification greatly improved the reliability of depressive disorder diagnosis by avoiding potentially gray areas. These include whether or not the condition is comprehensive in the individual's history of adversities. The only exception included in DSM-IV (5) refers to the two-month interval after the death of a loved one during which bereavement would be diagnosed.

As noted above, the ability to diagnose MDD has been greatly improved by the categorical approach. However, MDD tends to be a fairly heterogenous state with fluctuating symptoms over time, and a broader approach to phenomenology must be undertaken and appreciated to better treat our patients.

PHENOMENOLOGY OF DEPRESSIVE STATES

The psychic functional problems encountered by depressed individuals are extensive and not limited to the affective domain. For example, Jaspers (6) describes the archetypal features of depression as noted below, and he also recognizes the heterogeneity of depression and suggests that individual cases may not present with the same extent of disturbance in all categorical dimensions.

Its [depression] central core is formed from an equally unmotivated and profound sadness to which is added a retardation of psychic events, which is as subjectively painful as it is objectively visible. All instinctual activities are subjected to it. The patient does not want to do anything. The reduced impulse to move and to do things turns into complete immobility. No decision can be made and no activity begun. Associations are not available. Patients have no ideas. They complain of a complete disruption of memory. They feel their poverty of performance and complain of their inefficiency, lack of emotion, and emptiness. They feel profound gloom as a sensation in the chest or body as if it could be laid hold of there. The depth of their melancholy makes them see the world as grim and gray. They look for the unfavorable and unhappy elements in everything. They accuse themselves of much past guilt (self-accusations, notions of having sinned). The present has nothing for them (notion of worthlessness) and the future lies horrifyingly before them (notions of poverty etc.).

All these individual features described an extreme of pathology and distortion, and are meaningfully connected in the "symptom-complex" of depression. By examining in some detail the phenotypical dimensions of depressive states, we can focus on descriptive aspects of depression and not necessarily on ultimate diagnostic features. We will see that there is a wealth of possible descriptors of individual depressive states that are not necessarily diagnostic.

MDD's central descriptive features refer to the disturbance of feelings and affective states. Exhibiting a "depressed mood" may vary greatly in terms of individual experience. There may be alterations in the way one's body is experienced with regard to the "bodily feeling" or the "vital feeling." Sadness may be described at a very vague physical level such as the feeling of "pressure" or "misery." A common presentation is with "feelings of insufficiency," a sense of diminished capacity or "self-esteem." In addition, there is often a lowering of the "executive" abilities to understand, think, make decisions, and act with the emergence of the feeling of being incompetent, useless, or worthless.

In other cases, there may be an increased indifference to the environment with a decreased reactivity to stimuli, whether considered positive or negative by the patient. Striking in these descriptions is the inability to experience pleasurable events, called anhedonia. This particular condition needs to be seen in the continuum of human experience with varying degrees to which anhedonia is the extreme. Severe cases of anhedonia may be accompanied by apathy or an absence of any feeling. Apathy, in turn, may lead to abulia or lack of will to act. In these cases, the patient may passively endanger himself or herself by not eating, not avoiding possible noxious situations, nor looking out for his/her best interests. In a context of lack of joy (anhedonia), loss of feelings (apathy), and lack of will to act (abulia), the future is often construed as hopeless. This may be a particularly vulnerable period for the emergence of recurrent thoughts about death and possible suicidal activity.

The phenomenology of depression is not confined solely to disturbances of feelings and affective states. Often there are changes in other psychic phenomena such as perception (awareness of objects), experience of space and time, thinking (awareness of reality), and self-awareness. Alterations of the emotional tone of perception are relatively common experiences for the depressed individual. Habitual objects, the environment as a whole, or sometimes even the "self" may appear different, often with an unsatisfactory, frustrating quality. Things may not look the same as before, and a sense of derealization may emerge. It may seem as if time has stopped, and generally time-awareness may lose reliability. Hallucinations and delusions are possible. In severe cases, reality testing will be further affected and various cognitive distortions may be present affecting the patient's mental capacity. Spanning a large interval from transient thoughts of worthlessness and hopelessness to entrenched delusions of sin and guilt, emerging psychosis and thought disturbance may be comparable to that seen in schizophrenic spectrum disorders. Far from being exhaustive, this narrative description of the depressive state illustrates the potential heterogeneity of depressive disorders.

CLASSIFICATION OF THE DEPRESSIVE STATES

As discussed previously about the phenomenology of depressive states, individual clinical presentations may be quite different while still maintaining core features of depression. These cases can be not only clinically diverse, but also often have different courses and prognoses. Even the modalities of treatment may vary based on symptom heterogeneity. Now that we better understand the phenomenology of MDD, the ability to move toward a categorical and defining set of depressive symptoms is warranted. This may allow for a more accurate diagnosis that should ultimately improve patient outcomes, clinician communication regarding MDD, and facilitation of research in MDD.

Table 1 includes the categorical variants of depressive states included in DSM-IV-TR^{TM} (1). As you will note, even the categorical approach to

Table 1 DSM-IV-TR Depressive States

MDE (not a diagnostic per se)	
MDD (single episode or recurrent)	296.2x or 296.3x
Dysthymic disorder	300.4
Bipolar I disorder (most recent episode depressed or mixed)	296.5x, 296.6x
Bipolar II disorder (most recent episode depressed or mixed)	296.89
Cyclothymic disorder	301.13
Mood disorder due to general medical condition (with depressive features or with major depressive-like episode)	293.83
Substance-induced mood disorder (with depressive features or with mixed features)	
Bipolar disorder NOS	296.80
Depressive disorder NOS	311
Adjustment disorder (with depressed mood, with mixed anxiety and depressed mood, and with mixed disturbance of emotions and conduct)	309.0, 309.28, or 309.4
Comorbid conditions	

DSM-IV-TR Appendix B: Proposed new categories for depressive states
Postpsychotic depressive disorder of schizophrenia
Minor depressive disorder
Recurrent brief depressive disorder
Mixed anxiety–depressive disorder
Depressive personality disorder

Abbreviations: MDE, major depressive episode; MDD, major depressive disorder; NOS, not otherwise specified; DSM, Diagnostic and Statistical Manual of Mental Disorders.

depressive disorders has allowed some flexibility in diagnosis by creation of multiple categories.

DIFFERENTIAL DIAGNOSIS OF THE DEPRESSIVE STATES

In the DSM-IV-TR^{TM} (1), the central diagnostic building block is the major depressive episode (MDE). An MDE is present when the patient is exhibiting five out of the following nine symptoms as a discrete presentation lasting at least two weeks. The symptoms are depressed mood, diminished interest or pleasure in activities, loss of appetite or weight loss, sleep disturbance as insomnia or hypersomnia, psychomotor agitation or retardation, loss of energy, feelings of worthlessness or guilt, poor concentration, and recurrent thoughts about death or suicidal ideation, plan, or intent. Depressed mood or diminished interest (or pleasure in activities) must be one of the first symptoms. Defining the threshold for disorder would suggest that symptom severity be high enough to affect the patient's psychosocial functioning.

If a certain patient is experiencing the first MDE in his or her lifetime, MDD (single episode) is diagnosed. Conversely, if previous episodes have been present, MDD (recurrent) is considered. Additional specifiers will indicate the intensity of the condition (mild, moderate, severe, with or without psychotic features, etc.); the presence of particular clinical variants (catatonic, melancholic, atypical, and in postpartum), or the longitudinal variability (partial or full remission or the presence of seasonal patterns) may be used for a more accurate diagnosis.

If the MDE is experienced in the context of a history of at least one manic episode or hypomanic episode, then a diagnosis of bipolar I disorder or bipolar II disorder, respectively, may be made. Mixed states of combined (hypo) mania and depression may also occur in the realm of this set of disorders.

Dysthymic disorder is defined as having a depressed mood present, more days than not, for two years (one year in children and adolescents) in the presence of other associated symptoms of depression. The patient has to have at least two out of the following six symptoms: appetite disturbance, sleep disturbance, low energy, low self-esteem, poor concentration, and feelings of hopelessness.

Diagnostic considerations of special attention would include the presence of pertinent, clearly identifiable causes of distress like medical conditions, substance abuse or dependence, bereavement, or other stressors as in adjustment disorders. In these areas, treatment options and prognosis may differ widely. Residual categories are represented by depressive disorder and bipolar disorder not otherwise specified (NOS). Use of these "NOS" rubrics is indicated when ultimate diagnosis is unclear (including when it is not known if the condition is primary or secondary) or if key facets from categories overlap to make diagnosis difficult or impossible in the DSM-IV-TR categorical system.

A symptom-based approach to depression lends weight to the consideration that certain key symptoms may have more capacity to distinguish between MDD and other psychiatric conditions such as generalized anxiety disorder. "Guilt," "trouble concentrating," "lost appetite," and "wanting to die" were found to be more powerful in this regard (7). The clinical presentation of MDD may be further complicated by the presence of both psychological and medical comorbidities. The level of comorbidity in depression is often greater than 30% for anxiety disorders (8).

A solid working knowledge of the categorical DSM system, including areas outside of MDD, is warranted because anxiety disorders and substance use disorders are relatively common and relatively treatable conditions. Interest has also developed in some prognostically difficult areas, and research has been dedicated to the relationship between depression and somatization (9), trauma (10), dissociation (11), and borderline personality disorder (12). It may often be very difficult to tease out the medical symptomatology of the former from the enduring symptoms of chronic, empty depression and the self-injurious thoughts and behaviors of the latter.

EPIDEMIOLOGICAL INFORMATION

Now that we have reviewed the classic phenomenology and have discussed how the DSM-IV-TR (9–12) has better organized the diagnosis of MDD, the next step would be to discuss the frequency of this illness in the general population. The lifetime prevalence of MDD is 10% to 25% for women and between 5% and 12% in men (13,14). Nevertheless, after the first episode of depression, the female-to-male risk tends to become equal. These overall figures are significantly higher than the prevalence of bipolar disorders, which is roughly 0.4% to 1.6%. Bipolar illness is thought to be a more severe and pervasive illness, but MDD is also chronic and ultimately affects many more individuals. Most MDD patients will have an onset between the ages of 20 and 40 years. Today, depression is the second leading cause of burden of disease in the 15 to 44 years age category (15).

Some risk and predictive factors for MDD have been cited. Being admitted to a hospital or a long-term care facility, as well as having an increased number of outpatient visits for somatic reasons, tends to increase the risk for depression, or at least its detection (16,17). Other risk factors may be represented by lower socioeconomic status, separated and divorced status, and the presence of a relative excess of social stressors (18). Last but not least, correlations have been made regarding an increased risk for MDD with positive family history (19) the presence of early adverse experiences, and certain borderline personality attributes (20).

Generally, the prevalence of depression is thought to decrease after the age of 45; however, the diagnosis of depression in the elderly poses significant public health problems because this clinical population is expanding at a phenomenal rate. Risk factors in the geriatric population include female sex, low socioeconomical level, bereavement, prior depression, medical comorbidities and disability, cognitive deterioration, and vascular factors (21).

Finally, the greatest risk associated with MDD is the threat of suicide, both attempted and completed. Thirty percent of completed suicide cases have a mood disorder diagnosis (22,23). Moreover, MDD is associated with much social disability, and the lifetime risk of death by suicide may be as high as 15% (24). It seems increasingly important that we develop even more accurate diagnostic methods to allow us to choose the most appropriate treatment modality for our patients. Continuing work is warranted in order to better define the etiology of MDD. As mentioned above, the heterogenous mixture of symptoms that MDD patients experience points to a multifactorial etiology for this disorder, which makes research in this area more difficult. In our modern era, advanced techniques including neuroimaging, molecular genetics, and translational and solid clinical studies are helping to elucidate etiological factors, and thereby determine the ultimate causes of the MDD symptoms that we have discussed above. Improved treatment modalities will surely follow.

REFERENCES

1. Diagnostic and Statistical Manual of Mental Disorders. 4th ed Text Revision. American Psychiatric Association, 2000; 419–420.
2. Diagnostic and Statistical Manual of Mental Disorders. 2nd edition. American Psychiatric Association, 1968.
3. Diagnostic and Statistical Manual of Mental Disorders. 3rd edition. American Psychiatric Association, 1980.
4. Mayes R, Horwitz AV. DSM-III and the revolution in the classification of mental illness. J Hist Behav Sci 2005; 41(3):249–267.
5. Diagnostic and Statistical Manual of Mental Disorders. 4th ed Text Revision. American Psychiatric Association, 2000; 740–741
6. Jaspers K. General Psychopathology. Johns Hopkins University Press, 1997:596–597 (translation of the 1959 Springer-Verlag Berlin-Heidelberg edition of Allgemeine Psychopathologie).
7. Breslau N, Davis GC. Refining DSM-III criteria in major depression An assessment of the descriptive validity of criterion symptoms. J Affect Disord 1985; 9(3):199–206.
8. McLaughlin T, Geissler EC, Wan GJ. Comorbidities and associated treatment charges in patients with anxiety disorders. Pharmacotherapy 2003; 23(10): 1251–1256.
9. Lipsanen T, Saarijarvi S, Lauerma H. Exploring the relations between depression, somatization, dissociation and alexithymia–overlapping or independent constructs? Psychopathology 2004; 37(4):200–206.
10. Feeny NC, Zoellner LA, Fitzgibbons LA, Foa EB. Exploring the roles of emotional numbing, depression, and dissociation in PTSD. J Trauma Stress 2000; 13(3):489–498.

11. Fullerton CS, Ursano RJ, Epstein RS, et al. Peritraumatic dissociation following motor vehicle accidents: relationship to prior trauma and prior major depression. J Nerv Ment Dis 2000; 188(5):267–272.

12. Atlas JA, Wolfson MA. Depression and dissociation as features of borderline personality disorder in hospitalized adolescents. Psychol Rep 1996; 78(2): 624–626.

13. Blazer DG II. Mood disorders: epidemiology. In: Sadock VA, Sadock BJ, eds. Kaplan and Sadock's Comprehensive Textbook of Psychiatry. Philadelphia Lippincott: Williams and Wilkins, 2000:1299.

14. Kessler RC. Epidemiology of women and depression. J Affect Disord 2003; 74(1):5–13.

15. http://www.who.int/mental_health/management/depression/definition/en/ (accessed on 8th March 2005).

16. Battaglia A, Dubini A, Mannheimer R, Pancheri P. Depression in the Italian community: epidemiology and socio-economic implications. Int Clin Psychopharmacol 2004; 19(3):135–142.

17. Addington AM, Gallo JJ, Ford DE, Eaton WW. Epidemiology of unexplained fatigue and major depression in the community: the Baltimore ECA follow-up, 1981–1994. Psychol Med 2001; 31(6):1037–1044.

18. Lehtinen V, Joukamaa M. Epidemiology of depression: prevalence, risk factors and treatment situation. Acta Psychiatr Scand Suppl 1994; 377:7–10.

19. Sullivan PF, Neale MC, Kendler KS. Genetic epidemiology of major depression: review and meta-analysis. Am J Psychiat 2000; 157(10):1552–1562.

20. Bellino S, Patria L, Paradiso E, et al. Major depression in patients with borderline personality disorder: a clinical investigation. Can J Psychiat 2005; 50(4): 234–238.

21. Helmer C, Montagnier D, Peres K. Descriptive epidemiology and risk factors of depression in the elderly. Psychol Neuropsychiat Vieil 2004; 2(suppl 1):S7–S12.

22. Bertolote JM, Fleischmann A, De Leo D, Wasserman D. Psychiatric diagnoses and suicide: revisiting the evidence. Crisis 2004; 25(4):147–155.

23. Inskip HM, Harris EC, Barracough B. Lifetime risk of suicide for affective disorder, alcoholism, and schizophrenia. Br J Psychiat 1998; 172:35–37.

24. Kaplan HI, Sadock BJ. Synopsis of Psychiatry: Behavioral Sciences Clinical Psychiatry. 9th ed. Philadelphia: Lippincott, Williams and Wilkins, 2003.

2

Substrates of Sadness: The Pathophysiology of Depression

Boadie W. Dunlop

Department of Psychiatry and Behavioral Sciences, Emory University School of Medicine, Atlanta, Georgia, U.S.A.

Nikhil Nihalani

Department of Psychiatry, University of Rochester School of Medicine, Rochester, New York, U.S.A.

INTRODUCTION

Theories regarding the etiology of depressive states have been linked inextricably to models of treatment throughout medical history. The rationale for a healer's choice of treatment derives from the need to correct what has gone awry in the sufferer, according to the explanatory framework for the illness. In pre-scientific civilizations, mental illnesses were deemed to have resulted from some spiritual or magical force, thus requiring treatment through prayer, sacrifice, or other means (1). With the emergence of science under the civilizations of ancient Greece and Rome, theories changed from these ethereal concepts to those focused on the body and material causes. The methods of science have advanced tremendously over the past two millennia resulting in more numerous and effective treatments for depression and other mental illness. However, the etiology of major depression continues to be elusive despite the plethora of biological features found to differ between depressed and non-depressed people.

Part of the difficulty in determining the etiology of depression is the tendency of the illness to remit spontaneously, and its high level of responsiveness to placebo treatments. Through history, a number of interventions and compounds have been considered efficacious, though improvement likely stemmed simply from the natural history of the illness, or the common "placebo" components activated by administration of any treatment: instillation of hope, expression of concern, and an explanatory framework for the illness (2). While the tendency of depression to remit with time and care has and will always be a boon for care-providers, it has been a bane for researchers attempting to delineate the pathophysiology of the illness. Though researchers today have more tools than ever to investigate how depressed people differ from the non-depressed, the lessons from history have highlighted the challenge of pinpointing the biological basis of what is, at its core, a primarily subjective affective experience.

HISTORICAL DEVELOPMENT OF A BIOLOGICAL APPROACH TO DEPRESSION

The first recorded theories of a biological basis for major depression were developed by the ancient Greeks, through the theories of the four humors as outlined in the Corpus Hippocraticum in the fifth century B.C. (3). The humors corresponded to components of temperament, so that yellow bile was linked to a choleric or irritable temperament, blood to being sanguine or cheerful, phlegm to a phlegmatic style or stoicism, and black bile to melancholy or sadness. Applied to subjects experiencing depression, the theory identified "melancholia" or excessive black bile in the blood, as the root of the problem. Using the logic for which they are justly famous, Greek physicians applied the treatment of phlebotomy to lower the excessive levels of black bile. In a very real sense, these physicians were remedying what they perceived to be a "chemical imbalance." From today's perspective, we wonder how such treatment could have persisted for over a millennium, given the lowered levels of energy and vigor that must have resulted from such declines in hematocrit. Yet, we ought to pause to consider how is it that those physicians had such confidence in the treatment. Certainly it was dramatic, and thus may have induced additional effects in emotion-processing neurocircuits than the usual placebo treatments. The fatigue resulting from the treatment may have led to socially sanctioned relief from work or other stressors. But perhaps there were other biologic effects: an alteration in the stress response or immune-modulation systems, release of endogenous opioids or other neurotransmitters, or possibly altered signaling from the vagus nerve to the brain as a result of changes in cardiac functioning stemming from the bloodletting? While we no longer believe there is a black substance in the blood that directly lowers mood, the practice of bloodletting exemplifies how a theory of etiology (the four humors) can lead to an intervention (bloodletting) that may lead to improvement in illness, though perhaps for reasons completely unrelated to the theoretical and psychological model of the illness.

Of all the conditions identified in the Hippocratic classification scheme, melancholia is the only one to survive by the same name today, perhaps reflecting the ongoing challenge of adequately determining its etiology (4). The syndrome of melancholia continued to be described throughout the Dark and Middle Ages with little revision. However, St. Augustine's philosophical distinction between the origin of emotional functions and imagination in the "inferior soul," compared with the origin of higher mental functions such as intellect and will in the "superior soul," contributed to a greater level of moral theorizing about depression and mental illness in general (3,5).

It was not until the late 18th century, during the Age of Enlightenment, that humoral theories of melancholia gave way to a focus on the central nervous system (CNS). Wilhelm Griesinger (1817–1868) was perhaps the most important early contributor to the neurological investigation of psychiatric disorders. Griesinger argued that mental illness without exception stemmed from somatic changes and attempted to identify relationships between psychological symptoms and brain pathology (5).

While Griesinger contributed substantially to the concept of the neurobiological basis of mental illness, he held the view that the various forms of mental illness, including melancholia, simply reflected a unitary disease process at different levels of severity. It fell to Emil Kraepelin (1856–1926), through his dedicated long-term observation of thousands of patients, to lay the foundation for the current classification scheme for psychiatric disorders. Kraepelin grouped mental illnesses that preserved the premorbid personality of the individual under the category of manic-depressive illness, including what we today label bipolar disorder, major depression, and milder forms of mood disturbance (5). Dementia praecox (later renamed schizophrenia by Eugene Bleuler) was separated from the mood disorders because of its poor long-term prognosis, leading to personality decline. While many other eminent psychiatrists contributed to the formation of the neurobiological conceptualization of major depression, the work of Kraepelin and Griesinger founded the basic "what" and "how" to guide biological mood research to the present.

Sigmund Freud was a contemporary of Kraepelin who, though trained in the neurobiological approach to mental illness, came to focus his life's efforts on understanding the psychological processes at work in people. His seminal paper, Mourning and Melancholia, identified hostility against a psychologically internalized lost object as the root cause of depressive symptoms (6). The rise of psychodynamically focused psychiatry, particularly in the United States in the period around World War II, led to a substantial pause in biological exploration of major depression and other mental illnesses. It was not until the decade after the serendipitous discovery of the mood elevating effects of two medications that neurobiological investigation began in earnest again. The psychological theoretical approach is certainly worth review and study, but is outside the scope of this chapter. Key names and works that usually surface with regards to the psychological etiology of major depressive disorder (MDD) include Freud, Skinner, Beck, and Sullivan, to name a few. As we will see in following chapters, psychological as well as biological treatment are safe and effective in promoting resolution of depressive symptoms. Chapter 3 will explore the development of psychotherapy techniques and shed more light on the psychological etiologies of this disorder.

CLUES AND CHALLENGES TO EXPLORING THE NEUROBIOLOGICAL BASIS OF DEPRESSION

Observations of the natural course of various diseases provide some clues as to the biological cause of depression. For example, depressive symptoms emerging from the hypercortisolemia of Cushing's disease, the loss of dopaminergic function in Parkinson's disease, and the thyroid dysfunction in hypothyroidism all suggest a role for these elements in the pathophysiology of major depression.

Another source of clues is the biological effects induced by treatments that alleviate depressive symptoms. Indeed, the most influential theories of depressive pathophysiology derive from such observations. This approach, however, is fraught with the potential for etiological red herrings. Treatments may indeed correct the underlying source of an illness, as when an antibiotic kills the infectious germ. However, treatments may also induce improvement via mechanisms unrelated to the actual cause of the disease, such as diuretics in the treatment of essential hypertension. If a treatment reduces symptomatology without correcting the core pathologic process, it is possible that the disease may continue to progress until it reaches a point where such treatments are no longer effective. Finally, treatments may also cause measurable changes in aspects of biological systems unrelated to the pathophysiology of an illness, such as the cognitive slowing resulting from the use of nonselective beta-blockers in hypertension. In the relationship between treatment effects and disease pathophysiology, not all that can be counted counts and, perhaps, not all that counts can be counted (yet). In this light, it is helpful to recognize that the foci of biological research into depression pathophysiology have arisen largely from the discovery of effective pharmacologic treatments, more so than treatments have emerged from scientific investigation.

There are several great challenges facing those attempting to explore the origins of major depression. In addition to the previously mentioned placebo responsiveness and remitting nature of the illness, the clinical syndrome of major depression likely represents the final common phenotypic expression of several separate disease processes. The continuing limitations in adequately defining clinical subtypes of MDD are a significant hindrance to identifying homogeneous samples of patients who may share the same biological disturbances. Another ongoing challenge is to separate state effects (i.e., those features of the biology present only during the depressive episode) from trait effects (i.e., the biological features that are present before, during and after an episode of the illness, perhaps representing some aspect of vulnerability to depression).

The methods employed in exploring the neurobiology of depression in humans can be grouped into three main categories. First, the quantity or activity of a biological component or system can be compared in those affected by major depression and a group of "healthy controls" not afflicted with the illness. Second, a biological system may be challenged or stimulated through pharmacologic, psychologic, or social means, and the responses compared in depressed and nondepressed individuals. For both of these approaches, the ranges of the results typically overlap between the depressed and nondepressed groups, which limits their use as diagnostic tests, though insight into pathophysiology is possible. Another method is to explore the effects of treatment on biological systems of depressed patients. Measures that "normalize" to the levels of nonaffected individuals after remission from the episode identify state effects of the illness. Comparisons between subjects remitted from a depressive episode and "never-depressed" control groups are crucial for the identification of trait effects, which do not change significantly between ill and well phases of the illness.

Animal, in particular rodent, models of depression present their own challenges. Current models (e.g., learned helplessness, forced swim test, and chronic mild stress) all focus on inducing a state of persistant or inescapable stress. It is reasonable to wonder how much the experience of rodents, with their markedly less-developed prefrontal cortex, can model the profoundly painful and pessimistic thoughts about the self and the future that afflict humans experiencing depression. Despite this concern, these tests have been used to represent human depression and have subsequently demonstrated their worth through their success at identifying compounds that prove to have antidepressant effects in humans.

Another challenge is that excising CNS tissue samples from depressed patients is considered rather indecorous (at least while the brain's owner is still using it!). Because biopsy is not possible, researchers must study peripheral systems (such as lymphocytes or platelets) that may share similarities with the brain in some aspects of protein function, although the modulating factors affecting those systems may differ. Postmortem study of the brain is complicated by the uncertainties around the course of disease and the lifelong effects of treatments on the individual.

THE BIOGENIC AMINE HYPOTHESES: SIGNALING THE ASCENDANCY OF BIOLOGICAL MODELS OF DEPRESSION

The biogenic amines consist of naturally occurring biologically active compounds derived from the enzymatic decarboxylation of amino acids. Monoamines are a subset of the biogenic amines consisting of a single amine (NH_2) group bound to a carbon-containing side chain. The monoamines important in psychiatry are further subdivided into the catecholamines (epinephrine, norepinephrine, and dopamine), the indoleamines (serotonin and tryptophan), and the imidazoleamine, histamine. Acetylcholine, an ester of acetic acid and choline, is not a monoamine, but functions as a neurotransmitter in many regions of the CNS modulated by the monoamines. Neurons that produce these neurotransmitters are localized to specific nuclei in the brainstem: the locus coeruleus for norepinephrine, the raphe nuclei for serotonin, and the ventral tegmental area (VTA) and substantia nigra for dopamine. The tuberomamillary nucleus of the hypothalamus is the site of histaminergic neurons in the brain. Acetylcholine-producing neurons are located in the basal forebrain and pons.

Norepinephrine

In 1954, Bloch et al. reported the mood elevating effects of the monoamine oxidase inhibitor (MAOI) iproniazid, which was being used to treat tuberculosis (7). Monoamine oxidase (MAO) is an enzyme located on the outer mitochondrial membrane that acts to catabolize the monoamines by removing the amine group. By inhibiting the action of that enzyme, iproniazid slows the breakdown of the monoamine neurotransmitters: serotonin, norepinephrine, and dopamine. Subsequently, in 1958, there were three reports of the antidepressant activity of imipramine, an antihistamine being tried in the treatment of schizophrenia based on the benefits displayed by chlorpromazine in treating this illness (8–10). Imipramine was the first of the class of medications called tricyclic antidepressants (TCAs), acting primarily by inhibiting reuptake of norepinephrine from the synapse.

From the findings that these drugs were effective in treating depression, it was reasoned that they must affect a core aspect of the illness. Schildkraut proposed in 1965 that the monoamines are the key elements in the etiology of depression (11). Bunney and Davis proposed a similar hypothesis in the same year (12). Additional support to this hypothesis derived from the findings that the antihypertensive drug reserpine (which was used to treat hypertension by depleting stores of biogenic amines), could lower mood significantly in people and also induce sedation and motor retardation in animal models of depression. Amphetamine, which increases monoamine concentrations in the synapse, was also known to elevate mood. Norepinephrine, therefore, plays important roles in concentration, attention, memory, sleep, and appetite, which can all be disrupted in MDD. Stated simply, the catecholamine hypothesis proposed that depression may be related to a deficiency in cate-cholamines, in particular norepinephrine, at important receptor sites in the brain (11).

In the decades since the introduction of the catecholamine hypothesis, three principal components of the norepinephrine system have been explored in major depression: levels of norepinephrine and its metabolites, locus coeruleus activity, and responsiveness of adrenergic receptors. The findings of these investigations have supported the importance of norepi-nephrine functioning in depression, though not necessarily in ways that the original catecholamine hypothesis predicted.

Both elevations and reductions in norepinephrine and its primary CNS metabolite, 3-methoxy-4-hydroxyphenylglycol (MHPG), have been demon-strated in the cerebrospinal fluid (CSF), plasma, and urine of depressed patients (13). Unfortunately, interpreting measures of norepinephrine in per-ipheral fluids, such as plasma and urine, is confounded by difficulty in identi-fying the source of the transmitter, i.e., CNS or the sympathetic nervous system. Studies of the locus coeruleus suggest that there is dysregulation at this level of the system also, with the somewhat paradoxical findings of both decreased density of neurons, yet increased tyrosine hydroxylase activity (tyrosine hydroxylase is the enzyme active in the rate-limiting step in the pro-cess of converting the amino acid tyrosine into norepinephrine) (14,15).

The hypothesis of low norepinephrine in depressed subjects predicts that the postsynaptic beta adrenoreceptors should be upregulated (expressed in greater numbers) in the brain. While evidence exploring this prediction is mixed, a more consistent finding is the clear downregulation of beta recep-tors in the rat forebrain following longer term antidepressant treatment or electroconvulsive therapy (ECT) (16). The time required for this downregu-lation to occur in rats is similar to the delayed response to antidepressants in humans, leading to the hypothesis that downregulation of beta receptors is required for antidepressant efficacy.

Closely related to Schildkraut's hypothesis is the super-sensitivity hypothesis, positing that presynaptic α-2 receptors, which act to inhibit the release of norepinephrine, may be supersensitive in depressed subjects, result-ing in reduced overall release of norepinephrine from locus coeruleus neurons (17). Consistent with this hypothesis, levels of α-2 receptors in postmortem tissue from depressed patients are increased (18). The sensitivity of α-2 recep-tors can be explored by using clonidine, a centrally acting α-2 agonist. Activa-tion of postsynaptic α-2 receptors in the hypothalamus stimulates the release of growth hormone releasing hormone (GHRH), subsequently causing growth hormone (GH) secretion from the pituitary gland. Patients with depression are repeatedly found to have blunted GH release after receiving clonidine, suggesting a disruption in noradrenergic signaling (19,20). How-ever, other factors also regulate GH release, limiting the ability to draw conclusions from these findings.

While the precise role of norepinephrine in the pathophysiology of major depression remains unclear, there are consistent findings of disturbed norepinephrine turnover and receptor sensitivity. One model that attempts to integrate the various findings posits that under resting conditions norepinephrine concentrations may be lower than normal, but with stress there is an exaggerated norepinephrine signal, possibly secondary to supersensitive or upregulated receptors (21).

An offshoot of the catecholamine hypothesis incorporates a role for acetylcholine, as proposed by Janowsky et al. in 1972 (22). Their hypothesis postulates that depression results from an increase in the ratio of cholinergic to adrenergic signaling, and mania from a reverse of this ratio. As with the catecholamine hypothesis, this idea emerged from observations that depressed mood could occur following administration of cholinergic agonists or physostigmine (an inhibitor of cholinesterase, an enzyme that metabolizes acetylcholine). However, unlike the demonstrated effect of iproniazid and imipramine to elevate mood in support of the catecholamine hypothesis, administration of anticholinergic medications that lack effect on monoamine systems do not alleviate depression (23). While acetylcholine is no longer thought to play a central role in the etiology of depression, the consistently demonstrated supersensitivity of depressed subjects to cholinergic stimulation suggests that functioning of this system is disturbed in some manner in MDD (24).

Serotonin

Across the Atlantic in 1967, Coppen proposed that another monoamine, serotonin [also known as 5-hydroxytryptophan (5HT)], plays a more important role in major depression than norepinephrine (25). Relying on similar building blocks as Schildkraut (i.e., reserpine, iproniazid, and imipramine all alter levels of serotonin as well as norepinephrine), Coppen (later supported by two Russian pharmacologists, Lapin and Oxenkrug) demonstrated that the addition of tryptophan (the immediate precursor in the synthesis of serotonin) to an MAOI could improve mood in nondepressed subjects, and induce greater improvement in depressed subjects treated with an MAOI (26). Perhaps presaging today's cultural contrasts, the American conception of depression focused on disturbances in the neurotransmitter tied to vigilance and activity, while the European version centered on the transmitter associated with calm and patience.

The conceptualization of the role of serotonin in depression was modified in 1974 by Prange et al. with their influential permissive hypothesis of serotonergic function (27). Their formulation asserted that low central serotonergic function is present in both mania and depression, thus "permitting" a mood disturbance to occur, the form of which is determined by the overactivity (mania) or underactivity (depression) of noradrenergic systems.

In the decades following Coppen's hypothesis, a great deal of evidence emerged supporting the important role of serotonin in depression. Analogous to the study of the role of norepinephrine, investigations into serotonin functioning have explored levels of neurotransmitter metabolites, changes in receptor functioning, and neuroendocrine challenge testing. Similar to the lowered levels of CSF MHPG in the catecholamine hypothesis, lower levels of 5-hydroxyindoleacetic acid (5-HIAA, the primary metabolite of serotonin) are present in the CSF of some depressed patients (28,29). However, subsequent work demonstrated that low CSF 5-HIAA is strongly associated with impulsiveness in a variety of conditions including suicide, violent criminal behavior, and alcoholism, and is therefore not specific to major depression (30).

Of the 14 or more serotonin receptor subtypes characterized to date, only the $5HT_{1a}$ and $5HT_2$ receptors have thus far demonstrated a significant link to the pathophysiology of depression. As with the hypothesized upregulation of beta receptors in the face of reduced norepinephrine signaling in depression, postsynaptic expression of $5HT_{1a}$ and $5HT_2$ receptors may reflect an adaptation to reduced serotonin release. Post-mortem examination of tissue from the neocortex of depressed patients shows an increase in postsynaptic $5HT_2$ receptors, and less consistently similar findings for the $5HT_{1a}$ receptor (31,32). The main limitation of post-mortem studies of the brains of suicide victims is that the biology of suicide is not equivalent to that of depression; it is estimated that 30% of people who die by suicide are not depressed at the time of death (33,34).

More consistent findings have emerged from the study of serotonin uptake in platelets of depressed patients. Platelets are considered a good model for state-dependent brain serotonergic function as they express $5HT_2$ receptors and take up serotonin via the serotonin transporter (SERT) in a manner similar to CNS neurons (35). Most studies report SERT density to be reduced in platelets of depressed patients, though one large study did not find a difference between depressed subjects and controls (36,37). Reduced SERT density is also present in the cortex and midbrain of depressed subjects (38,39). The interpretation of these older findings of SERT density may need to be reconsidered in light of the recently identified polymorphism in the promoter region of the SERT gene (discussed below).

Just as clonidine-induced GH release can be used to explore noradrenergic functioning, the ability of fenfluramine (which increases serotonin release and reduces its reuptake) to stimulate prolactin secretion from the pituitary gland can be used to examine serotonergic function. In general, depressed subjects show blunted prolactin release in response to administration of fenfluramine and L-tryptophan compared to controls, indicating diminished integrity of the serotonin system (40). Some studies have demonstrate that this finding may persist in remitted patients, suggesting that the impaired serotonergic function is trait, rather than state related (41).

The strong preclinical and clinical data demonstrating a role for serotonin in the pathophysiology of depression led to the targeted development of selective serotonin reuptake inhibitors (SSRIs). This event marked the first time a treatment for depression was derived from scientific studies of the illness, rather than emerging from conjecture or serendipitous observations.

Dopamine

The forgotten "middle child" of the monoamine hypotheses for depression is dopamine. Unlike the diffuse projection pathways of the serotonin and norepinephrine systems, dopamine transmission in the brain is limited to four discrete paths. The nigrostriatal system projects from the substantia nigra in the midbrain to the basal ganglia, regulating motor control and some components of cognition, particularly those involved in the cortico-striatal-pallido-thalamo-cortical neuron loops. A second pathway important for reward, emotional expression, and motivation is the mesolimbic pathway, projecting from the VTA in the midbrain to the nucleus accumbens, amygdala and hippocampus. The third pathway, the mesocortical, also arises from the VTA and projects to the orbitofrontal and prefrontal cortex, regulating cognitive processing. Finally, the tuberoinfundibular pathway projects from the hypothalamus to the pituitary gland, where it inhibits the release of prolactin. The depressive symptoms of psychomotor slowing (nigrostriatal), impaired concentration (mesocortical), and anhedonia (mesolimbic) provide a compelling basis for considering dopaminergic dysfunction in depression.

In contrast to the substantial support for the involvement of norepinephrine and serotonin in the pathophysiology of depression, the evidence for a dopaminergic dysfunction in depression is derived almost exclusively from animal studies and observations of how pharmacologic agents affect the dopamine system. Although reserpine depletes dopamine in a manner similar to norepinephrine and serotonin, and MAO catabolizes dopamine in a manner similar to the other monoamines, it was not until the 1970s that Randrup et al. postulated a role for dopamine in depression (42a). The effects of cocaine and amphetamine, which block dopamine reuptake and can induce dopamine release, provided the first evidence that enhanced dopaminergic signaling could improve mood. Some antidepressants are thought to act in part through inhibiting dopamine reuptake, such as bupropion, amineptine, and nomifensine (no longer on the market in the United States). More recently, small studies have demonstrated the efficacy of pramipexole, a D2/D3 receptor agonist in both unipolar and bipolar depressed patients (42,43).

Studies in both animals and humans led to increasing interest in the role of D2 family of receptors (which includes the D2, D3, and D4 subtypes) in depression. Animal models of depression, such as the chronic mild stress model, demonstrate reduced sensitivity of D2/D3 receptors in the nucleus accumbens, with increases in the number of receptors following chronic antidepressant treatment (44,45). Treatment-refractory patients show lower concentrations than controls of the dopamine metabolite homo-vanillic acid (HVA) measured in internal jugular vein samples, with depression severity inversely related to HVA level (46). Interestingly, severely depressed and currently medication-free patients show a significantly greater hedonic response to orally, administered amphetamine than do mildly depressed or control subjects (47). Successful treatment with antidepressants in humans is associated with increased D3 gene expression in the shell of nucleus accumbens and increased D2 receptor density in the anterior cingulate cortex and striatum following chronic antidepressant treatment (48,49).

Lower levels of serum dopamine beta hydroxylase (which converts dopamine to norepinephrine) is the only component of the dopamine system found to differ consistently between depressed and control subjects, with this finding limited to patients with psychotic depression (50,51). Higher concentrations of plasma dopamine and increased CSF and plasma HVA are found in the psychotically depressed (29,52). In conclusion, while the evidence for altered dopaminergic signaling abnormalities among depressed patients considered as a whole is limited, this neurotransmitter may contribute significantly to depressive pathophysiology in a subset of patients, particularly those with severe illness or bipolar depression.

Changes in Monoamine Systems with Treatment

A significant challenge to the monoamine hypotheses of depression is the contrast between the rapid (within hours) changes in monoamine signaling induced by administration of antidepressants and the two to four weeks delay in treatment response to these agents. It is possible that the acute increases in transmitter synaptic concentrations induced by these drugs leads to an increase in feedback inhibition signals through presynaptic autorecep-tors, resulting in more gradual changes in signal transmission (53,54). Overall, chronic treatment with antidepressants appears to induce a reduction in norepinephrine signaling, as demonstrated by treatment-induced reductions in CSF norepinephrine and its metabolites, downregulation of beta recep-tors, and reduced tyrosine hydroxylase activity (21). In contrast, the seroto-nergic signal transmission appears to be enhanced by antidepressant treatment. The number and sensitivity of postsynaptic $5HT_{1a}$ receptors increase after effective antidepressant treatment, and animal models demon-strate increased serotonin levels after chronic exposure to antidepressants (54,55). The response of $5HT_2$ receptors to treatment is less clear, with anti-depressant medication inducing their downregulation, but ECT resulting in an increase in their expression (56). Less evidence is available for dopamine, but increased sensitivity of postsynaptic D2/D3 receptors in the ventral striatum has been demonstrated in animals treated with chronic antidepres-sants (57). These alterations in the monoamine systems have been shown to occur regardless of the identified mechanism of action of the antidepressant treatment employed. At this point, the salient effects of antidepressant treatment on monoamine signaling seem to be increased postsynaptic $5HT_{1a}$ sensitivity and reduced sensitivity of the postsynaptic beta-receptor, perhaps through $5HT_{1a}$ autoreceptor desensitization and/or α-2 autoreceptor desensitization (21).

Response to treatment with serotonin- or norepinephrine reuptake–inhibiting drugs appears to be dependent on the availability of the specific neurotransmitter targeted by the drug. Thus, dietary depletion of tryptophan (the amino acid precursor of serotonin) induces depressive relapse in the majority of patients treated with selective SSRIs, but not those treated with TCAs (58). Similarly, administration of α-methylparatyrosine, which reduces the level of catecholamines by inhibiting the action of tyrosine hydroxylase, induces the return of depressive symptoms in patients treated with a TCA, but not with an SSRI (59). In healthy subjects, depletion of these monoamine precursors does not lead to depression. Thus, monoamine levels do not seem to have a prime etiologic role in the development of depression, but rather serve an important role in modulating other neurobiologic systems involved in recovery from depression.

FAST-ACTING NEUROTRANSMITTERS: SMALL MOLECULES WITH BIG ROLES

The vast majority of synaptic signaling in the brain occurs via the effects of fast-acting neurotransmitters. Monoamine transmission is thought to exert its effects largely through its relative slow modulation of the activity of these fast neurotransmitters. Gamma-aminobutyric acid (GABA) is the predominant inhibitory neurotransmitter in the CNS, with GABAergic neurons constituting 20% to 40% of all neurons in the cortex and more than three quarters of all striatal neurons (60,61). Most GABAergic cells in the brain are interneurons, with short axons that form synapses within a few hundred micrometers of their cell body, connecting different neurons together and coordinating neuronal activity within local brain regions (62). Glutamate functions as the main excitatory transmitter of pyramidal neurons (63).

GABA and Neurosteroids

Projection neurons from the brainstem raphe nuclei to the cortex preferentially synapse on GABA interneurons (more so than pyramidal neurons), inducing their firing. As GABA interneurons typically synapse with large numbers of pyramidal neurons, this neuronal networking multiplies the impact of a single serotonergic projection neuron to the cortex (64). In animal studies involving treatment with antidepressants or electric shock, GABA receptor density is increased by antidepressants (65). Direct GABA injection into rodent hippocampus prevents the development of learned helplessness in rats (66). In humans, CSF and plasma GABA concentrations are lower in depressed than in control patients, with persistence of low plasma GABA levels for up to four years after remission, suggesting that low plasma GABA levels may be a trait marker for depression (67). Support for this idea emerges from the finding that plasma GABA levels are lower in non-depressed individuals who have a first-degree relative with a history of major depression than in those without such a family history (68). Recent studies employing magnetic resonance spectroscopy found reduced GABA levels in the occipital cortex of depressed subjects compared to controls, with increases in concentrations after successful treatment with medication or ECT (69,70). However, reduction in GABA concentrations is not specific to depression, having also been demonstrated in alcohol dependence and mania (71).

The neurosteroids 3α, 5α-tetrahydroprogesterone (allopregnanolone) and 3α, 5α-tetrahydrodeoxycorticosterone recently emerged as possible factors in the pathophysiology of major depression. These 3α-reduced metabolites of progesterone are produced by neurons and glial cells within the CNS and are believed to act in a paracrine manner as positive allosteric modulators at the GABA-A receptor, enhancing GABAergic transmission (72). Administration of neurosteroids in the mouse forced swim test model of depression demonstrates efficacy (73). Allopregnanolone can stimulate negative feedback on the hypothalamic–pituitary–adrenal (HPA) axis, as demonstrated by its ability to decrease plasma adrenocorticotropin hormone (ACTH) concentrations and release of corticotropin-releasing hormone (CRH) (74,75). In preliminary studies, depressed patients show significantly lower serum and CSF allopregnanolone levels compared to healthy controls, with normalization of these concentrations after successful treatment with medications, though not with ECT or transcranial magnetic stimulation (76,77). These discrepant results suggest that changes in neuroactive steroid levels following antidepressant therapy may reflect specific pharmacologic properties of the medication, rather than crucial changes in the biology of the depressed state.

Glutamate

Several different receptor subtypes mediate the effects of glutamate. In depression, the *N*-methyl-D-aspartate (NMDA) receptor may be of particular importance. NMDA signaling is crucial to many forms of learning, and in high concentrations glutamate can induce neurotoxicity. NMDA receptor antagonists have shown efficacy in an animal model of depression (78). Moreover, chronic treatment with antidepressants modulates NMDA receptor function (79). The reported loss of glial cells from various brain regions in depressed patients, theoretically may lead to an increase in glutamatergic transmission, as glial cells remove glutamate from the synapse via glutamate transporters (80). Elevated glutamate levels have been demonstrated in cortical regions where GABA levels are decreased, suggesting that both of the fast-acting neurotransmitter systems contribute to the pathophysiology of major depression. This finding also raises the possibility that a metabolic pathway common to both systems may be a primary site of dysfunction in MDD (81).

INTRACELLULAR SIGNAL TRANSDUCTION: TAKING IN THE MESSAGE

The binding of a neurotransmitter to its receptor is just the first step in a sequence of events in signal transduction, which may be ultimately needed for antidepressant efficacy to occur. A relatively simple type of receptor is the ligand-gated ion channel (e.g., the GABA-A receptor), which undergoes a conformational change after binding a neurotransmitter, resulting in the passage of ions (e.g., chloride) that stimulate or hyperpolarize (deactivate) the cell. However, other receptors that bind neurotransmitters function by activating a cascade of intracellular events. Many of these receptors are linked to G-proteins on the cytosolic surface of the plasma membrane that activate second messenger systems, such as cyclic adenosine monophosphate (cAMP), inositol triphosphate, or nitric oxide. Other types of receptors are coupled to tyrosine kinases, which add a phosphate moiety to intracellular proteins, leading to a chain of events that result in modifications of gene transcription.

The work of Duman et al. in exploring the intracellular signaling cascades occurring in depression and its treatment led to the neurotrophic hypothesis of depression (82). This hypothesis proposes that deficient neurotrophic activity contributes to disrupted functioning of the hippocampus in depression, and that recovery with antidepressant treatment is mediated in part by reversal of this deficit. The neurotrophins are a family of molecules, including brain-derived neurotrophic factor (BDNF), involved in the maintenance, growth, and survival of neurons and their synapses. cAMP response element binding protein (CREB) is a protein activated via G-protein systems that increases the expression of neurotrophic and neuroprotective proteins. Specifically, CREB increases the levels of BDNF and its receptor, tropomyosin receptor–related kinase B. BDNF is believed to regulate the survival of neurons via its interaction with the mitogen-activated protein kinases, which in turn can increase the expression of Bcl-2, a protein that acts to inhibit the programmed cell death of neurons. BDNF also regulates synaptic plasticity through its effects on the NMDA receptor, thus significantly affecting the way networks of neurons communicate (83).

To date, most of the evidence supporting a pathophysiologic role for BDNF in depression is derived from animal studies. Restraint stress in rats results in a reduction in BDNF expression in the hippocampus, suggesting a role for the HPA axis in suppressing BDNF levels (84). Direct injection of BDNF into the rat brain demonstrates efficacy in two animal models of depression (85,86). Many antidepressants increase CREB activity and BDNF levels in the hippocampus and prefrontal cortex, which occurs two to three weeks after initiating the antidepressant, consistent with the usual time course for clinical improvement (87,88). ECT also raises BDNF levels in the hippocampus (89). The few studies exploring BDNF levels in the post-mortem brains of depressed humans are inconclusive, with both increases and decreases reported (80). Several groups have reported decreased BDNF levels in the peripheral circulation of depressed subjects versus controls, though the degree to which plasma BDNF concentration reflects brain BDNF levels is uncertain (90). With the increasing evidence from neuro-imaging, animal models, and postmortem studies that major depression may be related to deficits in neuronal plasticity and survival, the actions and perturbations of BDNF and other neuroprotective proteins will certainly remain at the forefront of depression research efforts.

NEUROENDOCRINOLOGY: BRAIN–BODY INTERACTIONS

Stress Reactions and the HPA Axis

After the monoamines, the second major branch of biological investigation into depression is neuroendocrinology. The frequent observation that depressive episodes emerge in the wake of a significant life stressor provided the initial impetus, particularly, for research on the stress axis. The components of the stress response were initially identified in the 1930s by Selye, who grouped the bodily responses to stress into the "general adaptation syndrome," differentiating it from the physical symptoms produced by a specific disease process (91). Later work determined that the mobilization of bodily resources in the face of threat involved in the stress response was mediated by glucocorticoids (GCs) released from the adrenal cortex.

The HPA stress response system is a negative feedback system with a starting point in the paraventricular nucleus (PVN) of the hypothalamus. The PVN produces corticotropin-releasing hormone (CRH), sometimes referred to as corticotropin-releasing factor. In conjunction with arginine vasopressin, also released from the PVN, CRH induces the anterior pituitary to synthesize and release proopiomelanocortin-derived peptides, including ACTH and endorphins (endogenous opioids). The ACTH released into the peripheral circulation then acts at the adrenal cortex to stimulate the release of the GC cortisol from the adrenal cortex. Cortisol is the primary effector molecule of the HPA axis, inducing a variety of clinical effects seen in the stress response. In healthy individuals, cortisol induces negative feedback on its release through interaction with corticosteroid receptors in the pituitary, hypothalamus, hippocampus, amygdala, and septum. Thus, the system seems to have evolved to provide the organism with rapid, short-lived responses to acutely threatening situations.

The effects of cortisol on bodily systems are mediated primarily via intracellular receptors. There are two types of these corticosteroid receptors: type I [mineralocorticoid (MR)] and type II glucocorticoid (GR). The MR is thought to mediate the effects of cortisol under low-stress basal conditions, when the cortisol level is low. As cortisol levels increase, such as occurs during the circadian rhythm or in the face of stress, the MRs saturate and cortisol signaling occurs through GRs, including the negative feedback signal. Once bound with cortisol, both types of corticosteroid receptors translocate to the nucleus, where they act to induce changes in gene expression (92).

Interest in the role of the HPA axis in major depression stems from observing that patients with disorders of the HPA axis, such as the hyper-cortisolemic state found in Cushing's disease, often experience depression indistinguishable from patients with primary psychiatric illnesses. The usual secretion of cortisol follows a diurnal pattern, with a rapid rise to peak in the first two hours after awakening and with a gradual diminution of levels for the remainder of the 24-hour period. Beginning in the 1960s, several research groups reported that levels of cortisol are elevated in the CSF, plasma, and urine of depressed patients. The correlations are particularly strong among the most severely depressed subjects, especially those with psychotic features. Depressed patients tended not to show the same degree of decline in cortisol levels through the day as healthy control subjects, suggesting ongoing inappropriate activity of the stress response system (93).

These findings gave rise to the hope of developing an objective diagnostic test for major depression. Dexamethasone is a high-potency synthetic steroid that has been used to mimic the effects of stress-induced elevations of cortisol. Carroll initially reported the potential utility of the dexamethasone suppression test (DST) in diagnosing major depression (94,95). The DST is typically conducted by administering an oral dose of 1.0 or 1.5 mg of dexamethasone at 11 P.M., followed by plasma cortisol measurements at various times the following day. Individuals with normal HPA axis function should significantly suppress their endogenous cortisol production in response to the dexamethasone, owing to its negative feedback effects. In major depression, there is often a failure to suppress cortisol production; such subjects are referred to as "nonsuppressors." Unfortunately, the DST has a sensitivity too low for use as a screening test and insufficient specificity for use as a confirmatory test, because individuals with other types of illnesses and about 7% of normal controls are found to be nonsuppressors (96).

Despite its limitations as a diagnostic test, the DST continues to be of research value in exploring the biology of depression. Depressed subjects demonstrating nonsuppression on the DST usually become suppressors after recovery from depression, so the DST may play a role in prediction of depressive relapse (97). The sensitivity of the DST can be improved by administering 100 μg of CRH intravenously on the day following the dexamethasone dose, so as to further examine dysregulation of the HPA axis. This dexamethasone plus CRH test has become the standard challenge test for HPA functioning in patients with depression (98).

HPA axis functioning has direct effects on the monoamine systems. In animal models, chronic stress or exogenous GC administration induces a reduction in the expression of postsynaptic $5HT_{1a}$ and $5HT_{1b}$ receptors in the hippocampus, changes prevented by chronic antidepressant treatment (99). Reduced signaling through the $5HT_{1a}$ receptor in the hippocampus may underlie the impaired HPA inhibitory feedback in depression, resulting in the sustained overactivity of the HPA axis (100). GCs can increase levels of tyrosine hydroxylase, resulting in greater catecholamine production, thus linking the findings of both greater dopaminergic signaling and elevated HPA axis activity in psychotic versus nonpsychotic depressed subjects (101).

In the last decade, increasing consideration has been given to the idea that CRH may be the component of the HPA axis that is most central to the altered stress responsiveness seen in major depression. Depressed patients demonstrate elevated CSF CRH concentration with normalization of these levels on successful treatment (102). Intravenous administration of CRH produces blunted ACTH and endorphin release in depressed subjects compared to controls, suggesting that chronic oversecretion of CRH results in downregulation of CRH receptors in the pituitary gland (103). Oversecretion of CRH is consistent with the finding of increased numbers of CRH-containing cells in the PVN in subjects with depression (104). Although there is blunted responsiveness of ACTH release to CRH stimulation, overall cortisol levels remain elevated, probably secondary to the hypertrophy of the adrenal cortex that occurs in depression. In addition to the CRH neurons located in the hypothalamus, CRH neurons are found in a variety of cortical and subcortical brain regions, where CRH acts as a neurotransmitter. Centrally administered CRH (designed to mimic CRH neurotransmitter effects), severe depression, and the stress response all induce a similar symptom profile of reduced sleep, appetite, and sexual behavior, increased heart rate, blood pressure, and altered motor activity (105).

The overall picture that emerges is one of failure of the HPA feedback mechanism to terminate the stress response in patients with major depression. Instead of a short-lived activation in face of an acute threat, the HPA axis continues to function as if the stress or threat was ongoing, gradually resulting in chronic maladaptive changes. The specific reason for this feedback failure is still unclear. Possibilities include loss of number or function of corticosteroid receptor–containing neurons in the hippocampus, or dysregulation of some other factors involved in mediating the suppression of CRH neuronal firing.

Early Life Stress and Depression: The Stress-Diathesis Hypothesis

The inconsistent findings of HPA axis dysfunction among depressed patients as a whole has led to an effort to identify a biological subtype of depression, specifically one deriving from alterations in the development of the stress–response system that persist into adulthood among children exposed to stress early in life. In the stress-diathesis hypothesis of depression, childhood abuse or neglect, or loss of a parent are considered to constitute an early life stress (ELS). The increased risk for depression (and anxiety disorders) among adults who experienced ELS is well established (106,107). As demonstrated in the work of Caspi et al. (see below), the individual's genetic inheritance can protect against or increase the vulnerability for the later development of depression after experiencing ELS (108).

Many animal studies employing models of ELS, such as removal of rat pups from their mothers for various time periods demonstrate both acute and sustained changes in neuroendocrine and behavioral systems. In particular, rat pups exposed to maternal deprivation display hypersecretion of CRH and increased CRH signal transduction when exposed to psychological stressors as adults (109). Treatment with an SSRI or cross-fostering the rats results in improvements in these factors. In primate models of stress, mothers rearing their young in an environment of variable foraging demand (in which the food supply was unpredictable) provide less maternal care to their infants than mothers in situations where food supply was predictably plentiful or scarce. The offspring reared in the variable foraging demand condition have significantly elevated CRH concentrations and abnormal functioning of both norepinephrine and serotonin systems in adulthood (110).

Children exposed to ELS were found to have disturbed HPA axis activity, but the observed changes have not been uniform. Retrospective studies of adults who experienced ELS identified exaggerated levels of HPA activity when under stress (111). A recent groundbreaking study by Heim et al. examined HPA axis response to social stress in women with or without ELS exposure and with or without current major depression (112). Only women with a history of ELS demonstrated increased plasma ACTH and cortisol response to the stressor, and women with both ELS and depression had a sixfold greater ACTH response to stress compared to non-ELS, nondepressed control subjects. Another study that assessed HPA activity by administering intravenous CRH found greater ACTH response among nondepressed women with ELS, but depressed women showed blunted ACTH response regardless of presence or absence of ELS (113). While much work remains to be done to clarify the neurobiological consequences of ELS, these data suggest that there may be a permanent change in the set point for HPA activity in the face of stress among people exposed to ELS, perhaps forming the biological basis for a subtype of depression.

Hypothalamic–Pituitary–Thyroid Axis

The approach of observing the psychiatric effects of bodily illness led to interest in the role of thyroid hormones in major depression. Just as individuals with Cushing's disease are observed to develop depression in the setting of excess GC production, patients with poor thyroid hormone production (hypothyroidism) are frequently seen to develop severe depression.

The hypothalamic–pituitary–thyroid (HPT) axis is organized in a manner similar to the HPA axis, with thyrotropin releasing hormone (TRH) released from the median eminence of the hypothalamus and traveling through the hypothalamo–hypophysial portal system to induce the release of thyroid stimulating hormone (TSH) from the anterior pituitary gland into the peripheral circulation. TSH then induces the synthesis and release of the thyroid hormones, tri-iodothyronine (T3) and thyroxine (T4). T3 and T4 provide negative feedback at the hypothalamus and pituitary gland to inhibit the release of TRH and TSH, thus reducing the activity of the axis. T4 present in the brain is converted to T3 (considered the active form of thyroid hormone in the CNS) by the enzyme type II 5′-deiodinase. The action of this enzyme can be inhibited by cortisol, thus linking the HPT and HPA axes in depression (114). In rats, administration of antidepressants increases the activity of this enzyme (115).

In parallel to the findings of elevated CRH function in depression, the levels of TRH in CSF are higher in depressed subjects than healthy controls (116). TSH release in response to intravenous TRH stimulation is blunted in a minority of patients with major depression (117). Similar to the blunted response to CRH, the diminished response to TRH is thought to derive from downregulation of pituitary TRH receptors stemming from chronically elevated TRH levels. However, about 15% of patients with major depression display supersensitive TSH response to TRH stimulation (118). Unlike the HPA axis, the HPT axis can also be disrupted by two antithyroid antibodies, antithyroglobulin and antithyroid microsomal antibodies. These antibodies are found more frequently in depressed subjects than in the general population (119).

The evidence favoring an etiologic role for thyroid dysfunction in major depression is not as strong as the evidence for HPA axis and monoamine disruption. Early support for HPT dysfunction in depression came from the findings that augmentation of antidepressants with T3 could lead to faster and more complete improvement in depressive symptoms and response in patients previously not responding to medication (120). Confirmatory studies of these effects using larger samples and SSRIs instead of TCAs are currently underway. While severe thyroid dysfunction is one way by which a depressive syndrome can be induced, the contribution of milder, subclinical forms of thyroid dysfunction to depressive symptomatology is less clear. Apart from the question of pathophysiology, it is likely that major depression in the presence of thyroid dysfunction results in poorer response to standard treatments.

Growth Hormone and Somatostatin

GH is secreted from the anterior pituitary gland and may have a role in depression through its effects on the homeostasis of body fuel stores. Two hypothalamic peptides control secretion of GH: somatostatin inhibits and GHRH stimulates GH release. Dopamine, norepinephrine, and tryptophan also stimulate GH secretion. In healthy adults, GH secretion follows a circadian pattern, with peak levels in the first few hours of sleep. Depressed subjects, however, show diminished nocturnal GH levels and higher daylight GH levels (121,122). Adolescents demonstrating lower levels of GH release prior to sleep onset are at greater risk of developing depression as adults (123). Response to clonidine, a centrally acting α-2 agonist that normally stimulates GH release, is blunted in depressed patients (20).

Somatostatin is produced in the hypothalamus and has inhibitory effects on GABA activity and on the release of GH, CRH, ACTH, and TRH. This neuropeptide is, therefore, positioned to influence many of the factors implicated in the pathophysiology of depression. Several studies have demonstrated reduced levels of somatostatin in the CSF of depressed patients, which may stem from GC inhibition of somatostatin neurons (124,125). As with many other hypothalamic peptides, much remains to be determined about the role of somatostatin in depression.

Sleep

Sleep is of significance in the pathophysiology of depression in that sleep disruption can occur as part of the prodrome to a major depressive episode, as a symptom during the episode, or linger as a residual symptom in patients remitted from their illness. Depressed patients show three major changes in sleep pattern: reduced sleep maintenance, reduced latency to first episode of rapid eye movement (REM) sleep, and diminished slow wave sleep (SWS) (delta sleep or stage 3 and 4 sleep) (126). The latter two features often persist after achieving remission from the depressive episode. Remarkably, sleep deprivation (preventing the patient from falling asleep) acutely improves depressive symptoms, though there is a quick relapse back into depression following just one subsequent night of sleep (127). Theories about the pathophysiological relationship between sleep and depression focus primarily on REM sleep disturbances, supported by the finding that most antidepressants suppress REM sleep (126).

REM sleep occurs during periods of cholinergic activation, which is usually inhibited by serotonergic projections to the cholinergic nuclei in the pons. Thus, an imbalance of monoamine or cholinergic function, such as decreased serotonergic transmission or increased cholinergic activity or sensitivity can reduce SWS and increase REM sleep. REM suppression with antidepressant treatment may result from increased postsynaptic 5HT1a receptor activity or increased transmission of catecholamines (128). During REM sleep, depressed patients show greater activity in brainstem, limbic, and cortical regions than do controls, perhaps reflecting greater intensity of affective response to stimuli, such as dreams (129). Recent work also demonstrates abnormal brain activity in the period prior to the onset of non-REM sleep in depressed patients. During the transition from wakefulness to non-REM sleep, depressed subjects show greater persistence of waking state levels of high metabolic activity in the thalamus and frontal and parietal cortical regions compared to controls (130). These alterations in the sleep pattern are consistent with the concept of depression being a state of overarousal, and may underlie the subjective complaints of insomnia and nonrestorative sleep reported by depressed patients.

Cytokines

Several lines of evidence suggest that overexpression of pro-inflammatory cytokines may contribute to the pathophysiology of depression, which has led to the macrophage hypothesis of depression (131). First, many patients who receive interferon α (a cytokine used to treat hepatitis C and melanoma) or interleukin (IL)-2 develop depressive syndromes, and these symptoms of depression can be prevented and treated by standard antidepressant regimens (132,133). Second, depressed patients who are medically healthy often demonstrate elevated measures of proinflammatory cytokines, particularly tumor necrosis factor-α, IL-1 and IL-6 (134,135). Moreover, a positive relationship exists between severity of depression and serum levels of cytokines (136). Third, cytokines may alter the functioning of monoamine and HPA axis systems. Fourth, antidepressants exhibit anti-inflammatory activity, with clinical response correlating with reductions in cytokine levels (137). Finally, administration of an IL-1 receptor antagonist prevents the development of learned helplessness in rats (138). Women display higher immune activation levels than men, and experience a spike in secretion of cytokines with childbirth, providing a possible biological basis for the higher incidence of MDD in women (139,140). Elevated cytokine activity may also provide the epidemiological link between depression and increased rates of death after heart attack (141).

GENETIC CONTRIBUTIONS: RISK AND RESILIENCE

The contribution of genetic factors to the risk of an individual developing major depression is well accepted, though identification of the specific genes involved has so far made little headway. The genetics of depression will be fully covered in a later chapter. However, etiological factors are discussed briefly in this chapter.

Family-based studies have found that the relative risk for developing MDD in first-degree relatives of depressed individuals is nearly three times greater than in the general population. The heritability (i.e., the proportion of the variation in major depression attributable to genetic factors) is estimated to be 31% to 42%, and is likely higher for individuals with recurrent major depressive episodes (142). The genetic factors associated with depression risk appear to overlap with those for generalized anxiety disorder; the ultimate expression of illness (anxiety or depression) may depend on environmental factors.

Individuals sharing the same genotype can be discordant for developing MDD, pointing to the importance of the environment in the etiology of the illness. While the environmental contributions to MDD have long been recognized, only recently have studies demonstrated the interaction between life stress and genotype. In a groundbreaking study, Caspi et al. reported the effects of life stressors in a birth cohort of 847 Caucasian New Zealand children stratified into three groups on the basis of their genotype for the SERT (108). The SERT has two alleles for the promoter region of the gene (that part of the gene that enables a gene to be transcribed); the "short" or s-allele codes for lower transcriptional efficiency of the SERT and the "long" or l-allele codes for higher transcriptional efficiency of the SERT. Hence, individuals who carry two l-alleles produce more SERT than do individuals who carry two s-alleles, and those who carry one of each allele produce an amount somewhere in between.

In the study by Caspi et al., 17% of the subjects were s/s homozygotes [i.e., carried two copies of the s-allele (low activity)], 51% were heterozygotes (i.e., carried one copy each of the s- and the l-allele), and 31% were l/l homozygotes (high activity). Among all the study members, 17% met the criteria for major depression at some point 12 months prior to assessment at age 26. The members were also assessed for the number of stressful life events they had experienced between the ages of 21 and 26. There was no significant difference in the rates of major depression between the three groups among individuals who reported zero to two life stressors. However, with three, and particularly with four or more life stressors, the s/s homozygotes developed major depression at twice the rate of l/l homozygotes, with s/l heterozygotes in between. This study, for the first time, demonstrated an interaction between a specific genotype (the SERT promoter polymorphism) and the amount of life stress that resulted in a major depressive episode (phenotype). These findings have since been replicated in a sample from the United States (143). The results of these studies may be construed as the s/s SERT promoter polymorphism conferring a vulnerability for developing major depression, or conversely, that the l/l genotype provides a degree of resilience against life stress.

Similar to the findings of the SERT promoter polymorphism and risk for depression, the interaction between promoter region polymorphisms for MAO type A and the presence or absence of an adverse childhood environment may predict risk for conduct disorder in youth (144,145). Future exploration of the role of genes contributing to risk for major depression will certainly draw heavily on this paradigm of gene-by-environment interactions.

CONCLUSIONS

Despite MDD's position as a leading public health problem worldwide, our understanding of the etiology and pathophysiology of the illness has been remarkably limited. However, previously segregated approaches to exploring depression along the lines of monoamine functioning, neuroendocrine alterations, and psychological measures are becoming increasingly integrated. With the advancements of research methodologies in genetics, cell biology, and neuroimaging, a more comprehensive model of depression is taking the place of the older system-bound theories. Unfortunately, major aspects of the neurobiology of depression, particularly the substantial difference in incidence by gender, age, and socioeconomic and life stress status remain poorly understood.

Although we lack a definitive theory, several components of neurobiology discussed in this chapter are certain to have relevance to the etiology and pathophysiology of MDD. The genetic inheritance of the individual provides the basic components conveying vulnerability or resilience to the development of the illness. The rearing environment further modifies these characteristics, setting the stage for the potential of developing a mood disorder in adulthood. Later, psychological and social stressors may initiate cascades of events via the stress response system, affecting other neuroendocrine systems, monoamine activity, and the functioning of intracellular signaling pathways, such as CREB regulation of BDNF. This disruption of neurotrophin function in maintaining neuronal and synaptic integrity, particularly in the hippocampus, may lead to disruptions in the connectivity between brain regions identified in the neuroimaging studies of depressed subjects. This dysfunctional brain circuitry reveals itself in the symptoms of depression seen in the clinic, with phenotypic variability between individuals potentially stemming from the specificity and degree specificity of circuit disruption. While this model is complex and sure to become even more complicated with the findings of future studies, it reflects the astounding intricacy of the organ that forms the basis of our conscious experience.

REFERENCES

1. Alexander FG, Selesnick ST. The History of Psychiatry. Northvale, NJ: Aronson Inc., 1966.

2. Frank J, Frank J. Persuasion and Healing: A Comparative Study of Psychotherapy. London: Johns Hopkins University Press, 1991.
3. Glas G. A conceptual history of anxiety and depression. In: Kasper S, den Boer JA, Ad Sitsen JM, eds. Handbook of Depression and Anxiety. New York: Marcel Dekker Inc, 2003:1–47.
4. Wong ML, Licinio J. Research and treatment approaches to depression. Nat Rev Neurosci 2001; 2:343–351.
5. Stone MH. Healing the Mind. New York: W.W. Norton, 1997.
6. Freud S. Mourning and melancholia. In: Strachey J, ed. Standard Edition of the Complete Psychological Works of Sigmund Freud. Vol. 14. London: Hogarth Press, 1957:243–258.
7. Bloch RG, Dooneief AS, Buchberg AS, Spellman S. The clinical effect of iso-niazid and iproniazid in the treatment of pulmonary tuberculosis. Ann Int Med 1954; 40:881–900.
8. Kuhn R. The treatment of depressive states with G22355 (imipramine hydro-chloride). Am J Psychiat 1958; 115(5):459–464.
9. Azima H, Vispo RH. Imipramine; a potent new anti-depressant compound. Am J Psychiat 1958; 115(3):245–246.
10. Lehmann HE, Cahn CH, DeVerteuil RL. The treatment of depressive condi-tions with imipramine. Can Psychiatr Assoc J 1958; 3(4):155–164.
11. Schildkraut JJ. The catecholamine hypothesis of affective disorders: a review of supporting evidence. Am J Psychiat 1965; 122(5):509–522.
12. Bunney WE, Davis JM. Norepinephrine in depressive reactions: a review. Arch Gen Psychiat 1965; 13(6):483–493.
13. Potter W, Grossman G, Rudorfer M. Noradrenergic function in depressive disorders. In: Mann J, Jupter D, eds. Biology of Depressive Disorders. New York: Plenum Press, 1993:1–27.
14. Ordway G, Smith K, Haycock J. Elevated tyrosine hydroxylase in the locus coeruleus of suicide victims. J Neurochem 1994; 62:680–685.
15. Chan-Palay V, Asan E. Quantitation of catecholamine neurons in the locus coeruleus in human brains of normal young and older adults and in depres-sion. J Comp Neurol 1989; 287:357–372.
16. Duncan GE, Paul IA, Powell KR, Fassberg JB, Stumpf WE, Breese GR. Neu-roanatomically selective down-regulation of beta adrenergic receptors by chronic imipramine treatment: relationships to the topography of [3H] imipra-mine and [3H] desipramine binding sites. J Pharmacol Exp Ther 1989; 248(1):470–477.
17. Charney DS, Heninger GR, Sternberg DE, et al. Presynaptic adrenergic recep-tor sensitivity in depression. The effect of long-term desipramine treatment. Arch Gen Psychiat 1981; 38(12):1334–1340.
18. Meana J, Barturen F, Garcia-Sevilla JA. α-2 adrenoceptors in the brain of sui-cide victims: increased receptor density associated with major depression. Biol Psychiat 1992; 31(5):471–490.
19. Schatzberg A, Schildkraut JJ. Recent studies on norepinephrine systems in mood disorders. In: Bloom F, Kupfer D, eds. Psychopharmacology: The Fourth Generation of Progress. New York: Raven Press Ltd, 1995:911–920.

20. Matussek N, Ackenheil M, Hippius H, et al. Effects of clonidine on growth hormone release in psychiatric patients and controls. Psychiat Res 1980; 2:25–36.

21. Ressler KJ, Nemeroff CB. Role of serotonergic and noradrenergic systems in the pathophysiology of depression and anxiety disorders. Depress Anxiety 2000; 12(suppl 1):2–19.

22. Janowsky DS, el-Yousef MK, Davis JM, Sekerke HJ. A cholinergic-adrenergic hypothesis of mania and depression. Lancet 1972; 2(7778):632–635.

23. Janowsky DS, Risch SC. Cholinomimetic and anticholinergic drugs used to investigate an acetylcholine hypothesis of affective disorder and stress. Drug Dev Res 1984; 4:125–142.

24. Dube S, Kumar N, Ettedgui E, Pohl R, Jones D, Sitaram N. Cholinergic REM induction response: separation of anxiety and depression. Biol Psychiat 1985; 20(4):408–418.

25. Coppen A. The biochemistry of affective disorders. Br J Psychiat 1967; 113: 1237–1264.

26. Lapin IP, Oxenkrug GF. Intensification of central serotonergic process as a possible determinant of thymoleptic effect. Lancet 1969; 1(7586):132–136.

27. Prange AJ Jr, Wilson IC, Lynn CW, Alltop LB, Stikeleather RA. L-trypto-phan in mania. Contribution to a permissive hypothesis of affective disorders. Arch Gen Psychiat 1974; 30(1):56–62.

28. Roy A, De Jong J, Linnoila M. Cerebrospinal fluid monoamine metabolites and suicidal behavior in depressed patients. A 5-year follow-up study. Arch Gen Psychiat 1989; 46(7):609–612.

29. Asberg M, Traskman L, Thoren P. 5-HIAA in the cerebrospinal fluid: a biochemical suicide predictor? Arch Gen Psychiat 1976; 33:1193–1197.

30. Faustman WO, King RJ, Faull KF, et al. MMPI measures of impulsivity and depression correlate with CSF 5-HIAA and HVA in depression but not schizophrenia. J Affect Disord 1991; 22(4):235–239.

31. Mann J, Stanley M, McBride P, McEwen BS. Increased 5HT2 and Beta-adrenergic receptor binding in the frontal cortices of suicide victims. Arch Gen Psychiat 1986; 43:954–959.

32. Mattsubara S, Arora R, Meltzer H. Serotonergic measures in suicide brain: 5HT1a binding sites in frontal cortex of suicide victims. J Neural Transm 1991; 85:181–194.

33. Mann JJ, Waternaux C, Haas GL, Malone KM. Toward a clinical model of suicidal behavior in psychiatric patients. Am J Psychiat 1999; 156:181–189.

34. Beautrais AL, Joyce PR, Mulder RT, Fergusson DM, Deavoll BJ, Nightingale SK. Prevalence and comorbidity of mental disorders in persons making serious suicide attempts: a case–control study. Am J Psychiat 1996; 153(8):1009–1014.

35. Flores BH, Musselman DL, DeBattista C, Garlow SJ, Schatzberg AF, Nemeroff CB. Biology of mood disorders. In: Schatzberg AF, Nemeroff CB, eds. The American Psychiatric Publishing Textbook of Psychopharmacology. Washington, D.C.: American Psychiatric Press, 2004.

36. Mellerup E, Langer SZ. Validity of imipramine platelet binding sites as a biological marker for depression: A World Health Organization collaborative study. Pharmacopsychiatry 1990; 23:113–117.

37. Lewis DA, McChesney C. Tritiated imipramine binding distinguishes among subtypes of depression. Arch Gen Psychiat 1985; 42:485–488.
38. Malison RT, Price LH, Berman R, et al. Reduced brain serotonin transporter availability in major depression as measured by 123-I-2 beta-carbomethoxy-3 beta-(4-iodophenyl)tropane and single photon emission computed tomography. Biol Psychiat 1998; 44(11):1090–1098.
39. Stanley M, Virgilio J, Gershon S. Tritiated imipramine binding sites are decreased in the frontal cortex of suicides. Science 1982; 216(4552):1337–1339.
40. Newman M, Shapira B, Lerer B. Evaluation of central serotonergic function in affective and related disorders by the fenfluramine challenge test: a critical review. Int J Neuropsychopharmacol 1998; 1:49–69.
41. Flory J, Mann J, Manuck S, Muldoon M. Recovery from major depression is not associated with normalization of serotonergic function. Biol Psychiat 1998; 43:320–326.
42. Corrigan MH, Denahan AQ, Wright E, Ragual RJ, Evans DL. Comparison of pramipexole, fluoxetine, and placebo in patients with major depression. Depress Anxiety 2000; 11:58–65.
42a. Randrup A, Munkvad I, Fog R, et al. Mania, depression and brain dopamine. In: Essman WB and Valzelli S, eds. Current Developments in Psychopharmacology. New York: Spectrum Publications, 1975:206–248.
43. Zarate CA Jr, Payne JL, Singh J, et al. Pramipexole for Bipolar II Depression: a placebo-controlled proof of concept study. Biol Psychiat 2004; 56(1):54–60.
44. Papp M, Klimek V, Willner P. Parallel changes in dopamine D-sub-2 receptor binding in limbic forebrain associated with chronic mild stress-induced anhedonia and its reversal by imipramine. Psychopharmacology 1994; 115(4):441–446.
45. Ainsworth K, Smith SE, Sharp T. Repeated administration of fluoxetine, desipramine and tranylcypromine increases dopamine D2-like but not D1-like receptor function in the rat. J Psychopharmacol 1998; 140:470–477.
46. Lambert G, Johansson M, Agren H, Friberg P. Reduced brain norepinephrine and dopamine release in treatment-refractory depressive illness: evidence in support of the catecholamine hypothesis of mood disorders. Arch Gen Psychiat 2000; 57(8):787–793.
47. Tremblay LK, Naranjo CA, Cardenas L, Herrmann N, Busto UE. Probing brain reward system function in major depression. Arch Gen Psychiat 2002; 59:409–416.
48. Lammers CH, Diaz J, Schwartz JC, Sokoloff P. Selective increase of dopamine D3 receptor gene expression as a common effect of chronic antidepressant treatments. Mol Psychiat 2000; 5:378–388.
49. Larisch R, Klimke A, Vosberg H, Loffler S, Gaebel W, Muller-Gartner HW. In vivo evidence for the involvement of dopamine-D2 receptors in striatum and anterior cingulate gyrus in major depression. Neuroimage 1997; 5:251–260.
50. Cubells JF, Price LH, Meyers BS, et al. Genotype-controlled analysis of plasma dopamine beta-hydroxylase activity in psychotic unipolar major depression. Biol Psychiat 2002; 51(5):358–364.
51. Sapru MK, Rao B, Channabasavana SM. Serum beta-hydroxylase activity in classical subtypes of depression. Acta Psychiatr Scand 1989; 80:474–478.

52. Devanand DP, Bowers MB, Hoffman FJ, et al. Elevated plasma homovanillic acid levels in depressed females with melancholia and psychosis. Psychiat Res 1985; 15:1–4.

53. Blier P, de Montigny C. Serotonin and drug-induced therapeutic responses in major depression, obsessive-compulsive and panic disorders. Neuropsychopharmacology 1999; 21:91S–98S.

54. Blier P, Bouchard C. Modulation of 5HT release in the guinea pig brain following long-term administration of antidepressants. Br J Pharmacol 1994; 113–485.

55. Djicks F, Ruight G, DeGraaf J. Antidepressants affect amine modulation of neurotransmission in the rat hippocampal slice. Delayed effects. Neuropharmacol 1991; 30:1141–1150.

56. Gonzalez-Heydrich J, Peroutka SJ. Serotonin receptor and reuptake sites: pharmacologic significance. J Clin Psychiat 1990; 51(suppl):5–12.

57. Willner P. Sensitization to antidepressant drugs. In: Emmett-Oglesby MW, Goudie AJ, eds. Psychoactive Drugs: Tolerance and Sensitization. Clifton, New Jersey: Humana Press, 1989:407–459.

58. Delgado PL. Depression: the case for a monoamine deficiency. J Clin Psychiat 2000; 61(suppl 6):7–11.

59. Bremner JD, Vythilingam M, Ng CK, et al. Regional brain metabolic correlates of α-methylparatyrosine-induced depressive symptoms: implications for the neural circuitry of depression [see comment]. JAMA 2003; 289(23): 3125–3134.

60. Hendry SH, Schwark HD, Jones EG, Yan J. Numbers and proportions of GABA-immunoreactive neurons in different areas of monkey cerebral cortex. J Neurosci 1987; 7:1503–1509.

61. Tepper JM, Koos T, Wilson CJ. GABAergic microcircuits in the neostriatum. Trends Neurosci 2004; 11:662–669.

62. Kingsley RE. Concise Text of Neuroscience. Philadelphia: Lippincott Williams and Wilkins, 2000.

63. Fonnum F. Glutamate: a neurotransmitter in mammalian brain. J Neurochem 1984; 42(1):1–11.

64. Smiley JF, Goldman-Rakic PS. Serotonergic axons in monkey prefrontal cerebral cortex synapse predominantly on interneurons as demonstrated by serial section electron microscopy. J Comp Neurol 1996; 367(3):431–443.

65. Lloyd KG, Thuret F, Pilc A. Upregulation of gamma-aminobutyric acid (GABA) B binding sites in rat frontal cortex: a common action of repeated administration of different classes of antidepressants and electroshock. J Pharmacol Exp Therap 1985; 235(1):191–199.

66. Petty F, Sherman AD. A pharmacologically pertinent animal model of mania. J Affect Dis 1981; 3:381–387.

67. Gold BI, Bowers MB, Roth RH, Sweeney DW. GABA levels in CSF of patients with psychiatric disorders. Am J Psychiat 1980; 137(3):362–364.

68. Bjork JM, Moeller FG, Kramer GL, et al. Plasma GABA levels correlate with aggressiveness in relatives of patients with unipolar depressive disorder. Psychiat Res 2001; 101(2):131–136.

69. Sanacora G, Mason GF, Rothman DL, et al. Increased cortical GABA concentrations in depressed patients receiving ECT. Am J Psychiat 2003; 160(3):577–579.

70. Sanacora G, Mason GF, Rothman DL, Krystal JH. Increased occipital cortex GABA concentrations in depressed patients after therapy with selective serotonin reuptake inhibitors. Am J Psychiat 2002; 159(4):663–665.

71. Petty F. Plasma concentrations of GABA and mood disorders: a blood test for manic depressive disease? Clin Chem 1994; 40:296–302.

72. Belelli D, Lambert JJ. Neurosteroids: endogenous regulators of the GABA(A) receptor. Nat Rev Neurosci 2005; 6(7):565–575.

73. Khisti RT, Chopde CT, Jain SP. Antidepressant-like effect of the neurosteroid 3α-hydroxy-5α-pregnan-20-one in mice forced swim test. Pharmacol Biochem Behav 2000; 67(1):137–143.

74. Patchev VK, Shoaib M, Holsboer F, Almeida OF. The neurosteroid tetrahydroprogesterone counteracts corticotropin-releasing hormone-induced anxiety and alters the release and gene expression of corticotropin-releasing hormone in the rat hypothalamus. Neuroscience 1994; 62(1):265–271.

75. Patchev VK, Hassan AH, Holsboer DF, Almeida OF. The neurosteroid tetrahydroprogesterone attenuates the endocrine response to stress and exerts glucocorticoid-like effects on vasopressin gene transcription in the rat hypothalamus. Neuropsychopharmacology 1996; 15(6):533–540.

76. Baghai TC, di Michele F, Schule C, et al. Plasma concentrations of neuroactive steroids before and after electroconvulsive therapy in major depression. Neuropsychopharmacology 2005; 30:1181–1186.

77. Uzunova V, Sheline Y, Davis JM, et al. Increase in the cerebrospinal fluid content of neurosteroids in patients with unipolar major depression who are receiving fluoxetine or fluvoxamine. Proc Natl Acad Sci USA 1998; 95(6): 3239–3244.

78. Papp M, Moryl E. Antidepressant activity of non-competitive and competitive NMDA receptor antagonists in a chronic mild stress model of depression. Eur J Pharmacol 1994; 263:1–7.

79. Nowak G, Trullas R, Layer RT, Skolnick P, Paul IA. Adaptive changes in the N-methyl-D-aspartate receptor complex after chronic treatment with imipramine and 1-aminocyclopropanecarboxylic acid. J Pharmacol Exp Therap 1993; 265(3):1380–1386.

80. Slattery DA, Hudson AL, Nutt DJ. The evolution of antidepressant mechanisms. Fundam Clin Pharmacol 2004; 18:1–21.

81. Sanacora G, Gueorguieva R, Epperson N, et al. Subtype-specific alterations of gamma-aminobutyric acid and glutamate in patients with major depression. Arch Gen Psychiat 2004; 61(7):705–713.

82. Duman RS, Heninger GR, Nestler EJ. A molecular and cellular theory of depression. Arch Gen Psychiat 1997; 54:597–606.

83. Manji HK, Drevets WC, Charney DS. The cellular neurobiology of depression. Nat Med 2001; 7:541–547.

84. Smith MA, Makino S, Kvetnansky R, Post RM. Stress and glucocorticoids affect the expression of brain-derived neurotrophic factor and neurotrophin-3 mRNAs in the hippocampus. J Neurosci 1995; 15:1768–1777.

85. Siuciak JA, Lewis DR, Wiegand SJ, Lindsay RM. Antidepressant-like effect of brain-derived neurotrophic factor (BDNF). Pharmacol Biochem Behav 1997; 56(1):131–137.

86. Shirayama Y, Chen AC, Nakagawa S, Russell DS, Duman RS. Brain-derived neurotrophic factor produces antidepressant effects in behavioral models of depression. J Neurosci 2002; 22(8):3251–3261.

87. Nestler EJ, Terwilliger RZ, Duman RS. Chronic antidepressant administration alters the subcellular distribution of cyclic AMP-dependent protein kinase in rat frontal cortex. J Neurochem 1989; 53:1644–1647.

88. Nibuya M, Nestler EJ, Duman RS. Chronic antidepressant administration increases the expression of cAMP response element binding protein (CREB) in rat hippocampus. J Neurosci 1996; 6:2365–2372.

89. Vaidya VA, Siuciak JA, Du F, Duman RS. Hippocampal mossy fiber sprouting induced by chronic electroconvulsive seizures. Neuroscience 1999; 89(1): 157–166.

90. Karege F, Bondolfi G, Gervasoni N, Schwald M, Aubry JM, Bertschy G. Low brain-derived neurotrophic factor (BDNF) levels in serum of depressed patients probably results from lowered platelet BDNF release unrelated to platelet reactivity. Biol Psychiat 2005; 57(9):1068–1772.

91. Selye H. A syndrome produced by diverse nocuous agents. Nature 1936; 138–132.

92. Raison CL, Miller AH. When not enough is too much: the role of insufficient glucocorticoid signaling in the pathophysiology of stress-related disorders. Am J Psychiat 2003; 160(9):1554–1565.

93. Nemeroff CB. The neurobiology of depression. Sci Am 1998; 278(6):42–49.

94. Carroll BJ, Martin FI, Davies B. Pituitary-adrenal function in depression. Lancet 1968; 1(7556):1373–1374.

95. Carroll BJ. Use of the dexamethasone suppression test in depression. J Clin Psychiat 1982; 43:44–49.

96. Janicak PG, Davis JM, Preskorn SH, Ayd FJ. Principles and Practice of Psychopharmacotherapy. Philadelphia: Lippincott Williams and Wilkins, 1997.

97. Arana GW, Baldessarini RJ, Ornsteen M. The dexamethasone suppression test for diagnosis and prognosis in psychiatry. Arch Gen Psychiat 1985; 42:1193–1204.

98. Holsboer F, von Bardeleben U, Wiedemann K, Muller OA, Stalla GK. Serial assessment of corticotropin-releasing hormone response after dexamethasone in depression. Implications for pathophysiology of DST nonsuppression. Biol Psychiat 1987; 22(2):228–234.

99. Mendelson SD, McEwen BS. Autoradiographic analyses of the effects of adrenalectomy and corticosterone on 5-HT1A and 5-HT1B receptors in the dorsal hippocampus and cortex of the rat. Neuroendocrinology 1992; 55(4): 444–450.

100. McAllister-Williams RH, Ferrier IN, Young AH. Mood and neuropsychological function in depression: the role of corticosteroids and serotonin. Psychol Med 1998; 28:573–584.

101. Schatzberg AF, Rothschild AJ, Langlais PJ. A corticosteroid/dopamine hypothesis for psychotic depression and related states. J Psychiatr Res 1985; 19(1):57–64.

102. Banki CM, Karmacsi L, Bissette G, Nemeroff CB. CSF corticotropin-releasing hormone and somatostatin in major depression: response to antidepressant treatment and relapse. Eur Neuropsychopharmacol 1992; 2(2):107–113.
103. von Bardeleben U, Stalla GK, Muller OA, Holsboer F. Blunting of ACTH response to human CRH in depressed patients is avoided by metyrapone pretreatment. Biol Psychiat 1988; 24(7):782–786.
104. Raadsheer FC, Hoogendijk WJ, Stam FC, Tilders FJ, Swaab DF. Increased numbers of corticotropin-releasing hormone expressing neurons in the hypothalamic paraventricular nucleus of depressed patients. Neuroendocrinology 1994; 60(4):436–444.
105. Nemeroff CB. Neurobiological consequences of childhood trauma. J Clin Psychiat 2004; 65(suppl 1):18–28.
106. Mullen PE, Martin JL, Anderson JC, Romans SE, Herbison GP. The long-term impact of the physical, emotional, and sexual abuse of children: a community study. Child Abuse Negl 1996; 20(1):7–21.
107. McCauley J, Kern DE, Kolodner K, et al. Clinical characteristics of women with a history of childhood abuse: unhealed wounds [see comment]. JAMA 1997; 277(17):1362–1368.
108. Caspi A, Sugden K, Moffitt TE, et al. Influence of life stress on depression: moderation by a polymorphism in the 5-HTT gene. Science 2003; 301(5631): 386–389.
109. Newport D, Stowe ZN, Nemeroff CB. Parental depression: animal models of an adverse life event. Am J Psychiat 2002; 159(8):1265–1283.
110. Coplan JD, Andrews MW, Rosenblum LA, et al. Persistent elevations of cerebrospinal fluid concentrations of corticotropin-releasing factor in adult non-human primates exposed to early-life stressors: implications for the pathophysiology of mood and anxiety disorders. Proc Natl Acad Sci USA 1996; 93(4):1619–1623.
111. Lemieux AM, Coe CL. Abuse-related posttraumatic stress disorder: evidence for chronic neuroendocrine activation in women. Psychosom Med 1995; 57(2):105–115.
112. Heim C, Newport DJ, Heit S, et al. Pituitary-adrenal and autonomic responses to stress in women after sexual and physical abuse in childhood [see comment]. JAMA 2000; 284(5):592–597.
113. Heim C, Newport DJ, Bonsall R, Miller AH, Nemeroff CB. Altered pituitary-adrenal axis responses to provocative challenge tests in adult survivors of childhood abuse. Am J Psychiat 2001; 158(4):575–581.
114. Hindal JT, Kaplan MM. Inhibition of thyroxine 5'-deiodination type II in cultured human placental cells by cortisol, insulin, 3',5'-cyclic adenosine monophosphate and butyrate. Metabolism 1988; 37:664–668.
115. Campos-Barros A, Meinhold H, Stula M, et al. The influence of desipramine on thyroid hormone metabolism in rat brain. J Pharmacol Exp Therap 1994; 268(3):1143–1152.
116. Banki CM, Bissette G, Arato M, Nemeroff CB. Elevation of immunoreactive CSF TRH in depressed patients. Am J Psychiat 1988; 145(12):1526–1531.
117. Loosen P, Prange A. Serum thyrotropin response to thyrotropin-releasing hormone in psychiatric patients: a review. Am J Psychiat 1982; 139:405–416.

118. Extein I, Pottash AL, Gold MS. The thyrotropin-releasing hormone test in the diagnosis of unipolar depression. Psychiat Res 1981; 5(3):311–316.

119. Gold MS, Pottash AC, Extein I. Symptomless autoimmune thyroiditis in depression. Psychiat Res 1982; 6:261–269.

120. Wilson IC, Prange AJ Jr, McClane TK, Rabon AM, Lipton MA. Thyroid-hormone enhancement of imipramine in nonretarded depressions. N Engl J Med 1970; 282(19):1063–1067.

121. Mendlewicz J, Linkowski P, Kerkhofs M, et al. Diurnal hypersecretion of growth hormone in depression. J Clin Endocrinol Metab 1985; 60(3):505–512.

122. Schilkrut R, Chandra O, Osswald M, Ruther E, Baafusser B, Matussek. Growth hormone release during sleep and with thermal stimulation in depressed patients. Neuropsychobiology 1975; 1(2):70–79.

123. Coplan JD, Wolk SI, Goetz RR, et al. Nocturnal growth hormone secretion studies in adolescents with or without major depression re-examined: integration of adult clinical follow-up data. Biol Psychiat 2000; 47(7):594–604.

124. Bissette G, Widerlov E, Walleus H, et al. Alterations in cerebrospinal fluid concentrations of somatostatinlike immunoreactivity in neuropsychiatric disorders. Arch Gen Psychiat 1986; 43(12):1148–1151.

125. Wolkowitz OM, Rubinow DR, Breier A, Doran AR, Davis C, Pickar D. Prednisone decreases CSF somatostatin in healthy humans: implications for neuropsychiatric illness. Life Sci 1987; 41(16):1929–1933.

126. Winokur A, Gary KA, Rodner S, Rae-Red C, Fernando AT, Szuba MP. Depression, sleep physiology, and antidepressant drugs. Depress Anxiety 2001; 14(1):19–28.

127. Wirz-Justice A, Van den Hoofdakker RH. Sleep deprivation in depression: what do we know, where do we go? Biol Psychiat 1999; 46(4):445–453.

128. Seifritz E. Contribution of sleep physiology to depressive pathophysiology. Neuropsychopharmacol 2001; 25:S85–S88.

129. Nofzinger EA, Buysse DJ, Germain A, et al. Increased activation of anterior paralimbic and executive cortex from waking to rapid eye movement sleep in depression. Arch Gen Psychiat 2004; 61(7):695–702.

130. Germain A, Nofzinger EA, Kupfer DJ, Buysse DJ. Neurobiology of non-REM sleep in depression: further evidence for hypofrontality and thalamic dysregulation. Am J Psychiat 2004; 161(10):1856–1863.

131. Smith RS. Erratum: the macrophage theory of depression. Med Hypotheses 1991; 36:298–306.

132. Raison CL, Demetrashvili M, Capuron L, Miller AH. Neuropsychiatric side effects of interferon-α: recognition and management. CNS Drugs 2005; 19:1–19.

133. Musselman DL, Lawson DH, Gumnick JF, et al. Paroxetine for the prevention of depression induced by high-dose interferon alfa [see comment]. N Engl J Med 2001; 344(13):961–966.

134. Tuglu C, Kara SH, Caliyurt O, Vardar E, Abay E. Increased serum tumor necrosis factor-α levels and treatment response in major depressive disorder. Psychopharmacology 2003; 170(4):429–433.

135. Hestad KA, Tonseth S, Stoen CD, Ueland T, Aukrust P. Raised plasma levels of tumor necrosis factor α in patients with depression: normalization during electroconvulsive therapy [see comment]. J ECT 2003; 19(4):183–188.

136. Thomas AJ, Davis S, Morris C, Jackson E, Harrison R, O'Brien JT. Increase in interleukin-1-beta in late-life depression. Am J Psychiat 2005; 162:175–177.

137. Raison CL, Marcin M, Miller AH. Antidepressant treatment of cytokine-induced depression. Acta Neuropsychiatrica 2002; 4:18–25.

138. Maier SF, Watkins LR. Intracerebroventricular interleukin-1 receptor antagonist blocks the enhancement of fear conditioning and interference with escape produced by inescapable shock. Brain Res 1995; 695(2):279–282.

139. Grossman CJ. Interactions between the gonadal steroids and the immune system. Science 1985; 227:257–261.

140. Connor TJ, Leonard BE. Depression, stress and immunological activation: the role of cytokines in depressive disorders. Life Sci 1998; 62:583–606.

141. Frasure-Smith N, Lesperance F, Talajic M. Depression following myocardial infarction. Impact on 6-month survival [erratum appears in JAMA 1994 Apr 13; 271(14):1082]. JAMA 1993; 270(15):1819–1825.

142. Sullivan PF, Neale MC, Kendler KS. Genetic epidemiology of major depression: review and meta-analysis. Am J Psychiat 2000; 157:1552–1662.

143. Kendler KS, Kuhn JW, Vittum J, Prescott CA, Riley B. The interaction of stressful life events and a serotonin transporter polymorphism in the prediction of episodes of major depression. Arch Gen Psychiatr 2005; 62(5):529–535.

144. Foley DL, Eaves LJ, Wormley B, et al. Childhood adversity, monoamine oxidase A genotype, and risk for conduct disorder. Arch Gen Psychiatr 2004; 61(7):738–744.

145. Caspi A, McClay J, Moffitt TE, et al. Role of genotype in the cycle of violence in maltreated children. Science 2002; 297(5582):851–854.

3

Drug Development, Psychotherapy Development, and Clinical Use

Timothy J. Petersen

*Massachusetts General Hospital/Harvard Medical School,
Boston, Massachusetts, U.S.A.*

Geoffrey Hopkins, Arun Kunwar, and Thomas L. Schwartz

*Department of Psychiatry, SUNY Upstate Medical University,
Syracuse, New York, U.S.A.*

INTRODUCTION

This chapter has been developed to provide a brief yet historical account of the multiple achievements that have made treating major depressive disorder (MDD) safer, more efficient, and possibly more effective over time. Many of the treatments discussed below, albeit older, are still employed to gain remission from depressive symptoms. We will first review the history of anti-depressant development by way of the U.S. Food and Drug Administration's (FDA's) systematic approval of agents, dating back to the 1950s. Second, we will cover the development of psychotherapeutic techniques dating back to the 1800s. The thought behind this chapter is that we must know our history in regard to being aware of all of the potential treatments that may be used to better treat our MDD patients.

PHARMACOTHERAPY

Prior to 1980, the possibilities for treating depression included the use of tricyclics or tricyclic antidepressants (TCAs), the monamine oxidase inhibitors

(MAOIs), and electroconvulsive therapy (ECT). The antidepressant effect of these medications appears to be related to the modulation of both serotonergic and noradrenergic function within the brain, and, possibly, increased dopaminergic function with the MAOIs. Serious side effects of the TCAs are largely related to their blocking of a variety of other heterogeneous receptors namely H1 histaminic, cholinergic–muscarinic, alpha-1 adrenergic, thereby causing urinary retention, constipation, dry mouth, postural hypotension, sedation, and cardiotoxicity. MAOIs can cause the above-mentioned side effects, as well as hypertensive crisis, if tyramine products are consumed, necessitating dietary and medication restrictions. In the 1980s, the selective serotonin reuptake inhibitors (SSRIs) were introduced, and rapidly became the first choice in antidepressant pharmacotherapy owing to ease of dosing, tolerability, and safety. SSRIs, however, are not side effect free; nervousness and agitation, gastrointestinal (GI) complaints, weight gain, sexual side effects, headaches, and p450 drug–drug interactions with long-term use are all commonly encountered side effects. Just prior to the release of the first FDA-approved SSRI, the norepinephrine–dopamine reuptake inhibitor (NDRI), buproprion, was also released. Other modern classes of antidepressants exist as both serotonin–norepinephrine reuptake inhibitors (SNRIs) with venlafaxine and duloxetine being in this class, and mirtazapine being in the class of noradrenergic and specific serotonergic antidepressant (NaSSA). All of these agents manipulate the monoamines discussed in the etiology chapter of this book. The following paragraphs will discuss these medication classes historically in more detail.

TCA and Tetracyclic Antidepressants

TCAs, which are chemically related to phenothiazine antipsychotics, were initially investigated during the 1950s as neuroleptics to produce more effective and safer analogs of chlorpromazine, but instead they were observed to have remarkable antidepressant properties. Imipramine was the first antidepressant to be discovered in this process. TCAs are named after the drugs' molecular structure, which contains three rings of atoms; similarly, tetracyclics have four rings. Both TCAs and tetracyclics are discussed together because both are similar with regard to their properties (1).

For many years, TCAs were the first choice for pharmacological treatment of depression, and they remain effective for the treatment of a wide range of disorders including depression, panic disorder, generalized anxiety disorder, eating disorders, obsessive–compulsive disorder (OCD), and pain syndromes. Although they are effective, owing to their high toxicity, narrow therapeutic window, and potentially lethal outcome if used in suicide attempts, these drugs have been relegated to, at least, second-line treatment in most cases (2).

Mechanism of Action

TCAs generally block the reuptake of norepinephrine and serotonin, and this blockade is thought to account for the therapeutic actions of these drugs.

Though most of the TCAs block both norepinephrine and serotonin, some have higher affinity for serotonin blockade (clomipramine, amitryptiline, imipramine, etc.) and some (desipramine, maprotilene, nortryptyline, protriptyline, etc.) for norepinephrine blockade. Each TCA, therefore has a subtly unique pharmacodynamic profile. They are also competitive antagonists at the muscarinic–cholinergic receptors, histamine receptors, and alpha-1 adrenergic receptors. While blockade of norepinephrine and serotonin transporters accounts for their therapeutic actions, the blockade as competitive antagonists of these other receptors accounts for their side effects. Amoxapine, nortriptyline, desipramine, and maprotiline have the least anticholinergic activity, and doxepin has the most antihistaminergic activity. Amoxapine, through its metabolite, has potent dopamine-blocking activity, and has some antipsychotic-mimicking action and related side effects.

Typical dosing and adverse effect potential for the common TCAs are noted below in Table 1. Typically, doses are started low to minimize side effects, and are gradually increased over time to reach a steady state blood level consistent with those needed to achieve antidepressant efficacy. Agents may be chosen on the basis of the side effects that need to be avoided, or even on the basis of their particular affinity for serotonin or norepinephrine pumps, which may offer differential response on a case-by-case basis.

Pharmacological Actions

Most of the TCAs are completely absorbed after oral administration and undergo extensive metabolization. Half-life varies from 10 to 70 hours, and most of the TCAs can effectively be taken once daily. They are metabolized through cytochrome P450 2D6 pathways. Clinically significant drug interactions can occur when TCAs are used with other medications. Fluoxetine, duloxetine, paroxetine, and other drugs that are known to inhibit the P450 2D6 pathway may slow the metabolism of the TCAs and cause an increase in plasma level. This may increase risk of adverse events. Additionally, about 7% of the general population has a genetic variation that results in decreased activity of the P450 2D6 enzymes; these individuals metabolize TCAs much slower than usual, and this population may develop toxic drug levels at normally therapeutic doses. Owing to variability in absorption and metabolism of TCAs, there may be 30- to 50-fold differences in plasma concentration of the drug in persons receiving similar doses of medication. Because of this reason, some have recommended routine plasma drug monitoring. Of the TCAs, nortryptiline is unique, in that it has the clearest therapeutic window (plasma concentration above 150 ng/mL or below 50 ng/mL may reduce efficacy) (3).

Psychiatric Use

Owing to the side effects, TCAs are usually a clear second-line treatment for depression in individuals in whom, SSRIs failed (2). All TCAs are equally

Table 1 TCAs Dose and Side Effects

Drugs (Trade name)	Dose range (mg) [therapeutic plasma concentration (ng/mL)]	Anticholinergic effects	Sedation	Postural hypotension	Conduction abnormalities
Tertiary amines					
Amitryptiline (Elavil®, Endep®)	150–300 (100–250)	+ + + +	+ + + +	+ + +	+ + + +
Clomipramine (Anafranil®)	150–250 (?)	+ + + +	+ + + + +	+ + +	+ + + + +
Doxepin (Adapin®, Sinequan®)	150–300 (100–250)	+ + +	+ + + +	+ +	+ +
Imipramine (Tofranil®)	150–300 (150–300)	+ + +	+ + +	+ + + +	+ + + + +
Trimipramine (Surmontil®)	150–300 (?)	+ + + +	+ + + +	+ + +	+ + + + + +
Secondary amines					
Desipramine (Norpramin®)	150–300 (150–300)	+ +	+ +	+ + +	+ + +
Nortriptyline (Pamelor®, Aventyl®)	150–300 (50–150)	+ + +	+ + +	+	+ + +
Protriptyline (Vivactil®)	15–60 (75–250)	+ + +	+	+ +	+ + + +
Tetracyclics					
Amoxapine (Asendin®)	150–400 (?)	+ + +	+ +	+ +	+ +
Maprotiline (Ludiomil®)	150–225 (150–300)	+ +	+ + +	+ +	+ + +

Abbreviation: TCAs, tricyclic antidepressants.

effective in treatment of MDD and have been FDA approved for this purpose. TCAs usually take four to six weeks for full antidepressant effects, though some improvement may be observed as early as first week. Individuals who do not respond to one TCA may respond to another because their norepinephrine–serotonin binding profiles differ.

Adverse Reactions and Cautions

Sedation or drowsiness is one of the most common side effects of TCAs and it is mainly due to anticholinergic and antihistaminic properties (Table 1). Other adverse reactions include dry mouth, dizziness, constipation, blurred vision, palpations, orthostatic hypotension, tachycardia, incoordination, increase in appetite, nausea or vomiting, sweating, weakness, allergic exanthematous rashes, restlessness, insomnia, urinary frequency or retention, weight gain, libido changes, impotence, photosensitivity, and paresthesias. Clinical signs of toxicity include disorientation, confusion, lethargy, tremor, ataxia, thought disorder, hallucinations, delusions, and delirium. Fulminant acute hepatitis is rare, although a transient rise in serum transaminases is a noted occurrence. Rarely, agranulocytosis, leukocytosis, leukopenia, and eosinophilia can occur. Amoxapine with its dopamine blocking properties is more likely to cause extrapyramidal symptoms. All TCAs can reduce seizure threshold, but this effect is more common with the use of amoxapine and clomipramine.

TCAs should be avoided in people with known cardiac conduction defects because these medications are known to prolong cardiac conduction time. They should be used with extreme caution in anyone with heart disease because they can cause hypo or hypertension, syncope, QT prolongation, torsades de pointes, atrioventricular block, ischemia, and stroke. Sudden death has been reported with use of certain TCAs in children and adolescents; they should be used with caution in this population (4). TCAs should also be avoided in individuals with narrow-angle glaucoma because they can precipitate acute consequences.

TCAs are contraindicated within 14 days of use of any MAOIs owing to hypertensive crisis. Caution should be used when combining TCAs with SSRIs because some may increase TCA levels through P450 interactions, and may have additive central nervous system (CNS) side effects such as serotonin syndrome. Caution should also be taken when combining TCAs with other CNS depressants such as alcohol, hypnotics, opioids, anxiolytics, and over-the-counter medications because they all may have additive CNS depressant effects when combined with TCAs.

Like all other antidepressants, TCAs can induce a manic episode in individuals with or without a history of bipolar disorder. They are also more likely to cause rapid cycling in individuals with bipolar disorder, when used without mood stabilizer (5). A recent FDA warning states that, similar to other antidepressants, they may also cause worsening depression and suicidality, especially in the initial stages of pharmacotherapy in children, adolescents, and even adults (6).

MAOI Antidepressants

Introduction

The MAOI family of antidepressants was discovered by clinical observation of patients taking an early antituberculosis drug, iproniazid. Many of these patients were found to have become happy, energetic, and sometimes agitated. Later studies involving psychiatric patients given MAOI revealed mood improvement (7). Early MAOIs have been replaced by relatively safer versions, and currently two of these—phenelzine and tranylcypromine—are marketed in the United States for treatment of depression (8). Another MAOI, selegiline, is used in the United States for treatment of Parkinson's symptoms. MAOIs are now seldom, if ever, used as first-line antidepressants because of the risk of hypertensive crisis.

Mechanism of Action

MAOIs act by inhibiting the monamine oxidase enzyme. Neurons are unable to break down dopamine, norepinephrine, and serotonin. This causes an overall increase in the level of these biogenic amines that is thought to account for their antidepressant action as well as their side effects. The MAOIs marketed in the United States are "irreversible," i.e., they bind to the MAO enzyme and destroy its function permanently. Function returns only when new enzymes are synthesized. In the body, there are two major subtypes of MAO—A and B. The A form oxidizes serotonin and norepinepherine, while MAO B is involved in dopamine degradation.

Pharmacologic Action

MAOIs are well absorbed from the digestive tract. Part of their metabolism is via acetylation in the liver. Genetic subgroups in the population include both rapid and slow acetylators; rapid acetylators may require higher doses to achieve therapeutic effects and slow acetylators require lower doses and are at higher risk for toxicity (9). There is little data on MAOI distribution in the body and the elimination of this medication from the body. Like other antidepressants, the onset of action can take three to four weeks before symptom reduction can be noted.

Drug Interactions

MAOIs should not be used with reserpine, carbamazapine, TCAs, SSRIs, alcohol, methyldopa, levodopa, sympathomimetic agents, pseudoephedrine, phenylpropanolamine, dopamine, and inhaled anesthetics. CNS depressants, e.g., meperidine (Demerol), may have their effects prolonged and intensified. Similarly, hypertensive crisis can also occur when MAOIs are combined with drugs such as SSRIs, TCAs, or sympathomimetic drugs that increase monoamine activity. When MAOIs are concomitantly used with other antidepressants, there can be an increase of plasma serotonin concentration to toxic levels, leading to serotonin syndrome, as well as, a tyramine hypertensive crisis. For this reason, combining MAOIs and other antidepressants is generally avoided. Patients should have at least a few weeks of SSRI discontinuation before being started on an MAOI. It is one of the rare scenarios where a "washout" period is practiced while switching antidepressants.

Psychiatric Uses

MAOIs are not first-line agents for treatment of depression. Currently, they are used in patients who have not had a satisfactory response to SSRIs, NDRIs, SNRIs, or TCAs. MAOIs may be utilized before a trial of ECT in seemingly refractory depressed patients (10,11). Additionally, MAOIs have been shown to be effective in the treatment of various other psychiatric disorders including social phobia, panic disorder, and OCD. Table 2 outlines typical dosing guidelines for these agents.

Adverse Reaction and Cautions

MAOIs do pose hazards for patients when combined with certain foods and medications. Foods with high concentrations of the amino acid, tyramine, are potentially dangerous to patients taking MAOIs. The tyramine reaction manifests itself as a sudden and severe rise in blood pressure; in some cases, this leads to cerebrovascular accident and death. This reaction occurs in the context of inhibited MAO tyramine oxidation that leads to massive release of endogenous stores of norepinepherine, and subsequent hypertension. Mild hypertensive reactions can occur with consumption of as little as 6 mg of tyramine, while moderate to severe reactions can occur from consumption of 10 mg or more of tyramine (12,13). The clinical signs of acute hypertensive crisis include headache, flushing and sweating, light sensitivity,

Table 2 Typical Dosing Guidelines for MAOIs

Drug name (Trade name)	Enzyme inhibition	Initial dose (mg)	Dose range (mg)
Phenelzine (Nardil®)	MAOI A and B	45	45–90
Tranylcypromine (Parnate®)	MAOI A and B	20	20–30
Selegiline (Eldepryl®)	MAOI B	5	5–15

Abbreviation: MAOIs, monoamine oxidase inhibitors.

stiff neck, chest pain or abnormal heartbeat, nausea, and/or vomiting. Some of the most common tyramine-rich foods that need to be avoided are cheese, cured or spoiled meats, pickled herring, yeast extracts, soy sauce, beer, Chianti, and Vermouth. A full list of prohibited foods can be found in the package insert of each medication. Additionally, patients need to be told to avoid aspartame because it too has been noted to provoke hypertensive crisis in patients taking MAOIs (14).

Common Adverse Effects

Postural hypotension and dizziness, as well as drowsiness, blurred vision, dry mouth, constipation, flatulence, agitation, insomnia, headache, tremor, dry eyes, increased appetite, and weight gain are common adverse effects associated with MAOI use.

Contraindications

Severe hepatic or renal dysfunction, pheochromocytoma, active alcoholism, and inability to comprehend and/or follow cautions regarding dietary restrictions or medication are the absolute contraindications associated with the use of MAOIs. Asthmatics should not be prescribed MAOIs because they will occasionally need to utilize bronchodilators that can provoke a hypertensive crisis. MAOIs have been associated with increased risk of fetal malformation if they are taken in the first trimester (15).

NDRI Antidepressants

Bupropion (Wellbutrin) is a generally effective and well-tolerated antidepressant. In 1985, it was approved by the FDA for the treatment of depression. Its release actually preceded that of fluoxetine, the original SSRI. After a period of market removal, it was reintroduced to the U.S. market in 1989. This break in sales was due to a higher incidence of seizures in patients with comorbid eating disorder or seizure disorder. Resumption of sales coincided with findings that incidence of drug-induced seizures was not higher than that observed with the use of other antidepressants, when the medication was used within the recommended maximum dose range of 300 to 450 mg a day (total daily dose). In 1996, bupropion SR (Zyban) was approved for smoking cessation, when combined with behavioral modification techniques. Buproprion is a safe and effective antidepressant with mild psychostimulating effects. It can be considered as a possible first-line treatment option for depressed patients. It more recently has been approved in a once daily, better-tolerated "XL" preparation (16).

Mechanism of Action

The exact mechanism of antidepressant action of buproprion is unknown, but is thought to be due to its action on both dopaminergic and noradrenergic systems. This drug is therefore classified as an NDRI. Buproprion inhibits the pumps and a net increase of these monoamines is noted (16–18).

Pharmacolgic Action(s)

Bupropion is well absorbed from the GI tract and is primarily metabolized by the liver. It has three active metabolites, which have longer elimination half-lives than the parent compound. It may take up to 10 days for these metabolites to reach steady state in the plasma. The elimination half-life of the parent compound combined with its active metabolites ranges from 8 to 40 hours (19).

Psychiatric Uses

Buproprion is indicated for the treatment of depression and smoking cessation. It appears to be especially effective in those with prominent vegetative symptoms (20). It is also the only non-nicotine medication for smoking cessation (21).

The onset of antidepressant action typically occurs two to four weeks after initiation of treatment. The medication comes in three formulations: immediate release (IR) (75, 100 mg), slow release (SR) (100, 150, 200 mg), and extended release (XR) (150, 300 mg).

Dosing: The IR form of this medication is not typically used owing to the higher incidence of side effects. Generally, the SR version is initiated at 150 mg by mouth once a day for seven days, then at 150 mg by mouth twice a day as standing dose. If no efficacy is observed, the dose is increased to 400 mg total daily dose. The XR version of the medication can be taken once a day in the morning and comes in tablets of 150 and 300 mg strength. Effective dosing occurs between 300 and 400 mg/day (22).

Adverse Reactions and Cautions

Buproprion is an advantageous antidepressant because of its low incidence of cardiovascular effects, anticholergic effects, sedative effects, appetite stimulation effects, and sexual dysfunction effects (23). Most common side effects are headache, insomnia, dry mouth, anxiety, and nausea. Insomnia appears to be a dose-related side effect (24).

Of all the antidepressants, it has the least potential for causing sexual dysfunction because it does not increase serotonin levels (25). Buproprion does not alter cardiac rhythms (26). It does not contribute to weight gain as do many other antidepressants, and it can promote weight loss. Care should be taken in prescribing it to underweight patients (27,28). Buproprion is contraindicated in patients with a history of seizures (including febrile seizures), head injury, anorexia, or bulimia (16). It does lower the seizure threshold. However, seizure risk does not appear to be excessive when dosed below total daily dose of 450 mg/day. The risk of seizure appears to be higher from the use of the IR form of the drug (29).

SSRIs

SSRIs represent a relatively new class of antidepressant drugs. Fluoxetine was the first SSRI to be introduced, and was FDA approved for treatment of MDD in 1987. Because SSRIs affect only serotonin (in contrast to MAOIs and TCAs), they are associated with a lower incidence of certain side effects. They have thus become the antidepressant first-line drugs of choice. This shift away from the use of TCAs appears to be related to the better tolerability of the SSRIs, their cardiac safety, and to some extent, their simple dosing. An important reason for their current popularity is that SSRIs have less potential for lethal overdose and are therefore considered very safe medications for use in a population at risk for suicide.

Currently, in the United States, six SSRIs are available; they include fluoxetine, sertraline, paroxetine, fluvoxamine, citalopram, and escitalopram (in the order of FDA approvals). Although all have antidepressant efficacy, only citalopram, escitalopram, fluoxetine, paroxetine, and sertraline have received approval from the FDA for use as an antidepressant. Fluvoxamine has been approved for use in treating OCD but not MDD in the United States.

Mechanism of Action

Although all of the SSRIs belong to a chemically distinct family (except escitalopram which is an *S*-enantiomer of citalopram), they all share a common pharmacological characteristic. They all inhibit serotonin reuptake transporters, have only minimal effect on norepinephrine–dopamine reuptake, and cause minimal manipulation of muscarinic–cholinergic receptors, histamine receptors, and alpha-1 adnergic receptors. The net effect of transporter blockade is the elevation of serotonin concentration. They also have no effect on sodium channels, which allows for a safer cardiac profile. This selective blocking of serotonin helps with depression and anxiety, but without significant and serious undesired side effects of TCAs (30).

All of the SSRIs have very weak affinity for a variety of receptors including 5HT1a/2a, dopamine D1 and 2, adrenergic $\alpha 1/2$, β, histamine H1, γ-aminobenzoic acid, cholinergic and benzodiazepine receptors. These are usually of little importance, but in any given patient, there may be subtle clinical differences between the effects caused by the SSRIs. Citalopram or escitalopram is the most selective inhibitor of serotonin, fluoxetine weakly inhibits norepinephrine reuptake and binds to 5HT2c receptors, paroxetine has some anticholinergic activity and also binds to nitric oxide synthase, and sertraline weakly inhibits norepinephrine and dopamine reuptake. These subtle in vitro variations may explain why patients who fail to respond to one SSRI may respond to another (30).

Pharmacological Action

All of the SSRIs are well absorbed orally and have bioavailablity of more than 80%. Fluoxetine has the longest half-life of one to four days and its active metabolite norfluoxetine has a half-life that ranges between 7 and 15 days. Sertraline has a half-life of 26 hours and its less active metabolite *N*-desmethylsertraline has a half-life of 60 to 100 hours. The half-life of citalopram is 35 hours, while that of paroxetine and fluvoxamine are 21 and 15 hours, respectively; all three lack an active metabolite.

Fluoxetine, fluvoxamine, and citalopram are racemic mixtures of two enantiomers whereas paroxetine, sertraline, and escitalopram are made up of a single isomer (escitalopram is the pure *S*-enantiomer or single isomer of the racemic derivative citalopram). All of the SSRIs are primarily metabolized in the liver by cytochrome P450 enzyme system. Two enzymes, CYP 3A4 and 2D6, are mainly involved. Sertraline, citalopram, and fluvoxamine are substrates of CYP 3A4, which suggests potential drug interactions at this isoenzyme; however, it should be noted that all of the SSRIs inhibit this isoenzyme. Paroxetine is the most potent inhibitor of the CYP 2D6 isoenzyme followed by fluoxetine. All of the SSRIs may raise the serum concentrations of a number of drugs that are metabolized by CYP 2D6 such as TCAs, cyclobenzaprine, dextromethorphan, some of the atypical antipsychotics, and venlafaxine. Fluvoxamine is a potent inhibitor of several CYP isoenzymes including 1A2, 2D6, 2C9, 2C19, and 3A4, causing drug–drug interactions that are clinically more critical than those of other SSRIs (31).

Psychiatric Use

SSRIs are clearly considered the first-line agent for the treatment of MDD. All SSRIs are equally effective in treatment of MDD. No SSRI has ever been shown to be definitively superior in respect to efficacy or tolerability. It takes the SSRIs typically four to six weeks to realize their full antidepressant effect, although some improvement can be observed as early as first week. Individuals may respond subtly to different SSRIs, and those who do not respond to one SSRI may have a subtly different efficacy or tolerability response to another. Typical clinical guidelines suggest that one or two SSRIs should be tried before the patient is deemed refractory to this class of medication. SSRIs are as effective as any other antidepressants in treatment of mild to moderate depression (32). Some studies have suggested that SNRIs such as TCAs, venlafaxine, and mirtazapine may be slightly more effective than SSRIs in the treatment of severe depression and depression with melancholic features (33,34). Currently, there is not enough evidence to suggest that SSRIs should not be considered as first-line antidepressant.

SSRIs are also effective in the treatment of depression in special populations—children, older adults, medically ill, and pregnant women. Fluoxetine is the only SSRI that is approved for treatment of depression

Table 3 Pharmacokinetics and Dosing Guidelines for the SSRIs

Drug name (Trad name)	Half-life	Initial dose (mg)	Dose range (mg)
Citalopram (Celexa[R])	35 hr	10–20	10–80
Escitalopram (Lexapro[R])	27–32 hr	10	20–40
Fluoxetine (Prozac[R])	4–6 days	10–20	10–80
Fluvoxamine (Luvox[R])	15 hr	25–50	50–300
Paroxetine (Paxil[R], Paxil CR[R,a])	21 hr	10–20	10–50
Sertraline (Zoloft[R])	26 hr	25–50	50–200

[a]Paxil-controlled release.
Abbreviation: SSRIs, selective serotonin reuptake inhibitors.

in children, whereas both fluoxetine and sertraline are approved for the treatment of OCD in children. Fluoxetine is most studied in pregnant women, and various studies have failed to find any perinatal complication in children who are exposed to it in vivo. However, general warnings exist; some infants exposed to all SSRIs in utero may have a serotonin syndrome upon delivery (35). Emerging data also suggest that the use of other SSRIs may be safe in this population. Effects on breast-fed children are minimal, and available data suggest that exposure for the nursing child is lowest with the use of sertraline, fluvoxamine, and paroxetine (35). Table 3 outlines the typical pharmacokinetics and dosing guidelines for the SSRIs.

Adverse Reactions and Cautions

Nausea is the most common adverse effect and generally decreases over time. Vomiting, diarrhea, and constipation have been reported. Other common reactions include headache, insomnia, asthenia, dizziness, dry mouth, tremor, dyspepsia, flu-like syndrome, sweating, rash, and abnormal vision. Decreased libido and ejaculatory dysfunction can occur in up to one-third of the patients treated with SSRIs (32). All SSRIs can produce chronic weight gain, however transient weight loss has been reported with the use of fluoxetine within the first few weeks of dosing. All SSRIs can produce secretion of inappropriate antidiuretic hormone. Increased prolactin, galactorrhea, and decreased fasting glucose level (up to 30%) have also been reported.

Like all other antidepressants, SSRIs can precipitate mania or hypomania in individuals with or without history of bipolar disorder. They are also more likely to cause rapid cycling in individuals with bipolar disorder when used without a mood stabilizer. In general, SSRIs are considered safer for use in this population than MAOIs and TCAs (5). All SSRIs are likely to increase the risk of suicidal thinking and behavior (suicidality) in children, adolescents, and adults with MDD and other psychiatric disorders, especially in the initial stages of the treatment. Epidemiologically, use of antidepressants appears to be a preventative to suicidality, but in prospective clinical trials, increases in suicidal thinking have been noted. In child and adolescent studies, there have been no reported completed suicides (6,36).

Serotonin syndrome is a potentially problematic hypermetabolic reaction that can occur when SSRIs are used as monotherapy or even concurrently administered with an MAOI, l-tryptophan, lithium, or other antidepressants that can raise plasma serotonin concentration to toxic levels. Symptoms of serotonin syndrome include diarrhea, lethargy, restlessness, confusion, flushing, diaphoresis, tremor, autonomic instability, and myoclonic jerks. As the syndrome progresses, hyperthermia, rigidity, hypertonicity, myoclonus, delirium, coma, status epilepticus, and death may rarely occur. Treatment consists of removing offending agents and providing medical support as needed (37). Caution should also be taken when combining with other CNS depressants such as alcohol.

When abruptly discontinued, SSRIs can be associated with serotonin withdrawal symptoms. These include the following: dysphoric mood, irritability, agitation, dizziness, sensory disturbances (e.g., paresthesias such as electric shock sensations), anxiety, confusion, headache, lethargy, emotional lability, insomnia, and hypomania. While these events are generally self-limiting, there have been reports of serious discontinuation symptoms. The withdrawal symptoms are more common with shorter half-life drugs such as paroxetine and fluvoxamine and least likely with fluoxetine, which with its long half-life effectively tapers itself. Patients should be monitored for these symptoms when discontinuing treatment with SSRIs. A gradual reduction in the dose rather than abrupt cessation is recommended whenever possible (38).

Trazodone

Trazodone (Desyrel) is an antidepressant medication structurally unlike TCAs, MAOIs, SSRIs, or SNRIs. It is FDA approved to treat MDD.

Mechanism of Action

Trazodone blocks alpha adrenergic receptors and is a mild selective inhibitor of serotonin reuptake. It also has potential dopamine receptor binding activity (39). One of its active metabolites also has postsynaptic serotonin receptor action (40).

Pharmacolgic Actions

It is readily absorbed from the GI tract. The elimination half-life is approximately 6 to 11 hours. Metabolism is primarily by the liver with the majority of excretion via urine. It must be dosed multiple times per day.

Psychiatric Uses

Trazodone has been shown to be an effective antidepressant; it is often used in depressed patients with significant insomnia because it is markedly sedating. However, trazodone is also commonly used as a non-FDA approved hypnotic to improve sleep, at doses of 25 to 100 mg at bedtime (41,42). It has a wide dosing range (300–600 mg), making the optimal dose for depression treatment difficult to determine. Antidepressant effects of trazodone typically take two to four weeks to occur. Immediate sedating effects occur approximately one hour after oral administration. The starting antidepressant dose is 50 mg on day 1, 50 mg twice a day on day 2, and if tolerated, 50 mg three times a day on day 3. Increases in dose should then be guided by patient response and tolerability. Increases in dose by 50 mg every three to four days are typical. A typical target dose is 300 mg a day after which the patient is evaluated for antidepressant response and side effects for one to two weeks. If depressive symptoms continue, increases in dosing to 400 to 600 mg total daily dose are warranted. Observation for orthostatic hypotension and excessive sedation must be made throughout treatment. For insomnia, doses between 25 and 100 mg taken at bedtime are reported to be effective, although no major clinical trials are available (43–45).

Adverse Reactions/Cautions

The most common side effects are sedation, orthostatic hypotension, dizziness, and nausea; other less common side effects include blurred vision, lightheadedness, headache, nausea, dry mouth, and priapism (46,47). Priapism is an uncommon but serious adverse reaction to trazodone treatment (48). Rarely chorea and myoclonus can occur at higher dose therapy (49). Trazodone is not associated with anticholinergic side effects such as constipation or urinary retention (50). This medicine is felt to be safe in regard to cardiac functioning and overdose.

Nefazodone

Nefazodone (Serzone) was developed as a safer drug, relative to Trazodone. Nefazodone appears to be FDA approved to treat MDD and has comparable efficacy and tolerability of other modern antidepressants.

Mechanism of Action

Nefazodone is a potent serotonin $5HT_2$ receptor antagonist and a weak SNRI. Its antagonizing of the $5HT_2$ receptor results in greater $5HT_{1a}$ binding. Its most avid binding is to the $5HT_{2a}$ receptor, and at higher concentrations, it binds to alpha-1 adrenergic receptors and serotonin reuptake pumps as well (51). At low doses, the parent drug and its active metabolite can block the $5HT_{2a}$ receptor without necessarily blocking the serotonin reuptake pump. The low binding affinity of nefazodone for the 5HT reuptake pump may explain the necessity for higher concentrations of the drug to see an antidepressant effect (52).

Pharmacologic Action(s)

Nefazodone is well absorbed from the GI tract. It is an inhibitor of the p450 CYP 3A4 isoenzyme; therefore drug–drug interactions need to be considered. Significantly, alparazolam and triazolam are examples of medications that could cause unexpected rises in serum concentration owing to the inhibition of their metabolism. It is metabolized into triazolodine therefore examples of which itself is a potent $5HT_{2a}$ blocker (53). The average half-life of the parent compound and metabolites is averaged to be 11 to 24 hours. The wide range of half-lives of elimination of the parent compound and its active metabolites yields nonlinear pharmokinetics. Absorption is rapid after oral administration, with peak plasma concentrations of parent compound being achieved after 1.2 hours. It is excreted by both digestive and renal pathways (Package Insert).

Psychiatric Uses

Nefazodone is primarily used in the treatment of MDD. The usual starting dose is 100 mg twice a day, and it is upwardly titrated based upon patient response, with a typical target dose of 300 to 600 mg total daily dose. The rate of dose increase is 100 to 200 mg at one-week intervals, guided by patient clinical response and side effects. Among the elderly, the usual dose is halved (54).

Adverse Reactions/Cautions

Its complex and non-SSRI mechanism of action allows it to cause less activating insomnia and sexual side effects despite its elevating serotonin activity. Nefazodone has a relatively low incidence of anticholergic side effects due to its very low affinity for muscarinic–cholinergic receptors when compared to the TCAs.

Most common and dose-related side effects are nausea, drowsiness, fatigue, and dry mouth. Nausea typically decreases over time. Side effects appear to be dose related, increasing when doses over 300 mg/day are taken (55).

Rare but serious liver failure in patients treated with the drug has led to its removal from the market in Canada and Europe. Patients with active liver disease or elevated levels of liver transaminases should not ordinarily be treated with this medication. It appears that blood monitoring is not effective in predicting this side effect (56).

Selective SNRIs

Venlafaxine was first in the new class of drugs known as the SNRIs and was introduced into the market in 1993 (57). These modern "dual action" antidepressants offer the same mechanism and efficacy as the TCAs without many of the toxic side effects associated with the use of TCAs. In comparison to the SSRIs, which have a relatively narrow effect upon neurotransmitter systems, venlafaxine has effects upon multiple receptor systems (norepinephrine and serotonin). It is effective as an antidepressant in both the acute and long-term (6–12 months) setting. It is effective for the treatment of mild to severe depression, generalized anxiety disorder, as well as, social anxiety disorder for which, FDA approvals have been granted (58–61).

The most recent FDA-approved antidepressant is also an SNRI called duloxetine. It also is a dual mechanism drug. The two approved SNRIs are different in their affinity and capacity to block reuptake pumps. For example, venlafaxine is a full SSRI at lower doses and as the dose is increased, more of the norepinephrine is elevated. Duloxetine also favors serotonin elevation, but at initial doses, norepinephrine is somewhat elevated (62). Duloxetine is also FDA approved to treat pain associated with polyneuropathy and is in line for approval for use in the treatment of stress incontinence.

Mechanism of Action

At low doses, venlafaxine has an action of serotonin reuptake inhibition, and at higher doses (above 150 mg) it possesses norepinephrine reuptake inhibition (63). It has a mechanism of action similar to that of the TCA, imipramine, without anticholinergic, sedative, or hypotensive side effects. Most of its action occurs at the 5HT reuptake pump; it is five times more potent at this site than at the norepinephrine reuptake pump (51). This versatility allows a clinician to specifically target a transmitter system that needs to be manipulated in any given patient. It may be a weak inhibitor of dopamine reuptake, although this role is controversial. The net effect is that the drug increases serotonin and norepinephrine (64). The two approved SNRIs are different in regard to their affinity and capacity to block reuptake pumps. Like venlafaxine, duloxetine also favors serotonin elevation, but at initial doses, norepinephrine is somewhat elevated as well. This medication starts as "dual acting" from the start of clinical treatment. These differing ratios of transporter blockade also allow for subtly differing efficacy and tolerability profiles on a case-by-case basis. A clinician may choose one agent over the other depending on how much norepinephrine is desired, in a way comparable to the use of TCA in the past (62,65).

Pharmacologic Action(s)

Venlafaxine is a phenylethylamine compound, distinct from other antidepressants. Both the parent compound, venlafaxine, and its active metabolite, *O*-desmethylvenlafaxine are potent inhibitors of serotonin and norepinephrine reuptake and weaker inhibitors of dopamine reuptake. It does not have significant activity at histaminergic, muscarinic, nicotinic, or adrenergic receptors and is not a MAOI (66).

Venlafaxine is well absorbed from the GI system. The drug has linear kinetics over the normal dose range. Its elimination half-life is approximately five hours. It is primarily metabolized in the liver via the p450

2D6 isoenzyme system. It may have the lowest 2D6 and lowest protein binding capacity of modern antidepressants.

Formulation is as an IR or XR tablet or capsule. The XR formulation is more commonly used for both increased patient compliance and tolerability.

Dosing: The IR form is dosed at 37.5 mg twice a day with increases in dose of 75 mg no more than once every four days with target total daily dose of 150 to 375 mg a day. The XR formulation has a starting dose of 37.5 mg a day increased after four to five days to 75 mg, then up to 225 mg total daily dose with increases of dose no sooner than four days in-between dose escalation (67).

For duloxetine and its enteric coating of capsules, maximal serum concentrations are achieved approximately six hours after oral administration. The excretion half-life of the medication is approximately 12.5 hours, and steady state plasma levels are achieved after three days. Unlike venlafaxine, it is highly bound to proteins in plasma.

Both the oxidative and glucuronidation pathways are used in metabolism. It aggressively inhibits the p450 2D6 isoenzyme subsystem as a major drug interaction comparable to both fluoxetine and paroxetine. While smokers may see one-third less bioavailability of duloxetine due to CYP 1A2 induction, this represents a modest amount in relation to acceptable dosing ranges. Dose adjustment is not recommended for smokers (68,69).

The range of target dose is between 60 and 120 mg. No evidence exists in support of the opinon that doses above 60 mg a day will provide a clinically significant benefit (68,69).

Adverse Reactions/Cautions

Venlafaxine is a generally well-tolerated medication. It has little anticholergic side effects (minimal sedation or orthostatic hypotension) due to its low binding affinity to histaminic, muscarinc–cholinergic, or alpha-adrenergic receptors. At lower doses, side effects are similar to those associated with the use of SSRIs and at higher doses, those associated with the use of norepinephrine occur and there is an increase in the side effect rate, most notably nausea. The most commonly reported side effects are nausea, dry mouth, dizziness, restlessness, and insomnia. Venlafaline has low reported incidence of causing sexual dysfunction when compared to other antidepressants. At higher doses, mild increases in blood pressure may occur. Sustained hypertension occurs rarely, therefore regular blood pressure monitoring is recommended. This drug is also capable of inducing serotonin syndrome and serotonin withdrawal upon discontinuation (70–72).

For duloxetine, the most commonly experienced side effects are nausea, dry mouth, constipation, decreased appetite, fatigue, and increased sweating. Some patients may experience sexual side effects such as decreased libido, delayed orgasm, erectile dysfunction, delayed and/or abnormal ejaculation.

The risk of causing urinary retention is limited, but well noted. Some patients may experience weak obstructive voiding. As rare increases in liver function tests have been observed in patients treated with duloxetine, it is not recommended that it be prescribed to patients with substantial alcohol abuse. Also, patients with uncontrolled narrow angle glaucoma should not be prescribed this medication. It is not known to cause changes in electrocardiologic function. However, clinically significant increases in blood pressure have been observed in patients taking duloxetine, therefore regular monitoring of blood pressure and heart rate should occur during treatment (73–76). There have been no reports of symptoms associated with serotonin withdrawal, but the occurrence of serotonin syndrome is possible. The SNRIs, like all antidepressants, carry warnings about increased risk of suicide (65).

Mirtazapine

Mirtazapine has a unique pharmacological profile, unlike any previously mentioned drug. It is a dual action antidepressant with the coined term, "NaSSA." It has low toxicity, low drug–drug interactions. It appears particularly useful in depressed patients with prominent insomnia, anxiety, agitation, or anorexia.

Mechanism of Action

Mirtazapine is a potent antagonist of central alpha-2 adrenergic autoreceptors and heteroreceptors as well as an antagonist of postsynaptic serotonin 5HT2 and 5HT3 receptors. The use of mirtazapine results in increased serotonergic and noradrenergic transmission in a mechanism distinct from that of both TCAs and SNRIs. It is therefore termed as "NaSSA" (77). It also has potent binding to the H1 histamine receptor and may be quite sedating (78,79). Its sedative effect at lower doses is most likely due to histamine-1 receptor binding. The sedative effects can be present at doses below those that yield an antidepressant effect. As the dose is increased, the blockade of the alpha-2 adrenergic receptor occurs, and this may create an alerting effect (52).

Pharmacologic Action(s)

Typically used doses result in blockade of $5HT_{2a}$, $5HT_{2c}$, $5HT_3$, and alpha-2 adrenergic receptors. This combination offers a unique way of treating MDD (80,81). Mirtazapine has linear pharmacokinetics along its normal dose range.

Drug metabolism is by several p450 isoenzymes; however, it is not a potent inhibitor of any p450 isoenzyme. It is well absorbed in the GI tract, and is primarily excreted via the urine and, to a lesser extent, from the GI tract. Elimination half-life is 20 to 40 hours.

Mirtazapine is particularly useful for depressed patients who also have anxiety, sleep disturbance, somatization, and anorexia (82). It tends to be less activating and induces less insomnia and agitation than SSRI, SNRI, or TCA agents. There is also evidence supporting its long-term efficacy in preventing relapse of depression (83).

Adverse Reactions/Cautions

Common side effects include somnolence, appetite increase, and weight gain (84). Mirtazapine may be more sedating at lower doses (15 mg) than at higher doses (30 mg/day and up). This is likely due to its high affinity for histamine–H1 receptors. It is not associated with sexual dysfunction but may induce marked weight gain when compared with other older and modern antidepressants (85). There have been three reported cases of neutropenia that resolved after mirtazapine discontinuation (84).

Conclusions

This part of the chapter has covered the chronological history of drug development and FDA approval of antidepressants. It is clear that we have the ability to use multiple agents to treat MDD. Later in this book, we will discuss using multiple agents in a polypharmacy manner and how to mitigate antidepressant adverse effects. The final interesting area is in regard to the biological origins of MDD, in that drugs all elevate certain monoamines. These transmitters are elevated instantly, yet antidepressant effect is often delayed in patients. We do notice that the elevated transmitter leads to downregulation or lowering of the appropriate receptors on postsynaptic neurons. How does the neuron know to downregulate? We also note that there are often increases in neurotrophic factors that make neurons healthier (86). It is entirely possible that the initial elevation of monoamine transmitter(s), sets off a cascade of intraneuronal genetic events (transcription and translation of new proteins) that may signal receptor downregulation or increase neurotrophic factor output. In fact, our patients may not have a "chemical imbalance" but may have some genetic dysregulation, which will be discussed in a later chapter.

PSYCHOTHERAPY

In this section, we trace the development of psychotherapies for use in the treatment of depression and then provide an overview of the theoretical underpinnings, techniques, and purported mechanisms of change for each treatment. The therapies discussed here are often referred to as depression-focused psychotherapies and include a number of time-limited psychosocial treatments with varying degrees of empirical support. Broad categories of such treatments include behavior therapies (87), cognitive therapy (CT) (88), and interpersonal psychotherapy (IPT) (89). Each model of psychotherapy draws its name principally from the objectives of treatment.

One feature that these therapies hold in common is that they neither rely on psychodynamic formulations of depressive psychopathology nor emphasize more traditional methods centering on the therapeutic relationship to guide the process of therapy. Rather, each type of therapy emphasizes the use of model-specific formulations, psychoeducation, and procedurally guided interventions to help patients learn to cope with and, hopefully, recover from depression. Another common feature is that each of these psychotherapies has been subjected to empirical study using the methods of randomized clinical trials. In fact, these therapies are the best-studied nonsomatic treatments of MDD.

History of Depression-Focused Psychotherapies

A series of developments in the mental health field between the end of World War II and the early 1980s led to the development and ultimately acceptance of the aforementioned psychotherapeutic treatments for depression. First, there were increasingly significant doubts that more traditional psychodynamic approaches to psychotherapy were effective in the treatment of depression (90–93). For example, the reflective and nondirective methods commonly used in psychodynamic psychotherapy were viewed as, sometimes, counterproductive in work with more severely depressed patients, who seemed to benefit from more active therapeutic support, structure, and guidance (94,95). This was of particular concern because the field of psychopharmacotherapy had established antidepressants as providing reliably rapid relief from depressive symptoms (96,97). As a result, there was a great demand to find comparably effective treatments in the psychotherapeutic realm.

A second development that helped give rise to the development of the more time-limited, evidence-based psychotherapies was the lack of willingness of the thought leaders in the field of traditional psychotherapies to test the efficacy of their own treatment models. As a result, government research funds were earmarked for projects that involved testing the newer therapies. At completion of these studies, findings involving these newer therapies found their way to prestigious journals that were once mostly home to traditional therapy-related articles. Complicating the situation was the difficulty that traditional therapists had in operationalizing what took place during treatment—a problem that still exists today. One resulting shift that occurred as a result of the centering of empirical research on time-limited therapies was the loss of influence of academic psychiatrists and psychologists who espoused traditional therapies as the treatment of choice for depression.

Third is a development for the problem that involved a significant shortage of psychotherapists in the mental health community at large. More depressed patients were seeking outpatient treatment as a result of both deinstitutionalization and greater illness recognition. Given that a greater number of clinicians were required, it made sense to train at least some of these practitioners in schools of therapy that were growing in popularity and were becoming more affordable to patients and third-party insurers (98–100). As a result, a cadre of therapists trained in these new treatments began working in various mental health settings. Thus, the menu of psychotherapy options for the depressed patient increased.

Fourth, these trends coincided with the emergence of alternative, nonmedical paradigms to the problems of psychopathology and therapeutics. The behavioral approach, stemming largely from academic clinical psychology and work with animals, introduced models of treatment originating from research using classical (101) and operant (90) conditioning to change or modify overt behavior. CT, as best reflected in the clinical work of Beck (102), built upon behavioral formulations by incorporating similar attention to covert processes, such as thoughts, attitudes, and beliefs. The cognitive behavioral school of psychotherapy also was informed by new developments in the social psychology realm, notably the cognitive information processing models. From neoanalytic schools of psychotherapy, in addition to social psychiatry, marital counseling, and social work, came a growing appreciation of the interpersonal and relational contexts of depressions, culminating in the model of therapy developed by Klerman et al. (89).

Finally, as alluded to earlier, the issues of efficacy and reimbursement for health care services slowly but progressively became intertwined as concerns about the cost-effectiveness of mental health treatments mounted. The issue of reimbursement for psychotherapy is hardly a new one (103), and skepticism about the cost-effectiveness of psychotherapy has persisted for nearly 50 years (104). Research concerning the relative efficacy of various treatments has been stimulated by the need to demonstrate to third-party payers and governmental agencies that psychotherapy is a cost-effective endeavor. In addition, given that most points of contact for patients seeking mental health care are within primary care settings, the emphasis in this culture on cost containment, brief visits, and justification of continued treatment to third-party payers had considerable carry over into the mental health treatment realm.

The depression-focused psychotherapies share a number of features that include a short treatment duration (typically less than six months for a total of 16–24 sessions), specific linkage of a theoretical model of phenomenology with strategies for symptom reduction, specific methods to facilitate training of clinicians and enhance fidelity to the treatment model (105,106), and an emphasis on the identification and measurement of specific goals and outcomes of treatment. The latter two qualities are crucial advantages for empirical studies in that both independent (i.e., type of therapy) and dependent (i.e., symptom change) variables can be readily defined to ensure internal validity. The particular theoretical orientation of each model of treatment also yields predictions about specific outcomes, such as the effects of behavioral treatment on measures of social skill (107), CT on measures of dysfunctional attitudes (108), or IPT on measures of social adjustment (109). Finally, these therapies have several pragmatic features in common, including their compatibility for use in combination with pharmacotherapy and their suitability for use by selected nondoctoral therapists after appropriate training. Finally, all the depression-focused, time-limited therapies involve an alliance between patient and therapist that is based on mutual respect, genuineness, and empathy. The nature of this relationship is best described as collaborative as the therapist and patient work together toward a common goal—relief of symptoms and maximizing long-term wellness.

The current climate of depression-focused psychotherapy practice can best be characterized in the following manner. A significant percentage of practitioners (psychologists, social workers, and other therapist disciplines) who treat depressed patients identify themselves as practicing either cognitive-behavior therapy (CBT) or IPT. However, this percentage is likely higher in and near academic research centers and decreases as one moves into more isolated, nonacademic environments. There are still a substantial percentage of clinicians practicing psychodynamically oriented treatments, and another substantially sized group practicing some form of supportive therapy. Unfortunately, these latter two treatments do not have significant empirical support and thus are not considered front-line psychotherapeutic treatments for depression. One caveat to this description is that many practitioners practice something different from what they report to be practicing. Degree of fidelity to stated treatment orientation probably varies considerably, and this will likely be a phenomenon that we will face in the field for a long time. Nonetheless, increased dissemination of evidence-based treatment skills needs to be a priority for the field, and can be accomplished through continuing education programs, journal articles, and graduate training program enhancements. With these efforts, we can increase the number of clinicians providing state-of-the-art psychotherapeutic interventions.

Some significant developments that challenge some long-standing beliefs regarding how symptom reduction is attained within these treatment models have taken place during the last several years. Specifically, the development of mindfulness based CT (MBCT) by Segal et al. (110) as well as acceptance and commitment therapy (ACT) by Hayes et al. (111) represent significant paradigm shifts. MBCT, a group therapy for depressed patients, teaches patients to view negative thoughts as cognitive events, not reflective of necessary truths. Informed greatly by Jon Kabat Zinn's Mindfulness Meditation (112), MBCT does not aim to alter the content of cognitions, rather the way in which patients relate to them. Studies conducted to date, although pilot in nature, suggest that this treatment is quite efficacious. A larger, more pivotal study is now underway. ACT differs somewhat from MBCT in that it is mostly conducted in an individual format and emphasizes the reduction of avoidant behavior through increasing a patient's awareness of thoughts, feelings, memories, and physical sensations that have been feared and avoided. Practitioners emphasize that patients learn to accept internal events, and patients are also taught to develop greater clarity about personal values and to commit to needed behavior change.

Another significant change within the field has been modification of time-limited therapies to serve the needs of patients who are deemed responders or remitters to acute phase treatment. Several studies suggest that implementation of psychotherapy postacute phase treatment (typically an antidepressant) may confer a better long-term illness course than if these treatments are combined acutely (113). To address the needs of patients at this stage of treatment, some researchers have introduced a focus on relapse prevention through efforts to enhance well-being and eliminate residual depressive symptoms (114). Trials conducted to date using these therapies modified for illness stage show quite promising results. It could be that a sequential treatment strategy—acute phase pharmacotherapy followed by the continuation phase addition of these modified psychotherapies—may ultimately prove superior in preventing relapse and recurrence than using the traditional acute phase combination approach.

Finally, other noteworthy developments, reflecting findings published just before this writing, suggest potentially fruitful areas of further research. First, Hollon et al. (115,116) examined the effectiveness of CT versus antidepressant medication in the treatment of severe depression in a population for which antidepressant treatment is considered a necessary component of treatment. In the first study of its kind, Hollon et al. found CT alone to be as effective as antidepressant medication in the acute treatment of severe depression. This is a dramatic finding and one that suggests that CT, provided by well-trained therapists, can be used as a monotherapy for even the most depressed patients. In a companion study, Hollon et al. then compared relapse prevention effects of continuation CT versus antidepressant treatments and found that CT outperformed antidepressant treatment in relapse prevention. Patients receiving continuation CT had been tapered off antidepressant treatments taken during the acute phase of treatment. This study suggests that exposure to CT versus no exposure to CT is associated with a better long-term course. This was the first large-scale, multisite study to demonstrate this effect. In related work, Petersen et al. (117) demonstrated that exposure to continuation CT and antidepressant medications versus medications alone was associated with the maintenance of healthy gains in psychological constructs (e.g., attributional style) that are considered an important cognitive aspect of resolution of depressive symptoms. Taken together, these studies suggest that CT may have broader indications—even in severely depressed patients—than commonly thought, and may confer a better long-term illness course when added during the continuation phase of treatment.

A final area, also reflective of very recently published research, suggests that a psychotherapy system specifically designed to treat chronically depressed patients—the cognitive behavioral analysis system of psychotherapy (CBASP)—is quite efficacious in reducing symptoms in this subpopulation of depressed patients (118). Perhaps more intriguing is that CBASP, when combined in this study with nefazodone treatment, yielded response rates (greater than 70%) that are unheard of in acute phase clinical trials for MDD. A larger study is ongoing, and addresses the most glaring limitation of this study—lack of a placebo control group. From a broader perspective, the development of CBASP—a novel blend of interpersonal, cognitive, developmental, and psychodynamic conceptualization and techniques—suggests that more difficult-to-treat patients will respond to a psychotherapy that is customized to address the unique needs of this subgroup.

Overview of Depression-Focused Psychotherapies

IPT

IPT evolved between the late 1960s and early 1980s. The developers of IPT (119) trace its origins to the work of Meyer (120) that emphasizes the significance of psychosocial and interpersonal experiences within a more comprehensive psychobiological model of psychopathology. One of Meyer's associates, Sullivan (121), is similarly acknowledged for blending work from anthropology and sociology within a more interpersonally based approach to psychoanalysis. The interpersonal model of depression also draws upon the writings of Bowlby (122), Brown and Harris (123), Becker (124), and Chodoff (125), in which depression is viewed from relational and social perspectives.

IPT of depression was initially conceived as a brief psychological treatment for unipolar major depression. This outpatient therapy is typically provided over 12 to 16 weeks on an individual basis, although it has also been adapted for work with couples (126). It is readily used with or without concomitant antidepressant pharmacotherapy. A manual guiding individual therapy for patients with MDD is available (89), and various modifications of IPT for conditions such as dysthymia, depression in adolescents, and late-life depression have been described (126). When administered in research protocols, IPT is readily discriminated from CT and pharmacotherapy (127,128).

At the most basic level, IPT aims to improve the quality of a depressed patient's interpersonal world. Klerman and Weissman (119) emphasized that the premise of IPT is that regardless of its severity, phenomenology, or presumed etiology, depression occurs within an interpersonal context. The authors further proposed that helping patients to improve their understanding of and ability to modify the interpersonal context associated with depression facilitates the recovery process. Additional long-term benefits were proposed to include improved social function and prophylaxis against relapse. Original work utilizing IPT also drew heavily upon the methods and findings of social casework (129). As a result, the therapy was always intended to be feasible for social workers and other master's degree–prepared mental health workers, as well as psychologists and psychiatrists.

The social milieu of those suffering from depression is central to the IPT therapist's formulation of the treatment plan. Of particular importance are the high rates of life stressors temporally associated with the onset of unipolar depression, especially that arising from both acute and chronic marital difficulties (130–132). From this vantage point, a common theme in IPT centers on the relationship between the fragility of attachment bonds and vulnerability to depression. Conversely, the apparent protective or neutralizing role of social support (123) provides a potent avenue for therapy through efforts to help the patient strengthen his or her intimate relationships. Another important aspect of the depressed person's social milieu is his or her performance in social and interpersonal roles. Not only the depressed person's role functioning within his or her nuclear family, but also his or her social role performance at the workplace, with friends and peer groups, and in the broader sense of neighborhood or community are germane to IPT (119). Attention to social role performance thus includes the careful assessment of the individual's current and long-term patterns of functioning in diverse situations, as well as more recent or still-evolving role transitions.

IPT also may be considered a psychoeducational intervention because, in addition to laying strong social emphasis, therapists explicitly teach patients about depression and its treatment. This includes the therapist's willingness to provide practical advice or recommendations to help patients better tolerate the symptoms of depression (89). Although less structured than CT or behavior therapy, IPT similarly aims to help patients improve management of the symptoms and impairments associated with the depressive state. These efforts also serve to help lessen the demoralization and hopelessness experienced by most depressed people. The therapy may be quite active in this regard, by providing patients assistance using problem-solving strategies.

Treatment with IPT thus begins with an explanation of the diagnosis and treatment plan. Concurrently, the therapist establishes a working alliance and performs an assessment of current interpersonal relationships. Many therapeutic strategies used in IPT are based directly on core psychotherapy skills and processes, such as creating an environment in which there is nonjudgmental exploration and elicitation of feelings. In fact, the ability to become a competent IPT therapist is highly correlated with the therapist's ability to be empathic and genuine (89).

Next, the IPT therapist helps the patient to identify the common interpersonal theme areas that are associated with the depressive disorder. During the initial sessions of therapy, an interpersonal inventory is obtained to help guide treatment on one or two key problem areas. Four common theme areas generally serve as the focus for IPT: unresolved grief, role disputes, role transitions, and interpersonal deficits. The latter category incorporates areas such as the maladaptive interpersonal patterns associated with personality disorders, regression or deterioration in the patient's social role performance, social isolation, and/or decline of socioeconomic status (133).

Therapeutic interventions are guided by the manual of Klerman et al. (89). In cases of unresolved grief, explicit attention is provided to help the patient to mourn the lost loved one. Encouragement to begin to develop new relationships is also provided. When IPT centers on social role disputes, the therapist helps the patient to determine if his or her relationship difficulties might benefit from renegotiation (as when the conflict appears to be at an impasse) or dissolution (as when options might include separation or divorce). In states of role transition, the therapeutic strategies center on recognition of how the transition has affected the person's life, exploration of the likely consequences of these changes, and assistance in developing solutions to problems engendered by the transition. When interpersonal deficits are paramount, overcoming social isolation and lack of fulfillment is often emphasized. Regardless of the key theme area, the interpersonal therapist attends to the role of personality patterns in the genesis and maintenance of the problem. For example, the therapist may encourage the patient to try out a different way of interacting and to compare the outcome with his or her more habitual response (89). Patients who have difficulty engaging in such a productive relationship may have a harder time with IPT and, in turn, may elicit less competent interventions from otherwise well-trained therapists (134,135).

Some evidence suggests that IPT may be perceived as a more acceptable treatment for depression than either pharmacotherapy or cognitive-behavioral therapies, at least with respect to younger patients (136). Moreover, it has been suggested that it may be easier for traditionally trained therapists to master IPT than either behavioral or cognitive therapies (137).

Behavior Therapy

Behavioral treatments of depression are derived from operant conditioning, social learning theory, and, to a lesser extent, classical conditioning to various psychopathological states. These approaches share a common focus on changing observable, problematic behaviors and the use of functional analysis to modify the contingencies that shape and maintain the depressed patient's behavior.

From the vantage point of operant conditioning, the depressed patient is on a prolonged extinction schedule, in which there are fewer reinforcers and progressively fewer adaptive behaviors for which the patient will receive positive reinforcement (90). The despair experienced by the depressed person may be understood, in part, as being analogous to the emotional behaviors seen in a variety of organisms during extinction paradigms. Classical conditioning models, as best exemplified by Wolpe's (101,138) application of systematic desensitization, posit a relationship between sustained dysphoric arousal and induction of depressed mood and behavior. Incorporation of principles of social learning theory broadened behavior therapy to include cognitive or representational constructs, such as Bandura's (139) formulation of self-efficacy and Rehm's (140) concept of self-control. Thus, depressed persons' decreased confidence in their ability to solve their problems and minimization of their successes is posited to reduce the likelihood of coping behavior and worsen dysphoric emotional states.

The model of learned helplessness developed by Seligman (141) parallels the work of Wolpe (138) that was originally based on classical conditioning. For example, in animal studies, exposure to inescapable non-contingent shocks initially results in increased emotional arousal, with a more depressive-like state of passivity ultimately resulting from prolonged exposure. It is not clear, however, whether it is the neurochemical effects of prolonged stress or the perception that one's situation is hopeless that is more integral to the development of depression in humans.

Contemporary behavioral approaches also emphasize the reciprocity between the depressed patient's behavior and that of his or her significant others, friends, and coworkers. For example, research has shown that although acute changes in one's mood and behavior (i.e., crying or complaining) may evoke responses of support and sympathy from others, sustained contact with a depressed person typically results in avoidance and detachment on the part of the significant others (142,143). The depressed person may respond to such withdrawal with threats or demands to try to coerce the desired response from family members. Alternatively, the sick role may be adopted in which dependent, help-seeking behaviors are inadvertently reinforced by intermittently helpful loved ones. The dysfunctional communication patterns that characterize the relationships of many depressed patients create an environment that certainly maintains, and possibly triggers, some clinical depressions (131,142).

Behavioral treatments of depression include the social learning approaches of McLean (144) and Lewinsohn et al. (145), Rehm's (140) model of self-control therapy, social skills training (146), and Nezu's (147) structured problem-solving therapy. These approaches offer multicomponent treatment packages that have many more similarities than differences. Each model of therapy is time-limited, offering 8 to 16 weeks of therapy; all emphasize a functional analysis of the relationship between the presumed difficulty (i.e., deficient social reinforcement, poor social skills, or inefficient problem-solving strategies) and the onset and/or maintenance of the depressive syndrome. Each approach utilizes explicit, stepwise strategies to improve recognition of problem areas and to begin to implement the targeted changes in thoughts, feelings, or behavior. Behavioral therapies generally follow a model in which the desired behavior change is accomplished via education, observation, guided practice, social reinforcement of successive approximations, and individualized homework assignments.

Common strategies that are used in behavior therapy include self-monitoring, self-reinforcement, graded task assignments, activity scheduling, and targeted improvements in social skills through assertiveness training, modeling, and role playing. Relaxation training, which may be more parsimoniously viewed as a self-control skill rather than a counter-conditioning procedure (148), is also widely incorporated as a means to cope with anxiety or insomnia (145,149). Indeed, relaxation training may have a modest primary antidepressant effect, whether used alone (149,150) or in combination with pharmacotherapy (151).

Behavioral distraction techniques, such as thought stopping, are sometimes used to help patients gain some control over intrusive depressive ruminations. Behavioral therapies do not place a specific emphasis on the relationship between the therapist and the patient. Nevertheless, there is broad recognition that the core therapeutic qualities of empathy, genuineness, and respect help to strengthen the therapeutic alliance and to facilitate a treatment environment conducive to learning and mastery of the targeted therapeutic task.

Each form of behavior therapy emphasizes continued application of skills learned in treatment to reduce risk of relapse. More specific attention to relapse prevention is provided in several models of behavior therapy (98,145,149), in which patients may attend periodic booster sessions (149) or monthly sessions for continuation of therapy (146).

The behavior therapies have received much attention in group formats, which can be advocated as an efficient means to teach the model and strategies of relating to others (145,147,152). As in IPT, modifications for marital treatment are quite feasible (153,154).

Behavior therapy has largely been the domain of clinical psychologists, although not exclusively so (137,138). Nevertheless, many of the manual-guided behavioral therapies are easily learned by master's degree–prepared professionals of other disciplines (145). None of the treatment programs developed to date have been specifically intended for use in combination with pharmacotherapy, although their concomitant use is hardly contraindicated (146,149,155).

CT

CT developed between the late 1950s and mid-1970s as a result of the work of Beck (102,156). The cognitive theory of depression posits the involvement of three types of problems in cognition. The first type of cognitive dysfunction is reflected by the fact that depressed persons spend a disproportionate amount of time thinking gloomy or unpleasant thoughts about themselves, their world, and their future. Beck (102) has referred to the content of thoughts in these three domains—self, world, and future—as the cognitive triad. Cognitions that are particularly relevant are those that occur almost instantaneously with the worsening of depressed moods, which are referred to as automatic negative thoughts. These negative cognitions provide the gateway for the cognitive therapist to understand the depressed patient's phenomenological world.

The second type of cognitive dysfunction involves errors in information processing including over generalization, excessive personalization, selective abstraction, emotional reasoning, and all-or-none thinking (157). Such difficulties are characteristically state dependent, that is, only apparent during the depressive episode (158–160). Mood-dependent changes in information processing may be heuristically understood as serving to clarify and intensify the guiding beliefs that characterize the patient's phenomenological world (161,162). In this way, the mistaken conclusions resulting from errors in information processing serve to reinforce and maintain changes in self-esteem and pessimism that typify the depressive state.

The third type of cognitive dysfunction involves dysfunctional attitudes and depressogenic schema (102,163,164). Both attitudes and schema are considered to be ultimately accessible through questioning techniques, as illustrated by the use of the Socratic method or guided discovery (88). The personal meaning revealed in a series of automatic thoughts is thus used to infer deeper patterns of cognitive organization (102). Dysfunctional attitudes not only are associated with more extreme or intense reactions to life stress but also appear to confer a greater risk of encountering new adversities (165).

CT thus is more traditionally oriented than behavior therapy because dysfunctional attitudes and schema are unconscious and nonobservable constructs. These depressogenic structures are presumed to result from adverse early experiences (102,163). In persons prone to depression, schema representing excessive interpersonal dependence or perfectionistic demands are proposed to be silent during times of a stable romantic relationship or a high vocational attainment (166).

However, they are activated in response to specific, matching adversities (167,168). The activation of a pathological schema is hypothesized to induce mood-dependent changes in memory, information processing, and automatic negative thoughts (162,166). Stress–diathesis interactions may explain why only a portion of individuals becomes depressed following a stressor such as divorce or unemployment.

Like IPT and the behavioral therapies, CT was developed as a short-term model of treatment (88). More recent refinements in CT have been introduced in the areas of case formulation (169), treatment of personality pathology (164,170), inpatients (171,172), and chronic depression (118). Provisions are made for concomitant use of antidepressant medication in both outpatient (88) and inpatient (172) CT manuals. The technical fidelity and quality of CT sessions may be measured by an objective tool, the CT Scale (173), although the cross-site reliability of this scale needs to be ensured.

In addition to its more elaborate theoretical orientation, CT also differs from most forms of behavior therapy with respect to the detail of its guidelines for working with depressed patients (88,171). These guidelines include a unique approach to the therapeutic relationship, termed "collaborative empiricism"; this directs the therapist to assume the role of a coach or teacher in addition to his or her providing the more traditional nonspecific elements of understanding and support. Through this model of interaction the therapist and patient develop stepwise goals to reduce symptoms, improve management of pressing day-to-day problems, and increase morale. Collaboration is explicitly fostered via liberal use of feedback and questioning to ensure that the patient understands the material being covered. Compared with the process of more traditional dynamic therapies, CT requires therapists to be significantly more active within sessions (174), which may foster a stronger working alliance (175). Conversely, a premature or excess focus on correcting cognitive errors may strain the therapeutic alliance (176).

The therapist introduces each new technique or intervention as a hypothesized means to help bring about therapeutic change. Explicit homework assignments and the demonstration of methods and techniques within sessions are employed to facilitate the patient's participation. Each session utilizes a coherent structure in which an agenda is set, homework is reviewed, attention is given to one or two key problem areas, and feedback is obtained. Some evidence indicates that the therapist's ability to structure and pace sessions and to consistently integrate homework assignments are predictive of better outcomes (177,178).

Early in the course of therapy, particularly with more severely depressed patients, there is typically a greater emphasis on behavioral techniques. For example, daily monitoring of moods and activities is used to increase participation in rewarding behaviors and establish functional relationships between moods and automatic thoughts. Similarly, stepwise graded task assignments are used to address problems that are perceived as overwhelming.

Slowly, and at a pace appropriate to each patient's ability to use abstract thought, the therapy moves toward eliciting and testing the accuracy of automatic thoughts and developing rational alternatives. Therapeutic strategies, such as the use of written responses to stereotypic automatic negative thoughts, coping cards, and a printed, five-column form known as the Daily Record of Dysfunctional Thoughts are used to teach patients to begin to challenge their negative cognitions. Patients are also encouraged to keep their thought records as part of a journal or notebook so that a coherent summary of the course of therapy is readily available. Each session ends with a new homework assignment that builds logically on the material just covered.

It is important to distinguish the more simplistic models of cognitive intervention, such as verbal persuasion, from the actual process of CT. In contrast to persuasion, in which the expert advocates the correct position, CT emphasizes guided discovery of logical errors and alternate interpretations. That more positive alternative conclusions typically can be identified and validated is at the heart of CT.

One misperception about CT is that it minimizes affect and negates the personal significance of serious setbacks, recommending Pollyanna-like optimism in the face of adversity. Rather, when CT is conducted skillfully, the patient's emotional reaction to a significant event is respectfully and empathically understood in relation to his or her thoughts about self, world, and future (162). From the therapist's perspective, the personal meaning of the stressor may be found to be exaggerated when the patient's automatic negative thoughts are examined more objectively. Through the guided discovery process, the therapist helps the patient elicit the chain of associated thoughts to clarify a more exaggerated set of personal conclusions. This downward arrow technique may reveal, for example, that a person who has been fired from a job for poor performance has come to the following conclusion: I have failed at everything. Rather, objective examination of the situation might reveal that the job failure was partly attributable to being under poor training and partly the result of worsening depression. Previous examples of success in the workplace may be identified to help counteract depressive recall. The problems resulting from being fired also need to be assessed, and a plan to address these problems can be developed. CT thus differs from dynamic or experiential therapies in that affect is specifically used to lead to a cognitive process by which depressed patients learn to problem-solve and gain greater control over dysphoric moods (174,179).

It is also felt to be incumbent upon the cognitive therapist to help patients identify patterns and themes associated with depressive vulnerability prior to termination. In this regard, the final sessions of CT may be devoted to diagnosing pathological schemas and specific skills deficits and developing longer-range self-help plans to address these problems. Modification of such vulnerability is hypothesized to convey a more enduring prophylactic effect (88,162,180). It remains controversial whether such decreased vulnerability is better understood as the result of development of a compensatory set of skills (i.e., to offset a persistently pathological schema) or the actual revision of schema (180,181).

CONCLUSIONS

The depression-focused psychotherapies, as exemplified by IPT, several models of behavior therapy, and Beck's CT, are practical and effective outpatient treatments of mild to moderately severe MDD, and possibly more severe forms of depression. From differing vantage points, each therapy assesses the depressed patient's current state and problem areas, provides psychoeducation, explicitly instills hope, and guides selection of model-specific strategies to help patients reduce symptoms of the depressive episode. No one form of psychotherapy has emerged as superior to the others; interest, aptitude, and opportunities for supervised training may have more to do with a therapist's choice of a model than empirical evidence. It remains to be seen if an eclectic model of psychotherapy for depression will emerge, fusing the more clinically germane aspects of IPT, behavior therapy, and CT (182). Initial efforts to integrate these and components of more traditional therapies for the treatment of chronically depressed patients have thus far shown great promise (183). Caution should be exercised before automatically adopting such integrated therapies, however, because several studies have not established that combinations of various behavioral, marital, and cognitive strategies are more effective than single models of treatment (152,153,184,185).

The depression-focused psychotherapies probably work best when used alone, without concomitant pharmacotherapy, for more acutely depressed patients with higher levels of premorbid functioning and adequate social support (119,186,187). This indication should not be trivialized as a nonspecific response because these psychotherapies have been consistently shown to be superior to waiting-list or low-contact control conditions. In addition, a growing body of literature suggests that these time-limited therapies have mechanisms of action that are directly related to psychological constructs that are targets of treatment (117).

The greater initial cost of psychotherapy relative to pharmacotherapy is based on the assumption of a short course of treatment with a generic formulation of an older antidepressant (188). The actual greater cost of 16 weeks of psychotherapy is, in practice, largely offset by taking into account the expense of prescription of name-brand antidepressants and the necessary length of continuation and maintenance of pharmacotherapy. More difficult to factor into such equations are the possible benefits of late-emergent improvements in social adjustment of patients treated with IPT (109,129) or enduring prophylactic effects of CT (189). More recent literature suggests that this protective effect of CT may in fact be superior to prolonging medication as a monotherapy (114).

The depression-focused psychotherapies should be conducted by appropriately trained clinicians and, ideally, should be preferentially recommended for patients who are motivated to participate in a psychosocial treatment. When used as the primary treatment of MDD, clinicians would be wise to follow the suggestion of the Agency for Health Care Policy and Research (190) to re-evaluate the need for pharmacotherapy after several months of therapy. Unfortunately, this is not always done. For example, a survey by Kendall et al. (191) indicated that nonmedical psychotherapists typically wait for about 6 to 14 months before concluding that patients are not progressing in therapy. In such cases, months of unproductive suffering might have been circumvented by more timely use of antidepressant medication. For example, one group found that more than 70% of IPT nonresponders responded to a sequential trial of imipramine or fluoxetine (192).

Despite the strong evidence base supporting their efficacy, time-limited depression-focused psychotherapies are not practiced commonly across all treatment settings. Greater efforts should be made to require training in these therapies, both in psychology and psychiatry training programs. In addition, dissemination through continuing education programs that reach more isolated practice venues is critical to insure that state-of-the-art practices are available to all depressed patients. Practitioners with most frequent front line contact with depressed patients (e.g., primary-care settings) should be targeted for possible training in these therapies. Within research settings, further efforts need to be made to evaluate the use of these therapies in optimizing long-term outcome, and to determine how to best adapt these therapies for patients with unique clinical characteristics and/or comorbid conditions. With significant efforts made in the clinical and research realms, further refinement in how to best apply these depression-focused therapies can be achieved.

REFERENCES

1. Bernstein JG. Handbook of Drug Therapy in Psychiatry. 3rd ed. St. Louis, MI: Mosby-Year Book Inc., 1995:121.
2. Sadock BJ, Sadock VA, eds. Kaplan and Sadock's Pocket Handbook of Psychiatric Drug Treatment. 3rd ed. Philadelphia, PA: Lippincott Williams and Wilkins, 2001:241–251.
3. Murphy GE, Simons AD, Wetzel RD. Plasma nortriptyline and clinical response in depression. J Affect Disord 1985; 8(2):123–129.
4. Vieweg WV, Wood MA. Tricyclic antidepressants, QT interval prolongation, and torsade de pointes. Psychosomatics 2004; 45(5):371–377.
5. Calabrese JR, Rapport DJ, Kimmel SE, Shelton MD. Controlled trials in bipolar I depression: focus on switch rates and efficacy. Eur Neuropsychopharmacol 1999; 9(suppl 4):S109–S112.
6. FDA Public Health Advisory: Suicidality in Children and Adolescents Being Treated With Antidepressant Medications (issued 10/15/2004). Public access: http://www.fda.gov/cder/drug/antidepressants/SSRIPHA200410.htm.
7. Robinson DS, Nies A, Qavaries CL, et al. The monoamine oxidase inhibitor, phenelzine, in the treatment of depressive-anxiety states. Arch Gen Psychiat 1976; 33:347–350.
8. Thase ME, Trivedi MH, Rush AJ. MAOIs in the contemporary treatment of depression. Neuropsychopharmacology 1995; 12(3):185.
9. Davidson J, McLeod MN, Blum MR. Acetylation phenotype, platelet monoamine oxidase inhibition, and the effectiveness of phenelzine in depression. Am J Psychiat 1978; 135:467–469.
10. McGrath PJ, Stewart JW, Nunes EV, et al. A double blind crossover trial of imipramine and phenezine for outpatients with treatment refractory depression. Am J Psychiat 1993; 150:118–123.
11. Thase ME, Mallinger AG, McKnight D, et al. Treatment of imipramine–reistant recurrent depression. IV. A double-blind crossover study of tranylcypromine for anergic bipolar depression. Am J Psychiat 1992; 149:195–198.
12. McCabe BJ. Dietrary tyramine and other pressor amines in MAOI regimens: a review. J Am Diet Assoc 1986; 76:1059–1064.

13. Folks DF. Monamine oxidase inhibitors: reappraisal of dietary considerations. J Clin Psychopharmacol 1979; 40:33–37.
14. Ferguson JM. Interaction of aspartame and carbohydrates in an eating-disordered patient. Am J Psychiat 1985; 142:271.
15. Steward JW, Harrison AAW, Quitkin F, et al. Phe4nelzine-induced pyridoxine deficiency. J Clin Psychopharmacol 1984; 4:225–226.
16. Glaxo Smith Kline. Package Insert Wellbutrin SR, 2005.
17. Ascher JA, Cole JO, Colin JN, Feighner JP, Ferris RM, Fibiger HC. Buproprion: a review of its mechanism of antidepressant activity. J Clin Psychiat 1995; 56:395.
18. Preskorn SH. Buproprion: what mechanism of action? J Psychiatr Pract 2000; 6:39–44.
19. Goodnick PJ. Pharmacokinetics of second generation antidepressants: Buproprion. Psychopharmacol Bull 1991; 27:513.
20. Zisook S. Efficacy of buproprion. J Clin Psychiat Monogr 1993; 11(1):20–29.
21. Hayes JT, Ebbert JO. Buproprion sustained release for treatment of tobacco dependence. May Clin Proc 2003; 78(8):1020–1024.
22. Bernstein JG. Handbook of Drug Therapy in Psychiatry. 3rd ed. St Louis, MI: Mosby-Year Book Inc., 1995:134.
23. Settle EC. Buproprion: general side effects. J Clin Psychiat Monogr 1993; 11(1):33–39.
24. Johnston JA, Fiedler-KellyJ, Glover ED, Sachs DP, Grasela TH, DeVeaugh-Geiss J. Relationship between drug exposure and efficacy and safety of buproprion sustained release for smoking cessation. Nicotine Tob Res 2001; 3:131–140.
25. Segraves RT. Treatment-emergent sexual dysfunction in affective disorder: a review and management strategies. J Clin Psychiat Monogr 1993; 11(1):57–60.
26. Roose SP, Dalack GW, Glassman AH, et al. Cardiovascular effects of buproprion in depressed patients with heart disease. Am J Psychiat 1991; 148:512–516.
27. Gadde KM, Parker CB, Maner LG, et al. Bupropion for weight loss: an investication of efficacy and tolerability in overweight and obese women. Obes Res 2001; 9:544–551.
28. Reimherr FW, Cunningham LA, Batey SR, Hohnston JA, Ascher JA. A multicenter evaluation of the efficacy and safety of 150 and 300 mg/d-sustained–release buproprion tablets versus placebo in depressed outpatients. Clin Ther 1998; 20:505–516.
29. Rosenstein DL, Nelson JC, Jacobs SC. Seizures associated with antidepressants: a review. J Clin Psychiat 1993; 54:289–299.
30. Stalth SM. Essential Psychopharmacology. 2d ed. New York: Cambridge University Press, 2000:222–225.
31. Hiemke C, Hartter S. Pharmacokinetics of selective serotonin reuptake inhibitors. Pharmacol Ther 2000; 85(1):11–28.
32. Sadock BJ, Sadock VA, eds. Kaplan and Sadock's Pocket Handbook of Psychiatric Drug Treatment. 3rd ed. Philadelphia, PA: Lippincott Williams and Wilkins, 2001:186–203.
33. Stahl SM, Entsuah R, Rudolph RL. Comparative efficacy between venlafaxine and SSRIs: a pooled analysis of patients with depression. Biol Psychiat 2002; 52(12):1166–1174.

34. Perry PJ. Pharmacotherapy for major depression with melancholic features: relative efficacy of tricyclic versus selective serotonin reuptake inhibitor antidepressants. J Affect Disord 1996; 39(1):1–6.
35. Hallberg P, Sjoblom V. The use of selective serotonin reuptake inhibitors during pregnancy and breast-feeding: a review and clinical aspects. J Clin Psychopharmacol 2005; 25(1):59–73.
36. Fergusson D, Doucette S, Glass KC, et al. Association between suicide attempts and selective serotonin reuptake inhibitors: systematic review of randomized controlled trials. BMJ 2005; 330(7488):396.
37. Boyer EW, Shannon M. The serotonin syndrome. N Engl J Med 2005; 352(11):1112–1120.
38. Price JS, Waller PC, Wood SM, MacKay AV. A comparison of the post marketing safety of four selective serotonin re-uptake inhibitors including the investigation of symptoms occurring on withdrawal. Br J Clin Pharmacol 1996; 42(6):757–763.
39. Seeman P. Neuroleptics. In: Kalant H, Roschlan HE, Sellers EM, eds. Principles of Medical Pharmacology. Toronto: University of Toronto Press, 1985:329.
40. Otani K, Yasui N, Kaneko S, et al. Trazodone treatment increases plasma prolactin concentration in depressed patients. Int Clin Psychopharmacol 1995; 10(2):115.
41. Winokur A, Reynolds CF. The effects of antidepressants on sleep physiology. Prim Psychiat 1994; 1:22–27.
42. Schwartz T, Nihalani N, Virk S, et al. A comparison of the effectiveness of two hypnotic agents for the treatment of insomnia. Int J Psychiatr Nurs Res 2004; 10(1):1146–1150.
43. Cunningham LA, Borison RL, Carman JS, et al. A comparison of venlafaxine, trazadone and placebo in major depression. J Clin Psychopharmacol 1994;14:99.
44. Balon R. Sleep terror disorder and insomnia treated with trazodone: a case report. Ann Clin Psychiat 1994; 6:161.
45. Van Bemmel AL, Beersma DGM, Van den Hoofddakker RH. Changes in EEG power density of non-REM sleep in depressed patients during treatment with trazodone. J Affect Disorder 1995; 35(1–2):11.
46. Nierenberg AA, Adler LA, Peselow E, Zornberg G, Rosenthal M. Trazodone for antidepressant associated insomnia. Am J Psychiat 1994; 151:1069–1072.
47. Nemeroff CB. Evolutionary trends in the pharmacotheraputic management of depression. J Clin Psychiat 1994; 55(suppl 12):3–15.
48. Scher M, Frieger JN, Jeurgens S. Trazodone and priapism. Am J Psychiat 1983; 140:1362–1363.
49. Demuth GW, Breslow RE, Drescher J. The elicitation of a movement disorder by Trazodone: case report. J Clin Psychiat 1985; 46:535–536.
50. Swinkles JA, de Jonghe F. Safety of antidepressants. Int Clin Psychopharmacol 1995; 9(suppl 4):19.
51. Bolden-Watson C, Richardoon E. Blockade by newly developed antidepressants of biogenic amine uptake into rat brain synaptosomes. Life Sci 1993; 52:1023–1029.
52. Preskorn SH. Imiprimine, mirtazapine, and nefazodone: multiple targets. J Prac Psychiat Behav Health 2000; 97–102.

53. Taylor DR, Carter RB, Eison AS, et al. Pharmacology and neurochemistry of nefazodone, an novel antidepressant drug. J Clin Psychiat 1995; 56(suppl 6):3–11.
54. Rickels K, Robinson DS, Schweizer E, et al. Nefazodone: aspects of efficacy. J Clin Psychiat 1995; 56(suppl 6):43–46.
55. D'Amico MF, Roberts DL, Robinson DS, et al. Placebo controlled dose ranging trial designs in Phase II development of nefazodone. Psychoparmcol Bull 1990; 26:147–150.
56. Package insert. Serzone (nefazodone). Princeton, NJ: Bristol-Myers Squibb Company; Feb 2002.
57. Venlafaxine (Effexor). Package Insert. Philadelphia, PA: Wyeth-Ayerst Pharmaceuticals, 1993.
58. Clerc GE, Ruimy P, Verdeau-Palles J. A double-blind comparison of venlafaxine and fluoxetine in patients hospitalized for major depression and melancholia. Int Clin Psychopharmacol 1994; 9:139–143.
59. Dierick M, Realini R, et al. A double-blind comparison of venlafaxine and floxetine for treatment of major depression in outpatients. Prog Neuropsychopharmacol Biol Psychiat 1996; 20:57–71.
60. Mendlewicz J. Pharmacologic profile and efficacy of venlafaxine. Int Clin Psychopharmacol 1995; 10(suppl 2):5–13.
61. Entsuah AR, Rudolph RL, Hackett D, et al. Efficacy of venlafaxine and placebo during long-term treatment of depression: a pooled analysis of relapse rates. Int Clin Psychopharmcol 1996; 11:137–145.
62. Cowen PJ, Ogilvie AD, Gama J. Efficacy, safety and tolerability of duloxetine 60 mg once daily in major depression. Curr Med Res Opin 2005; 21(3):345–356.
63. Harvey AT, Rudolph RL, Preskorn SH. Evidence of the dual mechanisms of action of venlafaxine. Arch Gen Psychiat 2000; 57:503–509.
64. Muth EA, Moyer JA, Hasking JT, et al. Biochemical, neurophysiological and behavioral effects of Wy-45, 233 and other identified metabolites of the antidepressant venlafaxine. Drug Dev Res 1991; 23:191–199.
65. Bymaster FP, Dreshfield-Ahmad LJ, Threlkeld PG, et al. Comparative affinity of duloxetine and venlafaxine for serotonin and norepinephrine transporters in vitro and in vivo, herman suamn serotonin receptor subtypes and other neuronal receptors. Neuropsychopharmacology 2001; 25:871–880.
66. Klamerus KJ, Malone K, Rudolph RL, et al. Introduction of a composite parameter to the pharmakinetics of venlafaxine and its active O-desmethyl metabolite. J Clin Pharmacol 1992; 32:716–724.
67. Venlafaxine (Effexor XR). Package Insert. Philadelphia, PA: Wyeth-Ayerst Pharmaceuticals, 2005.
68. Sharma A, Goldberg MJ, Cerimele BJ. Pharmacokinetics and safety of duloxetine, a dual-serotonin and norepinephrine reuptake inhibitor. J Clin Pharmacol 2000; 40:161–167.
69. Lantz RJ, Gillespie TA, Rash TJ, et al. Metabolism, exceteion and pharmacokinetics of duloxetine in healthy human subjects. Drug Metab Dispos 2003; 31:1142–1150.
70. Schweitzer E, Feighner J, Mandos LA, Rickels K. Comparison of venlafaxine and imipramine in acute treatment of major depression in outpatients. J Clin Psychiat 1994; 55:104–108.

71. Montgomery SA. Venlafaxine: a new dimension in antidepressant pharmacotherapy. J Clin Psychat 1993; 54:119–126.

72. Venlafaxine. Package Insert. Wyeth Ayerst, 1999.

73. Detke MJ, Lu Y, Goldstein DJ, et al. Duloxetine 60 mg once daily dosing versus placebo in the acute treatment of major depression. J Psychiat Res 2002; 36:383.

74. Goldstein DJ, Mallinckrodt C, Lu Y, et al. Duloxetine in the treatment of major depressive disorder: a double-blind clinical trial. J Clin Psychiat 2002; 63:225–231.

75. Berk M, du Pless AD, Birkett M, et al. An open-label study of duloxetine hydrochloride, a mixed serotonin and noradrenaline reuptake inhibitor, in patients with DSM-III-R major depressive disorder. Lilly Duloxetine Depression Study Group. Int Clin Psychopharmacol 1997; 12:137–140.

76. Viktrup L, Pangallo B, Detke MJ, et al. Urinary side effects of duloxetine in the treatment of depression and stress urinary incontinence. Prim Care Compan J Clin Psychiat 2004; 6:65–73.

77. Stahl SM. Essential Psychopharmacology Neuroscientific Basis and Practical Applications. 2d ed. Cambridge University Press, 2000:255.

78. de Boer TH, Maura G, Raiteri M, de Vos CJ, Wieringa J, Pinder RM. Neurochemical and autonomic pharmacological profiles of the 6-aza-analogue of mianserin, Org 3770 and its enantiomers. Neuropharmacology 1988; 27: 399–408.

79. de Boer T, Ruigt G, Berendsen H. The alpha 2-selective adrenoceptor antagonist Org 3770 (mirtazapine remeron) enhances noradrenergic and serotonergic transmission. Hum Psychopharmacol 1995; 10:107s–118s.

80. Catterson M, Preskorn SH, Bremner JD, Dessain EC. Double-blind crossover study of mirtazapine, amitriptyline and placebo in patients with major depression. Poster presentation at the 36th annual meeting of the American Psychiatric Association for New York 1996:7.

81. Preskorn SH, Omo K, Magnus RD, Shad MU. Assessment of potential drug-drug interactions following immediate crossover from fluoxetine to mirtazapine. Poster session, San Diego: American Psychiatric Association Meeting, 1998.

82. Kasper S. Clinical efficacy of mirtazapine: a review of meta-analysis of pooled data. Int Clin Psychopharmcol 1995; 10(suppl 4):25–35.

83. Montgomery SA, Reimitz PE, Zivkov M. Mirtazapine versus amitriptyline in the long term treatment of depression: a double-blind, placebo-controlled study. Int Clin Psychopharmcol 1998; 18:63–73.

84. Mirtazapine, Package Insert. Organon, 1998.

85. Mongomery SA. Safety of mirtazapine: a review. Int Clin Psychopharmacol 1995; 10(suppl 4):37–45.

86. Stephen M. Stahl. In: Essential Psychopharmacology: Neuroscientific Basis and Practical Applications. Cambridge and New York: Cambridge University Press, 2000.

87. Hoberman H, Lewinsohn PM. Behavioral approaches to the treatment of unipolar depression. In: Klerman GL, ed. Treatment of Psychiatric Disorders. Vol 3. Washington, D.C.: American Psychiatric Association, 1989:1846–1862.

88. Beck AT, Rush AJ, Shaw BF, Emery G. Cognitive Therapy of Depression. New York: Guilford Press, 1979.
89. Klerman GL, Weissman MM, Rounsaville BJ, Chevron E. Interpersonal Psychotherapy of Depression. New York: Basic Books, 1984.
90. Ferster CB. A functional analysis of depression. Am Psychol 1973; 28: 857–870.
91. Liberman RP, Raskin DE. Depression: a behavioral formulation. Arch Gen Psychiat 1971; 24:515–523.
92. Rush AT. Psychotherapy of the affective psychoses. Am J Psychoanal 1980; 40:99–123.
93. Weissman MM. The psychological treatment of depression: research evidence for the efficacy of psychotherapy alone, in comparison and in combination with pharmacotherapy. Arch Gen Psychiat 1979; 36:1261–1269.
94. Arieti S. Affective disorders: manic-depressive psychosis and psychotic depression: manifest symptomatology, psychodynamics, sociological factors and psychotherapy. In: Arieti S, ed. American Handbook of Psychiatry. Vol. 3. New York: Basic Books, 1976.
95. Jacobson E. Depression. New York: International Universities Press, 1964.
96. Cole JO. Therapeutic efficacy of antidepressant drugs. JAMA 1964; 190:448.
97. Davis JM. Efficacy of tranquilizing and antidepressant drugs. Arch Gen Psychiat 1965; 13:552.
98. Olfson M, Klerman GL, Pincus HA. The roles of psychiatrists in organized outpatient mental health settings. Am J Psychiat 1993; 150:625–631.
99. Windle C, Poppen PJ, Thompson JW, Marvelle K. Types of patients served by various providers of outpatient care in CMHCs. Am J Psychiat 1998; 145: 457–463.
100. Scott J. Social and community approaches. In: Paykel ES, ed. Handbook of Affective Disorders. New York: Guilford Press, 1992.
101. Wolpe J. Psychotherapy by Reciprocal Inhibition. Stanford, California: Stanford University Press, 1958.
102. Beck AT. Cognitive Therapy and the Emotional Disorders. New York: International Universities Press, 1976.
103. Parloff MB. Psychotherapy research evidence and reimbursement decisions: Bambi meets Godzilla. Am J Psychiat 19982; 139:718–727.
104. Eysenck HJ. The effects of psychotherapy: an evaluation. J Consult Psychol 1952; 16:319–324.
105. Dobson KS, Shaw BF. The training of cognitive therapists: what have we learned from treatment manuals? Psychotherapy 1993; 30:573–577.
106. Luborsky L, DeRubeis RJ. The use of psychotherapy treatment manuals: a small revolution in psychotherapy research style. Clin Psychol Rev 1984; 4:5–11.
107. Bellack AS, Hersen M, Himmelhoch JM. A comparison of social-skills training, pharmacotherapy, and psychotherapy for depression. Behav Res Ther 10:101–107.
108. Whisman MA, Miller IW, Norman WH, Keitner GI. Cognitive therapy with depressed inpatients: specific effects on dysfunctional cognitions. J Consult Clin Psychol 1991; 59:282–288.

109. Weissman MM, Klerman GL, Prusoff BA, Sholomskas D, Padian N. Depressed outpatients. Results one year after treatment with drugs and/or interpersonal psychotherapy. Arch Gen Psychiat 1981; 38:51–55.
110. Segal ZV, Teasdale JD, Williams MG. Mindfulness-Based Cognitive Therapy for Depression: A New Approach to Preventing Relapse. Guilford Publications, 2001.
111. Hayes SC, Strosahl K, Wilson KG. Acceptance and Commitment Therapy: An Experiential Approach to Behavior Change. New York: Guilford Press, 1999.
112. Kabat-Zinn J. Wherever You Go There You Are: Mindfulness Meditation In Everyday Life.: Hyperion Press, 1994.
113. Fava GA. Sequential treatment: a new way of integrating pharmacotherapy and psychotherapy. Psychother Psychosom 1999; 68(5):227–229.
114. Fava GA, Ruini C. Development and characteristics of a well-being enhancing psychotherapeutic strategy: well-being therapy. J Behav Ther Exp Psychiat 2003; 34(1):45–63.
115. Hollon SD, DeRubeis RJ, Shelton RC, et al. Prevention of relapse following cognitive therapy versus medications in moderate to severe depression. Arch Gen Psychiat 2005; 62:417–422.
116. Hollon SD, Jarrett RB, Nierenberg AA, Thase ME, Trivedi M, Rush AJ. Psychotherapy and medication in the treatment of adult and geriatric depression: which monotherapy or combined treatment? J Clin Psychiat 2005; 66:455–468.
117. Petersen T, Harley R, Papakostas GI, Montoya HD, Fava M, Alpert JE. Continuation cognitive-behavioral therapy maintains attributional style improvement in depressed patients responding acutely to fluoxetine. Psychol Med 2004; 34:555–561.
118. McCullough JP. Cognitive Behavioral Analysis System of Psychotherapy: Treatment of Chronic Depression. New York: Guilford Press, 2000.
119. Klerman GL, Weissman MM. Interpersonal psychotherapy: theory and research. In: Rush AJ, ed. Short-Term Psychotherapies for Depression. New York: Guilford Press, 1982:88–106.
120. Meyer A. Psychobiology: A Science of Man. Springfield, IL: Charles C. Thomas Publishing, 1957.
121. Sullivan HS. The Interpersonal Theory of Psychiatry. New York: Norton, 1953.
122. Bowlby J. Attachment and Loss. London: Hogarth Press, 1969; Psychopharmacol 1995; 10(2):115.
123. Brown GW, Harris T. Social Origins of Depression: A Study of Psychiatric Disorders in Women. London: Tavistock Press, 1978.
124. Becker J. Depressive Theory and Research. New York: Wiley, 1974.
125. Chodoff P. The depressive personality: a critical review. Arch Gen Psychiat 1972; 27:665–673.
126. Klerman GL, Weissman MM, eds. New Applications of Interpersonal Psychotherapy. Washington D.C.: American Psychiatric Press, 1993.
127. DeRubeis RJ, Hollon SD, Evans MD, Bemis KM. Can psychotherapies for depression be discriminated? A systematic investigation of cognitive therapy and interpersonal therapy. J Consult Clin Psychol 1982; 50:744–756.

128. Hill CE, O'Grady KE, Elkin I. Applying the Collaborative Study Psychotherapy Rating Scale to rate therapist adherence in cognitive-behavior therapy, interpersonal therapy, and clinical management. J Consult Clin Psych 1992; 60:73–79.

129. Weissman MM, Paykel ES. The Depressed Women: A Study of Social Relationships. Chicago: University of Chicago Press, 1974.

130. Beach SR, Arias H, O'Leary KD. The relationship of marital satisfaction and social support to depressive symptomatology. J Psychopathol Behav Assess 1986; 8:305–316.

131. Coyne JC, Downey G. Social factors and psychopathology: stress, social support, and coping processes. Annu Rev Psychol 1991; 42:401–425.

132. Rounsaville BJ, Prusoff BA, Weissman MM. The course of marital disputes in depressed women: a 48 month follow-up study. Compr Psychiat 1980; 21:111–118.

133. Markowitz JC. Psychotherapy of the post-dynamic patient. J Psychother Prct Res 1993; 2:157–163.

134. Barber JP, Muenz LR. The role of avoidance and obsessiveness in matching patients to cognitive and interpersonal psychotherapy: empirical findings from the treatment for depression collaborative research program. J Consult Clin Psychol 1996; 64:951–958.

135. Foley SH, O'Malley S, Rounsaville B, Prusoff BA, Weissman MM. The relationship of patient difficulty to therapist performance in interpersonal psychotherapy of depression. J Affect Disord 1987; 12:207–217.

136. Banken DM, Wilson GL. Treatment acceptability of alternative therapies for depression: a comparative analysis. Psychotherapy 1992; 29:610–619.

137. Thase ME, Hersen M, Bellack AS, Himmelhoch JM, Kornblith SJ, Greenwald DP. Social skills training and endogenous depression. J Behav Ther Exp Psychiat 1984; 15:101–108.

138. Wolpe J. The experimental model and treatment of neurotic depression. Behav Res Ther 1979; 17:555–565.

139. Bandura A. Self-efficacy: toward a unifying theory of behavioral change. Psychol Rev 1977; 84:191–215.

140. Rehm LP. A self-control model of depression. Behav Ther 1977; 8:787–804.

141. Seligman MEP. Helplessness: on Depression, Development, and Death. San Francisco: Freeman, 1975.

142. Barnett PA, Gotlib IH. Psychosocial functioning and depression: distinguishing among antecedents, concomitants, and consequences. Psychol Bull 1988; 104:97–126.

143. Coyne JC. Depression and the response of others. J Abnorm Psychol 1976; 85:186–193.

144. McLean P. Behavior therapy: theory and research. In: Rush AJ, ed. Short-Term Psychotherapies for Depression. New York: Guilford Press, 1982:19–49.

145. Lewinsohn PM, Antonuccio DA, Steinmetz JL, Teri L. The Coping with Depression Course: A Psychoeducational Intervention for Unipolar Depression. Eugene, Oregon: Castalia Publishing, 1984.

146. Hersen M, Bellack AS, Himmelhoch JM, Thase ME. Effects of social skills training, amitriptyline, and psychotherapy in unipolar depressed women. Behav Ther 1984; 15:21–40.

147. Nezu AM. Efficacy of a social problem-solving therapy approach for unipolar depression. J Consult Clin Psychol 1986; 54:196–202.

148. Goldfried MR, Davison GC. Clinical Behavior Therapy. New York: Holt, Rinehart, and Winston, 1976.

149. Wilson PH. Combined pharmacological and behavioral treatment of depression. Behav Res Ther 1982; 20:173–184.

150. McLean PD, Hakstian AR. Clinical depression: comparative efficacy of outpatient treatments. J Consult Clin Psychol 1979; 47:818–836.

151. Bowers WA. Treatment of depressed inpatients. Cognitive therapy plus medication, relaxation plus medication, and medication alone. Br J Psychiat 1990; 156:73–78.

152. Rehm LP, Kaslow NJ, Rabin AS. Cognitive and behavioral targets in a self-control therapy program for depression. J Consult Clin Psychol 1987; 55:60–67.

153. Jacobson NS, Dobson KS, Fruzzetti AE, Schmaling KB, Salusky S. Marital therapy as a treatment for depression. J Consult Clin Psychol 1991; 59: 547–557.

154. O'Leary KD, Beach SRH. Marital therapy: a viable treatment for depression and marital discord. Am J Psychiat 1990; 147:183–186.

155. Roth D, Bielski R, Jones M, Parker W, Osborn G. A comparison of self-control therapy and combined self-control therapy and antidepressant medication in the treatment of depression. Behav Ther 1982; 13:133–144.

156. Beck AT. Depression. New York: Harper and Row, 1967.

157. Burns D. Feeling Good: The New Mood Therapy. New York: William Morrow, 1980.

158. Coyne JC, Gotlib IH. The role of cognition in depression: a critical appraisal. Psychol Bull 1983; 94:472–505.

159. Haaga DA, Dyck MJ, Ernst D. Empirical status of cognitive theory of depression. Psychol Bull 1991; 110:215–236.

160. Robins CJ, Hayes AM. An appraisal of cognitive therapy. J Consult Clin Psychol 1993; 61:205–214.

161. Teasdale JD. Emotion and two kinds of meaning: cognitive therapy and applied cognitive science. Behav Res Ther 1993; 31:339–354.

162. Thase ME. Transition and aftercare. In: Wright JH, Thase ME, Beck AT, Ludgate JW, eds. Cognitive Therapy with Inpatients: Developing a Cognitive Milieu. New York: Guilford Press, 1993:414–435.

163. Segal ZV. Appraisal of the self-schema construct in cognitive models of depression. Psychol Bull 1988; 102:147–162.

164. Young JE, Lindemann MD. An integrative schema-focused model for personality disorders. J Cog Psychother 1992; 6:11–23.

165. Simons AD, Angell KL, Monroe SM, Thase ME. Cognition and life stress in depression: cognitive factors and the definition, rating, and generation of negative life events. J Abnorm Psych 1993; 102:584–591.

166. Persons JB, Miranda J. Cognitive theories of vulnerability to depression: reconciling negative evidence. Cogn Ther Res 1992; 16:484–502.

167. Hammen C, Ellicott A, Gitlin M, Jamison KR. Sociotropy/autonomy and vulnerability to specific life events in patients with unipolar depression and bipolar disorders. J Abnorm Psychol 1989; 98:154–160.

168. Segal ZV, Vella DD, Shaw BF, Katz R. Cognitive and life stress predictors of relapse in remitted unipolar depressed patients: test of the congruency hypothesis. J Abnorm Psychol 1992; 101:26–36.
169. Persons JB. Cognitive Therapy in Practice: A Case Formulation Approach. New York: WW Norton & Company, 1989.
170. Beck AT, Freeman A, Pretzer J, et al. Cognitive Therapy of Personality Disorders. New York: Guilford Press, 1990.
171. Thase ME, Wright JH. Cognitive behavior therapy manual for depressed inpatients: a treatment protocol outline. Behav Ther 1991; 22:579–595.
172. Wright J, Thase M, Beck A, et al. Cognitive therapy with inpatients. Depression 1993; 1:329–330.
173. Vallis TM, Shaw BF, Dobson KS. The cognitive therapy scale: psychometric properties. J Consult Clin Psychol 1986; 54:381–385.
174. Jones EE, Pulos SM. Comparing the process in psychodynamic and cognitive-behavioral therapies. J Consult Clin Psychol 1993; 61:306–316.
175. Raue PJ, Castonguay LG, Goldfried MR. The working alliance: a comparison of two therapies. Psychother Res 1993; 3:197–207.
176. Hayes AM, Castonguay LG, Goldfried MR. Effectiveness of targeting the vulnerability factors of depression in cognitive therapy. J Consult Clin Psychol 1996; 64:623–627.
177. Bryant MJ, Simons AD, Thase ME. Therapist skill and patient variables in homework compliance: controlling an uncontrolled variable in cognitive therapy outcome research. Cognit Ther Res 1999; 23:381–399.
178. Persons JB, Burns DD, Perloff JM. Predictors of dropout and outcome in cognitive therapy for depression in a private practice setting. Cognit Ther Res 1988; 12:557–575.
179. Wiser S, Goldfried MR. Comparative study of emotional experiencing in psychodynamic-interpersonal and cognitive-behavioral therapies. J Consult Clin Psychol 1993; 61:892–895.
180. Persons JB. The process of change in cognitive therapy: schema change or acquisition of compensatory skills? Cognit Ther Res 1993; 17:123–137.
181. Barber JP, DeRubeis RJ. On second thought: where the action is in cognitive therapy for depression. Cognit Ther Res 1989; 13:441–457.
182. Karasu TB. Toward a clinical model of psychotherapy for depression, II: an integrative and selective treatment approach. Am J Psychiat 1990; 147:269–278.
183. Keller MB, McCullough JP, Klein DN, et al. A comparison of nefazodone, the cognitive behavioral-analysis system of psychotherapy, and their combination for the treatment of chronic depression. N Engl J Med 2000; 342(20):1462–1470.
184. Jacobson NS, Hollon SD. Prospects for future comparisons between drugs and psychotherapy: lessons from the CBT-versus pharmacotherapy exchange. J Consult Clin Psychol 1996; 64:104–108.
185. Rude SS. Relative benefits of assertion or cognitive self-control treatment for depression as a function of proficiency in each domain. J Consult Clin Psychol 1986; 54:390–394.
186. Safran JD, Segal ZV, Vallis TM, Shaw BF, Samstag LW. Assessing patient suitability for short-term cognitive therapy with an interpersonal focus. Cognit Ther Res 1993; 17:23–28.

187. Teri L, Lewinsohn PM. Individual and group treatment of unipolar depression: comparison of treatment outcome and identification of predictors of successful treatment outcome. Behav Ther 1986; 17:215–228.

188. Lave JR, Frank RG, Schulberg HC, et al. Cost-effectiveness of treatments for major depression in primary care patients. Arch Gen Psychiat 1998; 55:645–651.

189. Hollon SD, DeRubeis RJ, Evans MD, et al. Cognitive therapy and pharma-cotherapy for depression. Singly and in combination. Arch Gen Psychiat 1992; 49:774–781.

190. Depression Guideline Panel, 1993.

191. Kendall et al, 2004.

192. Thase ME, Buysse DJ, Frank E, et al. Which depressed patients will respond to interpersonal psychotherapy? The role of abnormal electroencephalo-graphic sleep profiles. Am J Psychiat 1997; 154:502–509; 148:512–516.

4

Treatment Outcomes with Acute Pharmacotherapy/Psychotherapy

Thomas L. Schwartz and Lynn Stormon

Department of Psychiatry, SUNY Upstate Medical University, Syracuse, New York, U.S.A.

Michael E. Thase

University of Pittsburgh Medical Center, Western Psychiatric Institute and Clinic, Pittsburgh, Pennsylvania, U.S.A.

INTRODUCTION

As discussed in Chapter 1, depression is an illness that has been prevalent and has been impacting the quality of life for many years. The original treatment was for family, friends, and clinicians to be empathic, supportive, and compassionate. These are some of the hallmarks of all major applied psychotherapies. Initially, the organized works and theories of Sigmund Freud allowed clinicians to follow a theoretical approach toward the treatment of depression. This has been followed up with other forms of psychotherapy, which are effective in treating major depressive disorder (MDD). Likewise, in the 1950s the monoamine hypotheses behind the etiology of MDD utilized reverse engineering when researchers discovered that the tricyclic antidepressants (TCAs) elevated certain monoamines and caused depression symptoms to lift. This allowed for the development of the drugs outlined in Chapter 3. This chapter is designed to provide the reader with the current evidence base in regard to acute treatment outcomes of pharmacotherapy and psychotherapy as individual treatments for MDD. Longer term and maintenance outcomes will be covered in the following chapter.

ACUTE TREATMENT OUTCOMES WITH ANTIDEPRESSANT PHARMACOTHERAPY

Over the last few decades a series of antidepressants have been developed, studied, and deemed approved for use in MDD patients. The selective serotonin reuptake inhibitors (SSRIs), serotonin–norepinephrine reuptake inhibitors (SNRIs), and norepinephrine and serotonin selective receptor antagonists include multiple medications. The norepinephrine–dopamine reuptake inhibitor (NDRI) is represented by only a single U.S. marketed antidepressant. These newer medications, non-TCAs and non–monoamine oxidase inhibitors (MAOIs) generally have not increased efficacy in regard to the treatment of depression. However, the newer antidepressants noted above have collectively resulted in improvements in the pharmacotherapy of depression in terms of ease of use by clinicians, increased tolerability for patients, and greater safety following overdose (1). Theoretically, this expansion of relative neurotransmitter-specific products allows for more precise treatment of target-specific depressive symptoms (2). The first part of this chapter will discuss the methods to establish efficacy of these newer antidepressants and also the comparative acute efficacy of these newer antidepressants.

Measuring Antidepressant Efficacy

Randomized controlled trials (RCTs) have been the gold standard for evaluation of medical therapies, including the use of antidepressants, for over 40 years. On the basis of these results, it has been suggested for decades that all U.S. Food and Drug Administration (FDA)–approved antidepressants are roughly equal in treating MDD to a reasonable "response" (3–6). The clinical caveat that individual patients may differ remarkably in their responses to any particular antidepressant should be noted. This difference between research subject populations compared to the relatively comorbid and heterogenous clinical patient population and a research tendency toward underpowered RCTs continues to suggest that all antidepressants may be equal in the face of differences noted in clinical practice (7,8).

Statistically with respect to clinical trials of antidepressants, it has been presumed since the 1960s that an effective medication can be expected to deliver a response rate of approximately 67%, as compared to a placebo response rate of about only 33%. The advantage of the active drug in this case could be expressed as an absolute value of only $+34\%$, as a relative benefit ($+100\%$ or a twofold advantage), or as an Odds Ratio (OR) (OR; computed as $0.67/0.33$ divided by $0.33/0.67 = 2$ divided by $0.5 = +4.0$). Alternatively, the effect could be described by a difference in scores on a standard depression rating scale such as the Hamilton Rating Scale for Depression (HAM-D) (9) or the Montgomery–Asberg Depression Rating Scale (MADRS) (10). In this case, a 33% advantage in response rates would correspond to about a six-point difference on the HAM-D. Such a difference can be expressed with the standardized term "effect size" (referred to as d). An effect size is calculated by dividing the difference in change scores by the pooled standard deviation of the change scores in the two groups, which for the HAM-D is usually about 10 points. Thus, d in this case is calculated as 6 divided by 10 or $d = 0.6$. Regardless how a difference of this magnitude is expressed, these are relatively large effects in the world of behavioral sciences (11), and an investigation planned to detect such a difference would need to enroll only 30 to 50 patients per arm to have the requisite 80% statistical power. But, if smaller drug–placebo differences were observed, proportionally larger sample sizes would need to be enrolled to obtain 80% power. The need for larger sample sizes would be clearly required to show minor, symptom-relief differences between antidepressants. This size of study is relatively unseen in the literature and difficult to complete due to the number of subjects and the finances needed to complete such a study. This may explain why no RCT literature exists that can definitively show superiority of one drug over another despite real-world clinicians anecdotally noting clear differences between agents.

Type 2 bias errors in antidepressant clinical trials have increased over time (7). "Intent-to-treat" principle in analyzing study results, decisions to conduct longer trials, and completing trials in ambulatory settings have resulted in higher attrition (5,12). Another contributor is an increase in placebo response rates up to approximately 40% (13). These errors in modern-day depression studies would suggest, or even necessitate, that an investigator enroll 300 to 500 patients per arm to have 80% statistical power (14,15). It is commonplace in RCTs designed to investigate nonpsychiatric medications (antihypertensives and anticholesterolemics) to enroll thousands of subjects to avoid such errors.

In the absence of appropriate large-scale studies, we may use meta-analytic techniques to make comparisons on the basis of all available data. There are two principal types of meta-analysis: one type uses summary data extracted from published papers, abstracts, or study reports; the other type pools the raw data (via validated rating scales like the Hamilton) from each participant in a series of studies. The former method is more widely used, in part because the individual patients' data are usually not readily available. In a meta-analysis of studies, "N" is the number of trials and the dependent variable is either a categorical (i.e., response rate) or a continuous (i.e., change in HAM-D) outcome extracted from the study report. In a "pooled" meta-analysis, raw individual patient data, "N," and the number of participants are available; because the source data are available, a better range of outcomes can be examined.

Now that we understand how antidepressant research is conducted and know some of the limitations of this approach, we can begin to discuss how antidepressants differ based on the literature that is in the public domain and is available for quantitative and qualitative analyses. We must operationalize our definition of what a good outcome would be for an MDD patient who is taking an antidepressant. Until the early 1990s, treatment researchers inconsistently applied the terms "response" and "remission." In 1991, a task force consensus recommended using the term response to describe a significant (i.e., ≥50%) reduction in depressive symptoms, and recommended that the term "remission" be reserved to describe a higher grade of improvement (16). From this vantage point, remission was virtually defined by a complete relief of depressive symptoms, i.e., to a level that would be essentially indistinguishable from that of a healthy control group. Although the task force's recommendation to use a specific low score on the first 17 items of the HAM-D scale (i.e., ≤7) was certainly arbitrary, subsequent research (17,18) has confirmed the validity of this threshold. Clinical validity to obtain full remission may be found in studies linking the presence of untreated depressive symptoms to higher risk of relapse (19,20) and poorer social and vocational functioning (21). Most recent RCTs will now report "response" and " remission" rates. The evaluation of remission rates may help to overcome the RCT errors noted above as it is a more stringent clinical variable and, in theory, a drug would need a greater effect to create this greater clinical difference.

This chapter will focus primarily on newer antidepressants as they are clearly in wider clinical use. However, some quick comments about older TCA and MAO agents are required for the sake of continuity with Chapter 3. As the definition of depression and the measurement of depressive symptoms have been evolving since the introduction of the first antidepressants in the 1950s, we must rely on meta-analyses if we want to compare the older and newer antidepressants. Thase et al. (22) conducted a meta-analysis of all published reports comparing TCAs and MAOs. This meta-analysis was commissioned for use by the U.S. Federal Government's Agency for Health Care Planning and Research Depression Guideline Panel (1993). It should be kept in mind that this meta-analysis was completed several years before controversies about the relative efficacy of newer antidepressants emerged. Thase et al. (22) found that although the MAOIs phenelzine and isocarboxazid were more effective than placebo in studies of hospitalized depressed patients they were significantly less effective than the TCAs. Tranylcypromine could not be evaluated because only a single inpatient study was completed. By contrast, they found trends favoring all three MAOIs in the more numerous studies of depressed outpatients. In fact, although the TCAs were effective compared to placebo, phenelzine and tranylcypromine were significantly more effective than the TCA comparators in outpatients. Thus, the idea that these two classes of antidepressants were equally effective was true only when the studies were grouped together without regard for the inpatient–outpatient distinction. This fact again illustrates that underpowered RCTs may be heavily dependent upon patient population variables.

Similar findings were reported by Stewart et al. (23) in a pooled analysis of eight controlled outpatient studies comparing the MAOI, phenelzine, and the TCA, imipramine, which focused on treatment of atypical depression. Stewart et al. (23) found that the MAOIs were superior to TCAs, which in turn were more effective than placebo in regard to this depressive subtype. In summary, there is strong evidence from both forms of meta-analysis that the TCAs and MAOIs were not equivalently effective but, rather, these older antidepressants treated different patient groups with differing degrees of efficacy. Again, despite FDA-level data showing antidepressants to be equal, they clearly manifest differences in acute outcomes.

We will now discuss and compare the effectiveness of the antidepressants introduced in the 1980s to the present in treating MDD. Following this discussion, we will discuss outcomes with psychotherapy. SSRIs are a class, unlike the TCAs, and are grouped together by a common chemical profile, namely, potent inhibition of the serotonin (5-HT) uptake transporter and relatively low affinities for other receptors. The SSRI class includes five distinct antidepressants: fluoxetine, fluvoxamine, sertraline, paroxetine, and citalopram. A sixth drug, escitalopram, is the active stereoisomer of citalopram. The SSRIs have been the most widely used antidepressants throughout most of the world for more than 15 years (1). This safer and more tolerable class of agents has allowed more depressed patients to receive treatment when compared to previous decades.

The relative efficacy of the SSRIs was first established in comparison to the TCAs, which were the standard for antidepressant therapies during the 1950s to the 1970s. Independent of efficacy and tolerability, the SSRIs had collectively two important advantages relative to TCAs. First, the SSRIs generally could be started at relative therapeutic doses, which reduced the need for titration. Second, the SSRIs have much greater safety in overdose (24,25). Better cost effectiveness was initially the major non-empirical advantage of the TCAs, but this advantage has recently diminished because various SSRIs have become available in generic formulations.

With respect to relative efficacy and tolerability, a large number of RCTs have compared the SSRIs to the TCAs, particularly imipramine and amitriptyline, and several meta-analyses have been also performed (5,26–30). One should note that the manufacturers of the SSRIs conducted the majority of these comparative studies and, it is likely that at least some relevant studies have not been published as a result of the "File Drawer Effect." The major clinical advantage favoring the SSRIs over the TCAs in RCTs has been its superior tolerability. Montgomery et al. (31) conducted a meta-analysis of 42 comparative studies and reported that 27% of patients discontinued TCAs due to adverse side effects compared with only 19% of patients receiving SSRIs. The advantage in tolerability favoring the SSRIs is even larger in some subpopulations of depressed patients. For example, Roose et al. (32) conducted a 12-week study comparing paroxetine and nortriptyline in 116 depressed elders. They found that the rate of discontinuation due to side effects in the group treated with the TCA was double (33%) that of those treated with the SSRI (16%). Kornstein et al. (33) also observed a comparable tolerability advantage among the subset of women treated in a double-blind study comparing sertraline and imipramine therapies for chronic depression.

Meta-analyses comparing SSRIs and TCAs have generally demonstrated comparable efficacy (5,26–30). However, there is evidence that TCAs are often more effective in the treatment of major depression (6,27), particularly where more severely acute and chronic patients are concerned. These patients are often classified as melancholic and are often hospitalized (22,34).

Anderson (34) advanced this work one step further by dividing the 25 available inpatient studies into two subgroups: one consisting of the 15 studies comparing SSRIs with amitriptyline or clomipramine (i.e., the so-called "dual-action" reuptake blockading TCAs) and the second consisting of the 10 studies comparing SSRIs versus the more noradrenergically specific and active TCAs (in which he grouped imipramine, desipramine, and nortriptyline together with the tetracyclic compound maprotilene). A clear advantage in this analysis was determined to exist for the first group of agents, which would allow two neurotransmitter systems to be facilitated. In fact, if one would recalibrate effect sizes in terms of average TCA versus SSRI differences, the results of Anderson (34) would suggest that amitriptyline and clomipramine also are significantly more effective therapies for depressed inpatients than the remainder of the TCA class.

Ever since the approval of sertraline in the late 1980s, the attempts to compare effectiveness of the newer antidepressants to deem superiority of efficacy and tolerability have grown exponentially. There are of course differences between these "classmates" with respect to effects on other receptors or transporters, which may account for subtle differences in tolerability as well as differences in pharmacokinetics that affect the time to attain steady state and the risk of discontinuation symptoms following abrupt discontinuation (1,35). So, it is possible that there could be modest differences in efficacy as well among the various SSRIs. Unfortunately, few high-powered RCTs have been performed to capitalize on the power of meta-analysis (35). More often drugs are compared in a "head-to-head" fashion, and use of a placebo control is relatively nonexistent in the literature. This often makes it difficult to determine if either comparative agent is truly effective. Nonetheless, some evidence is less stringent and may be used in an evidence-based fashion.

Some differences have emerged by way of this data. The therapeutic effects of fluoxetine, for example, tend to emerge more slowly than those of other SSRIs (36). Perhaps a controversial piece of evidence of a possible within-class difference arises from studies comparing the racemic drug citalopram with its active stereoisomer, escitalopram (37,38). Specifically, Gorman et al. (37) reported that escitalopram, 10 to 20 mg/day, had certain efficacy advantages compared to citalopram, 20 to 40 mg/day, in a pooled analysis of three double-blind clinical trials. The advantages, which were evident as numeric trends but not consistently statistically significant, were particularly apparent among the subset of patients with moderate-to-severe depressive syndromes (i.e., pretreatment MADRS scores >25).

At first glance, the mechanism underlying efficacy differences between a racemic drug and its active stereoisomer may be difficult to fathom, especially considering that the drugs were proportionately dosed. After all, a patient taking 40 mg/day of citalopram is really taking 20 mg/day of escitalopram. However, some evidence has emerged recently to suggest that the inactive stereoisomer, R-citalopram, may actually have some effects that antagonize the activity of escitalopram (39). If true, this might mean that the two drugs' doses were actually not comparable.

A few years after SSRIs became available, a newer class of novel antidepressants emerged called the SNRIs. The drugs that are referred to as SNRIs or dual-reuptake inhibitors are venlafaxine and duloxetine. A third, milnacipran, is available in Europe but not in the United States. Comparable to the relatively "dual-acting" TCAs noted above, these SNRIs also directly modulate two relevant neurotransmitter systems, serotonin and norepinephrine. Each of these agents possesses a differential ability to facilitate these two systems by way of reuptake pump blockade. Given this similar mechanism of action to the TCAs, the data supporting some TCA superiority, and a safer SNRI adverse effect profile, these medications should have the potential for greater antidepressant efficacy than SSRIs on the basis of exerting either a broader spectrum of efficacy or at a neuronal level a synergistic effect (15,40).

Venlafaxine was the first SNRI to be introduced and is the most extensively studied. There has been evidence of an efficacy advantage for venlafaxine over fluoxetine for nearly a decade (41,42). However, both scientific and marketplace issues have precluded the field's uniform acceptance that venlafaxine has stronger therapeutic advantages. Venlafaxine, immediate and sustained preparations, and its major metabolite, O-desmethylvenlafaxine, are substantially more potent inhibitors of serotonin reuptake transporters than norepinephrine transporters (43). There has been legitimate concern that the drug is not an SNRI at lower therapeutic doses, but is all SSRI at that dose level (44,45). Moreover, the initial immediate formulation of venlafaxine was viewed as harder to use than the SSRIs due to dosing, titration, and increased adverse effects (1,46), and as a result, was often reserved for second- or third-line use (47). Although the introduction of extended release formulation made venlafaxine more like an SSRI in terms of simplicity of prescription and tolerability (46), questions persisted about the dosing threshold at which venlafaxine causes sufficient inhibition of norepinephrine reuptake. This point is particularly important because, although the antidepressant effects of venlafaxine show some degree of dose dependence (48,49), the manufacturer did not obtain FDA regulatory approval to use the extended release formulation in 300 and 375 mg/day doses. The use of this SNRI allows for some versatility, comparable to some TCA predecessors, where a clinician may tailor the dose used to accommodate greater or lesser facilitation of serotonin or norepinephrine based on patient symptomatology.

There are at least 45 RCTs comparing venlafaxine and various SSRIs and a number of meta-analyses examining the efficacy of venlafaxine have been completed, including meta-analyses of study summary results (50,51) and of original data sets (15,52,53). Collectively, these meta-analyses document a reliable, albeit, modest advantage favoring venlafaxine over the SSRI comparators. In absolute terms, the difference in remission rates ranges from 5% to 10% (52,53) and a potential difference in change on the HAM-D ranges from 1 to 2 points (15,51). These effects are relatively small (i.e., $d = 0.14$), but they do amount to about 70% of the real magnitude of the advantage of SSRIs over placebo. Again, many of these studies have limits and have been underpowered given the use of relatively small sample sizes and lack of placebo.

In a recent and comprehensive meta-analysis, Nemeroff (54) examined the impact of various design characteristics and alternate definitions of outcome in 33 double-blind, head-to-head studies, including more than 7500 depressed patients. This meta-analysis was based on the entire set of double-blind SSRI-venlafaxine–controlled studies completed by Wyeth (the manufacturer of venlafaxine) worldwide prior to January 2003. Across all studies, the advantage in remission rates favoring venlafaxine over SSRIs was 6.6% (OR: 1.3). A series of sensitivity analyses demonstrated that the advantage of venlafaxine relative to the SSRIs was not dependent on any one subgroup of studies (e.g., placebo controlled vs. not placebo controlled, inpatient vs. outpatient, etc.) or any particular definition of response or remission. Moreover, although they found that the effect size favoring venlafaxine over fluoxetine (19 studies) was larger than that observed in the 14 RCTs using other SSRIs, both comparisons were statistically significant. They did not find superiority versus each particular SSRI, and at times, the comparisons versus paroxetine, sertraline, fluvoxamine, and citalopram were not statistically significant.

Wyeth has conducted at least two other studies comparing venlafaxine with various SSRIs since completion of the meta-analysis by Nemeroff et al., and the results of several studies funded by the manufacturers of SSRIs have been presented or published (54a,54b). In addition, several more studies have been completed or are ongoing with funding from other, nonpharmaceutical sources. Two recent comparative, nonplacebo studies completed by the manufacturers of sertraline and escitalopram have revealed no efficacy advantage of venlafaxine over the first agent and poorer efficacy compared to the latter agent (55,56). Assuming that data from all public and private funding sources are eventually made available, it should be possible to resolve, once and for all, whether the overall pattern of results favors this particular SNRI over the SSRIs.

It should be noted that several criticisms have been raised about the venlafaxine meta-analyses. Most broadly, it is true that the first pooled analyses (52) were heavily dependent on the venlafaxine versus fluoxetine comparisons (i.e., five of the eight original studies used that specific SSRI as the comparator). Even in the more recent meta-analysis of Nemeroff et al., nearly 60% of the participants in the SSRI arm were treated with fluoxetine. It is also true that the six- to eight-week time frame of standard RCTs is not adequate to determine if the advantage of venlafaxine may have persisted longitudinally. A third criticism is that some patients who previously had not responded to another member of the SSRI class were included in these trials. If this subgroup accounted for one-third of the participants, for example, and the prior nonresponders to SSRIs were 30% more likely to remit with venlafaxine therapy (57), the apparent advantage in the overall group would be artifactual. This issue would similarly need to apply to the earlier generation of studies that contrasted the then novel SSRIs versus TCA comparators.

Milnacipran, which has been available in France, Japan, and several other countries, was the second SNRI to come to the international marketplace. Milnacipran can be thought of as the mirror image of venlafaxine as a dual-reuptake inhibitor, namely, a drug that is more noradrenergic at minimum therapeutic doses (i.e., 25 mg twice daily) and may "recruit" serotoninergic effects at higher therapeutic doses (i.e., up to 100 mg twice daily) (58,59). One would expect that, as a relatively well-tolerated dual-reuptake inhibitor, milnacipran might be found to share with venlafaxine and TCAs an efficacy advantage over the SSRIs. Although some data suggest that this may be the case (60–64), other individual studies have not found differences (65,66). To date, a comprehensive meta-analysis has not been undertaken, as there are generally too few comparative studies at this time.

The most recent SNRI to be developed is duloxetine, which is currently available in the United States. The manufacturer has described this drug as the "balanced SNRI," referring to the fact that duloxetine is a significantly more potent norepinephrine reuptake inhibitor than venlafaxine, as well as a significantly more potent serotonin reuptake inhibitor than milnacipran. As such, it is believed that duloxetine will exert a clinically relevant effect on both neuronal systems at the minimum therapeutic dose (i.e., 60 mg) (67). It should be noted that this drug is still preferential and has higher affinity for serotonin, but incorporates more norepinephrine activity at the minimal therapeutic dose. It appears that fewer titrations will be necessary than with milnacipran or venlafaxine, but at the cost of manipulating each transmitter system for fine tuning patient responses and alleviating tolerability issues. A potential advantage relative to venlafaxine is that duloxetine has shown a potentially less marked effect on blood pressure in some trials, even at the highest doses (i.e., 60 mg b.i.d.) (68).

Although clinical experience is still limited with duloxetine, six double-blind, placebo-controlled trials have been completed using SSRIs as comparators: two with fluoxetine and four with paroxetine.

The individual patient data from these trials have been made available and a meta-analysis has been completed (69). The results in the overall study group ($n = 1656$) suggest that this SNRI had a greater antidepressant effect, although the 5% absolute difference in remission rates was not statistically significant. It is noteworthy that these studies utilized a relatively low inclusion severity score on the HAM-D (patients with scores >14 were eligible) and, among the subgroup of 750 patients who scored 19 and higher on the HAM-D prior to treatment, the advantage of duloxetine therapy versus the SSRIs was almost identical to that reported by Thase et al. (52) in the initial eight FDA approved studies of venlafaxine. This is also comparable to the TCA versus SSRI analyses discussed above.

Three characteristics of this initial group of duloxetine RCTs warrant additional comment. First, the SSRI versus placebo difference in remission rates in these trials is identical to that reported by Thase et al. (52) and Nemeroff et al. (53) for venlafaxine. Thus, the advantage of the SNRI was not the result of the inefficacy of the comparator. Second, all six of the duloxetine studies used fixed dose designs, which are somewhat less sensitive in detecting drug–placebo differences than a flexible dose design (70). Third, none of the trials used the minimum therapeutic dose of duloxetine, whereas all six of the trials used the minimum therapeutic dose of the SSRI comparator (i.e., 20 mg/day of fluoxetine and paroxetine). Additional RCTs are therefore needed to evaluate the relative efficacy of the 60-mg dose of duloxetine to the full dose range of the comparator SSRI.

There are two drugs currently available that we should call norepinephrine and serotonin receptor modulators, nefazodone and mirtazapine. Nefazodone is a potent $5\text{-}HT_2$ inhibitor and a weak and transient inhibitor of 5-HT and NE uptake. The concerns about hepatotoxicity have led to the withdrawal of nefazodone from the markets in Europe, the United Kingdom, and Canada, the relative efficacy versus the SSRIs may be moot as a result. The manufacturer of nefazodone has conducted at least five head-to-head, nonplacebo comparisons versus SSRIs. However, they have not made original data available for a meta-analysis, nor have they disclosed whether other unpublished studies have been withheld. Nefazodone appears to have acute-phase antidepressant efficacy comparable to the SSRIs (71–73).

Mirtazapine, which has virtually no inhibitory effects on any monoamine uptake transporters, is thought to potentiate norepinephrine and serotonin neurotransmission by blocking presynaptic alpha$_2$ autoreceptors on norepinephrine neurons and alpha$_2$ heteroceptors located on serotonin neurons.

Several preliminary studies suggested that mirtazapine may have a more rapid onset of antidepressant activity than SSRIs (74,75). A total of 12 head-to-head RCTs have now been completed contrasting mirtazapine versus SSRIs; the original data from more than 2400 participants have been made available, and a meta-analysis has been completed in similar fashion to those concerning venlafaxine and duloxetine (69). The SSRI comparators include fluoxetine (four studies), sertraline (two studies), paroxetine (three studies), citalopram (one study), and fluvoxamine (two studies). The results confirm the early evidence of differences in the temporal pattern of response in relation to the SSRIs. Specifically, mirtazapine therapy differentiated the best from the SSRI comparators between the second and fourth weeks of therapy, with only a 6% difference in remission rates at week 6 and a 4% difference at week 8. This suggests an "accelerant" response whereby mirtazapine patients tend to respond faster while the SSRI patients respond equally well but at a later time. Subanalyses indicated that this temporal difference was largely, although not entirely, mediated by greater effects on sleep (early) in the course of therapy. The ability to induce sleep and possibly anxiolysis by way of histamine-1 receptor blockade would account for a several-point decline in HAM-D scores within the early weeks of the study. This drug's pharmacodynamic profile also makes it less likely to cause activation or agitation, which is another way to rapidly lower HAM-D scores. The single inpatient trial that contrasted mirtazapine and the immediate release formulation of venlafaxine yielded findings of equal efficacy (76), although that study did not have adequate power to conclude that the temporal difference was statistically significant.

The remaining three internationally marketed newer antidepressants, bupropion, reboxetine, and moclobemide, are not as widely available as the SSRIs, and they are grouped together here for convenience. Of these three, only bupropion is available in the United States. Nevertheless, all share the specific tolerability advantage of a low incidence of sexual and weight gain–related side effects and any of the three might be considered for a patient who was intolerant to the serotonin-mediated side effects of an SSRI or SNRI.

As noted earlier, bupropion is classified as an NDRI; it is available in the United States and Canada, but has not yet been introduced in Europe. It is less widely prescribed compared to fluoxetine, sertraline, or paroxetine, but nevertheless has more than a decade of data and clinical use in the United States, and sales have continued to grow at a slow but steady pace. A total of seven, double-blind head-to-head comparisons have been completed using fluoxetine (two studies), sertraline (four studies), and paroxetine (one study) as comparators. The manufacturer has made the original data available for study participants, and a meta-analysis has been completed

(68). The findings document almost exact parity with the SSRIs. These findings, therefore, are dissimilar to those mentioned for TCAs and SNRIs versus the SSRI class. Moreover, the drug–placebo differences in these trials are, again, exactly as predicted from the previous meta-analyses: both bupropion and the SSRIs had remission rates of 10% compared to placebo (d = 0.2). It is possible that the strongest pharmacodynamic property in the treatment of depression is the synergistic effect between serotonin and nor-epinephrine, as offered by some TCAs and the SNRIs. Bupropion is a dual-acting drug in the dopamine and norepinephrine system, but may carry less efficacy than the SNRIs or TCAs, relatively speaking.

In conclusion, there are numerous problems that impair the statistical sensitivity of RCTs to detect sometimes subtle, but clinically relevant differences between the newer antidepressants. Among the host of medications now available to treat depression, there is evidence of differences in tolerability and efficacy. The SSRIs are the new standard of efficacy, largely because of their better tolerability and superior safety profiles as well as, across the board, comparable trial-by-trial efficacy when compared to the previous standards, the TCAs. Some of the SSRIs carry multiple FDA approvals in the areas of depression, anxiety, eating disorder, and menstrual disorders. Sertraline carries a safety approval in postmyocardial infarction patients. The TCAs tend to show greater efficacy when compared to the SSRIs mainly in studies of more severely depressed and often hospitalized patients and, even then, the advantage was limited to just two TCAs, amitriptyline and clomipramine. Following the hypothesis that these TCAs have greater efficacy in severe depression because of "dual mechanism" potentiation of norepinephrine and serotonin, meta-analyses of studies of venlafaxine, duloxetine, and mirtazapine have documented evidence of greater efficacy in comparison to SSRIs. In the case of the dual-reuptake inhibitors, the advantage emerges across the first several weeks of acute-phase therapy, whereas the advantage in mirtazapine was greatest within weeks of therapy and diminished thereafter. By contrast, newer medications that do not simultaneously affect norepinephrine and serotonin, such as bupropion, have not shown greater efficacy in head-to-head trials with the SSRIs. No confirmatory meta-analyses exist to support these comparative claims however. As with any clinical disease state, at any given time, any patient may preferentially respond to one agent over another. These would be considered studies with a "sample size of 1." Our ability to use genetic and imaging techniques in the future may allow us to pick the agent with the highest likelihood of remission. These techniques will be discussed in later chapters. In the interim, "Patient Symptom Profiling" or assuming that certain symptoms may relate to poorly functioning neurotransmitter systems (15) may be a useful clinical technique that utilizes pharmacodynamic theory to help support the evidence base noted above when choosing medications for individual patients. This would suggest that certain symptoms are derived from the faltering norepinephrine system; for example, if an MDD patient cannot focus, pay attention, and is fatigued, it would make clinical sense to choose one of the antidepressants with noradrenergic activity, even if studies do not exist to show preferential treatment response.

ACUTE TREATMENT OUTCOME WITH PSYCHOTHERAPY

Analytical psychotherapies have been the dominant form of psychotherapy since the late 1800s. There are several dynamic theories, which have been applied to the treatment of MDD. Newer, depression-focused psychotherapies grew out of a series of developments in the mental health field between the late 1950s and the early 1980s. First, there was the slowly growing perception that more traditional psychodynamic approaches to psychotherapy were not well suited for the treatment of depression (77–80). For example, the reflective and nondirective methods commonly used in psychodynamic psychotherapy were viewed as sometimes counterproductive in work with more severely depressed patients, who seemed to benefit from more active, directive therapeutic support, structure, and guidance (81,82).

From an evidence-based point of view, the newer, focused psychotherapies have a greater database of outcome information. Dynamic clinicians and researchers often could not lend their work to the empirical scrutiny of randomized controlled clinical trials, especially because the training and use of systematic, calibrated dynamic techniques was not possible or available. This ultimately served to undermine the power base of psychodynamic psychotherapy in terms of allocation of research funds and publication in peer-reviewed general psychiatry journals (83).

Focused therapies also arose out of the ability to categorically diagnose the higher prevalence of mild-to-moderate, ambulatory cases of depression. This increase in diagnostic ability provided a compelling rationale for training larger numbers of mental health specialists of diverse disciplines. This supply and demand issue drove the need for easier learning curve therapies and manualized therapies. This would improve the efficiency of training and the ability to measure competence and calibrate the ability of individual therapists. The availability of ambulatory mental health services included the growth of community mental health services and outpatient private practices (84,85). There were simply not enough traditionally trained analytical psychotherapists to treat all persons seeking services. The newer, focused therapies could be provided by therapists with less training, which would help patients who could not afford the types of psychotherapy performed by dynamically trained or analytical private practitioners (86).

Focused therapies also emerged when nondynamic theoretical approaches gained notoriety. The behavioral approach, stemming largely from academic clinical psychology, introduced models of treatment originating from research using classical (87) and operant (77) conditioning models to change or modify overt behavior. Cognitive theory, influenced mostly by Beck (88), built upon behavioral formulations by incorporating similar attention to covert cognitive processes, such as thoughts, attitudes, and beliefs. From neoanalytic schools of psychotherapy, social psychiatry, marital counseling, and social work also came a growing appreciation of the interpersonal and relational contexts of depression, culminating in the model of therapy developed by Klerman et al. (89). With the advent of focused psychotherapies in MDD, there has been a marked increase in research in regard to acute outcomes and long-term outcomes. This chapter will focus on psychotherapy's ability to treat MDD acutely, and the following chapter will consider chronic outcomes separately.

We will now proceed with a thorough discussion of how effective these therapies are in alleviating depression in regard to acute outcomes. Randomized clinical trials have compared the depression-focused psychotherapies with both psychosocial and pharmacological control conditions. Literature published prior to 1995 has been reviewed extensively (5,22,90–92), and the major published controlled studies are summarized below in decreasing order of the available evidence base.

Cognitive Therapy

Cognitive therapy (CT) was first introduced by Beck and is the best studied psychological treatment of major depression when compared to the reasonable interpersonal therapy (IPT) evidence base and the less stringent behavioral therapy (BT) evidence base (5,91,93). CT has been extensively studied in comparison with both waiting-list control conditions and other forms of psychotherapy, as well as pharmacotherapy. However, despite such intensive study, only two published trials of CT have included a placebo–clinical management condition (94,95).

There is no doubt about the efficacy of CT as an acute-phase treatment for MDD when compared with waiting-list control conditions (96–103). In the Agency for Health Care Policy and Research (AHCPR) meta-analysis (5), CT had an overall efficacy rate of 46.6% with an advantage of 30% when compared with waiting-list control conditions. Although CT was not consistently superior to the placebo plus clinical management condition in the Treatment of Depression Collaborative Research Program (TDCRP) study (94), a recent subanalysis did suggest efficacy in the subset of patients with features of atypical depression (104). Moreover, Jarrett et al. (95) found CT to be equal to phenelzine and superior to pill placebo in a well-controlled 10-week double-blind study of 108 patients with atypical depression. Both active treatments yielded 58% intent-to-treat response rate, compared to 28% in the pill placebo group. Differential attrition from the pill placebo condition hampered interpretation of these data, although significant differences were apparent at week 4, i.e., before there was a pronounced difference in drop-out rates.

With respect to comparisons with pharmacotherapy, results of four studies indicate that CT is superior to treatment-as-usual (TAU) medication control conditions, whether CT is administered alone (105) or in combination with TAU (99,101,106,107). In each of these studies, a primary care provider prescribed the pharmacotherapy. Results from studies utilizing more rigorous pharmacotherapy conditions (94,95,105,108–111) have yielded more consistent evidence of parity. Exceptions to such parity include an initial study by Beck's group, in which results favored CT over imipramine hydrochloride (112), Murphy et al. (113) a small study of depressed outpatients (in which both CT and relaxation training were significantly more effective than desipramine), Markowitz et al. (114) study of mildly depressed HIV seropositive men, in which imipramine was more effective than CT, and the TDCRP study. In the TDCRP study, pharmacotherapy was more effective than CT in a more severely depressed subgroup of patients (94,115) and with respect to rapidity of improvement (116,117). The AHCPR meta-analysis, which did not include the studies of Hollon et al. (109), McKnight et al. (110), Murphy et al. (113), Blackburn and Moore (108), and Jarrett et al. (95), revealed a modest 15% advantage for CT over pharmacotherapy on the basis of three suitable studies. Inclusion of the five more recent studies probably would eliminate the difference between CT and pharmacotherapy.

Recently, Keller and coworkers (118) studied a modified form of CT and the antidepressant nefazodone singly and in combination, in a large ($n = 681$) multicenter trial of patients with chronic major or "double" depressive disorders. The modification of CT, developed by McCullough (119), emphasized the use of situational analysis of interpersonal interchanges to help chronically depressed patients learn more specific, goal-directed approaches to improving relationships. The two monotherapies were comparably effective at week 12, although nefazodone was more rapidly effective. The combination of CT and pharmacotherapy was markedly more effective than both of the monotherapies (e.g., intent-to-treat response rates: CT alone, 48%; nefazodone alone, 48%; combination, 73%). Analyses of the rates of change in symptoms suggested that the combined condition benefited by having the early effects of nefazodone as well as the later emerging effects of psychotherapy.

CT generally has been found to have an efficacy comparable to that of other active psychotherapies, including behavioral marital therapy (96,120), BT (121,122), IPT (94), brief dynamic therapy (121,123,124), pastoral counseling (98), and nondirective group therapy (125). In the Murphy et al. (113) study, CT was not significantly more effective than relaxation training (e.g., patients receiving a final BDI < 9; CT, 82%, RT, 73%), although the latter therapy was intended to serve as a nonspecific control group. As discussed previously, CT was less effective than IPT in the Markowitz et al. (114) study of mildly depressed HIV seropositive men. In the Jacobson et al. (120) first study, individual CT appeared to be more effective than behavioral marital therapy in a subset of patients with satisfactory marriages, whereas the latter treatment produced greater gains on measures of marital satisfaction in maritally distressed couples.

The Sheffield project compared cognitive-behavioral and dynamic-interpersonal therapies, each provided for either 8 or 16 weeks (123). Although neither treatment was identical to the models of CT and IPT described previously, they are sufficiently similar to be relevant. At the end of acute treatment, the two therapies were comparably effective. There was an interaction between pretreatment symptom severity and duration of therapy, with more severely symptomatic patients benefiting more from longer courses of treatment (123).

In the AHCPR meta-analysis, individual CT [50.1%] appeared somewhat more effective than group CT [39.2%]. Published comparative studies have similarly documented a slight advantage for individual CT compared to group CT (99,126). When CT has been compared with other group therapies, both positive (127,128) and negative (125) findings have been reported. Ravindran et al. (129) recently found that group CT added little symptomatic benefit when combined with sertraline in a study of 97 patients with primary dysthymic disorder.

CT is the only form of individual psychological treatment to be specifically modified for treatment of hospitalized depressed patients (130,131). Initial treatment experiences were described by Shaw (132) and Scott (133). In a small but controlled study of 30 antidepressant-resistant, "neurotic," major depression patients, deJong et al. (134) reported inpatient CT to be significantly more effective than either low-contact inpatient or outpatient comparison conditions. In an open-label study of 16 unmedicated patients with features of endogenous depression, Thase et al. reported an 81% response rate after up to four weeks of CT. A subsequent report expanded the series to 30 patients, with nine of the next 14 patients also responding (135). Poorer outcomes were observed among cases with significant comorbidity (136) and/or a prior history of nonresponse to antidepressant medication (137). In two controlled studies of combined treatment (138,139), some evidence favored CT plus antidepressants when compared with antidepressants alone. In Bowers's (138) study, however, the advantage of adding CT to standard inpatient treatment was significantly greater than that observed in the attention-control group that received relaxation training only. In the Miller et al. study, the additive benefit was largely limited to a subgroup of patients with high levels of dysfunctional attitudes (139).

One advantage of the relatively large number of studies of CT is that evidence about correlates or predictors of response has emerged (140). Specifically, single or unmarried status, high pretreatment levels of dysfunctional attitudes, chronicity, and increased initial symptomatic severity have been associated with poorer outcomes following 10 to 16 weeks of treatment with CT (141–143). Men and women appear to be equally responsive to CT (142,144), although more severely depressed women may have somewhat poorer outcomes (144). Patients with certain comorbid personality disorders appear to respond as well to CT as do patients with no personality disorders (145), although Barber and Muenz (141) found that those with obsessive compulsive traits were less responsive to CT than IPT. It should be noted that research trials of MDD typically have excluded patients with more severe Axis II psychopathology. Such patients are more likely to drop out of CT in a private practice study (146).

Positive correlates of CT outcome may include high pretreatment levels of learned resourcefulness (147,148) or self-efficacy (149), optimism (150), motivation (151), and homework compliance (152). The relationship between learned resourcefulness and CT outcome has not been replicated by all groups (142,153) and may be relevant to only more severely depressed patients (154). High levels of therapist core skills have been associated with favorable outcomes in one study (147) but not in others (155). Years of therapeutic experience (147) and technical competence in structuring therapy (152,156) also have been associated with better outcomes. Nevertheless, this line of research warrants further attention, particularly in trying to understand the results of studies such as the TDCRP in which the performance of CT varied across sites (157).

Interpersonal Psychotherapy (IPT)

IPT has been studied as an acute-phase treatment in at least five randomized clinical trials of outpatients with nonpsychotic MDD (80,94,158,159). In the initial study, IPT was superior to a triage-based supportive treatment and comparable to treatment with therapeutic amitriptyline monotherapy during a 12-week clinical trial (80,160). Some evidence from this trial suggested that IPT was more effective than amitriptyline in terms of improvements in mood, suicidal ideation, and interest, whereas the pharmacotherapy was superior in terms of resolution of appetite and sleep disturbances (160). Combined treatment had additive benefit compared with either IPT or amitriptyline alone (160).

The general equivalence of IPT and pharmacotherapy was reported in one 16-week study of elderly depressed outpatients (159,161). IPT and nortriptyline were equally effective for those patients who completed the protocol, although IPT was associated with a significantly greater retention of patients in the trial (16 out of 17 vs. 10 out of 18) (159). Among patients who completed the protocol, both treatments resulted in 50% to 60% reductions in mean depression symptom scores. By contrast, Reynolds et al. (158) found that IPT plus pill placebo was significantly less effective than pharmacotherapy with nortriptyline and no more effective than pill placebo alone. Patients receiving the combination of IPT and nortriptyline were not significantly more likely to remit when compared to the nortriptyline monotherapy condition. The study of Reynolds et al. (158) was unique in that all patients had bereavement-related depressive syndromes.

In a multicenter investigation sponsored by the National Institute of Mental Health, the TDCRP, IPT was compared with CT, active imipramine plus clinical management, and inert placebo plus clinical management. The efficacy of IPT was found to be comparable to that of both imipramine and CT by the end of a 16-week acute-phase protocol (94), although imipramine was more rapidly effective (116,117). Unlike imipramine, IPT was as effective for patients with atypical depression as for those with more classic neurovegetative profiles (104). Within the IPT group, subsequent analyses suggested that patients with less pronounced interpersonal problems did better (162), and patients with personality disorders did worse (145). Barber and Muenz (141) further examined specific personality traits. They found that IPT (in comparison to CT) was significantly more effective for patients with obsessive compulsive traits and significantly less effective for those with avoidant traits. Two other groups have reported an association between depression with anxiety symptoms and poorer IPT response (163,164).

The study of Schulberg et al. (165) tested IPT against both therapeutic nortriptyline and an unstructured therapy TAU condition among patients treated in four urban primary care clinics. Results indicated that nortriptyline was significantly more rapidly effective but that IPT became equally effective by the end of the trial; both interventions were significantly more effective than the TAU control condition. A subsequent analysis suggested that standardized pharmacotherapy with nortriptyline was more cost effective (166).

In the original study of DiMascio et al. (160), IPT was less effective than amitriptyline among patients who met the Research Diagnostic Criteria (RDC) for the endogenous depression subtype, whereas IPT was more effective in situational nonendogenous depression (167). These relationships were not confirmed in the subsequent TDCRP trial, in which IPT and imipramine were comparably effective in patients who met the RDC criteria for the endogenous or situational subtypes (162). Moreover, IPT did relatively well in subsequent analyses of the TDCRP focusing on pretreatment symptom severity (115,168). IPT response also was not associated with pretreatment symptom severity response in several other studies (169,170). Finally, IPT also showed a relatively late-emerging advantage in terms of patients' improved social adjustment (171). However, there was little evidence of selective or specific effects for IPT at the end of the acute-phase treatment of the TDCRP trial (172).

Markowitz et al. (114) completed a study of 101 depressed men who were seropositive for human immunodeficiency virus. Patients were randomly assigned to one of four conditions: IPT ($n = 24$), cognitive-behavioral therapy (CBT) ($n = 27$), or supportive psychotherapy with ($n = 26$) or without ($n = 24$) imipramine monotherapy. At the end of the 17-week protocol, IPT and the supportive therapy plus active imipramine were equally effective and, on most analyses, both conditions were more effective than the CBT or supportive therapy–alone conditions. The authors speculated that IPT may be a better fit than CBT for the real-world concerns of the depressed HIV seropositive patient.

IPT techniques have been studied in acute depression (as above), in maintenance and prophylaxis against depressive relapse (158,173,174), in adolescent depression (175), in PTSD (176), in depression in pregnancy and postpartum (177–179), and in eating disorder patients (180). In conclusion, there is broad empirical support for the use of IPT in MDD patients. Overall, these effects are similar in magnitude to acute-phase antidepressant pharmacotherapy, although the time course of symptom reduction appears to be slower. IPT may be less effective for patients with prominent anxiety, certain types of personality pathology, and more pronounced interpersonal difficulties. Such patients may do better if treated with the combination of IPT and pharmacotherapy.

Behavior Therapy

BT is one of the oldest forms of focused psychotherapy, and a good number of older studies have examined the efficacy of various forms of BT in relation to either waiting-list control conditions or TCAs (5,181). In the AHCPR meta-analysis, an overall intention-to-treat efficacy rate of 55.3% was observed for BT, based on 10 suitable studies. Moreover, BT appeared to have a small advantage in relation to dynamic psychotherapies (182,183). When each particular model of BT is considered separately, the strength of the evidence becomes less robust. For example, only one controlled study has evaluated the efficacy of social skills training (184) and social learning therapy (185). In a controlled trial of 120 female outpatients with MDD, Hersen et al. (184) found social skills training (plus placebo) to be no more or less effective than either amitriptyline hydrochloride or short-term dynamic psychotherapy (plus placebo). Skills training did provide a significant advantage on several behavioral indices of assertiveness (186), but the real-world benefits of these differences have not been established. McLean and Hakstian (185) reported the results of a study of 178 depressed outpatients. Patients were randomly assigned to 10 weeks of acute-phase treatment with a BT program or one of three comparison conditions: amitriptyline, relaxation training, or nondirective psychotherapy. The pattern of results generally favored BT over the other treatments, with the behavioral control condition—relaxation training—making a surprisingly strong intermediate showing. Interestingly, the advantage for the BT condition dissipated somewhat by the three-month follow-up (185).

Results of randomized controlled clinical trials generally suggest that BT produces symptomatic improvements comparable to those seen with other active psychological treatments, including Beck's model of CT (96,120,121) and nondirective or psychodynamically oriented therapies (121,187,188). When subtle differences are observed, results have favored BT (185,189,190). The best studied behavioral treatments are Rehm's self-control therapy (191–195) and psychoeducational model of treatment (187,196).

Most recently, Jacobson et al. (122) conducted a study comparing a relatively simple treatment, behavioral activation, with both the full model of CT and a cognitive-behavioral intervention minus the focus on core schema. The same therapists conducted all three conditions. The study group consisted of 38 men and 113 women with mild-to-moderate MDD. About 80% of the patients were referred from a health maintenance organization. The acute phase included 20 sessions, with six months of additional follow-up. They found that the three treatments were equally effective, with response rates ranging from 58% to 68%. Pretreatment symptom severity did not predict differential response, and relapse rates were similar across the six months of follow-up. The most important aspect of this study is that behavioral activation appears well suited for use by relatively junior, non-doctoral therapists.

Another more recent study contrasted a brief model of problem-solving therapy, consisting of only six sessions, against clinical management and either amitriptyline (mean dose: 139 mg/day) or pill placebo (197). The study was conducted in primary care clinics. The problem-solving intervention was so brief that the amount of clinical contact did not differ significantly across conditions. Both active treatments were significantly more effective than the pill placebo condition after 6 and 12 weeks of treatment. Remission rates at week 12 were as follows: problem-solving therapy, 60% (18/30), amitriptyline, 52% (16/31), and placebo, 27% (8/30).

Meta-analysis indicates that group (51%) and individual (58%) BT are roughly comparable in efficacy in the treatment of depressed outpatients (5). This conclusion is supported by the results of one randomized clinical trial directly comparing group and individual modalities (187). Behavioral marital therapy also has shown promise in two controlled trials (96,120). In summary, an older literature review suggests that BT is a credible treatment for depressed outpatients, although the most compelling evidence of efficacy arises from studies using waiting-list control groups.

Psychodynamic Psychotherapy

Psychoanalysis serves as the foundation for long-term and short-term dynamic therapies for a wide range of mental disorders and is the origin of many "common factor" concepts such as the therapeutic alliance (198–200). A voluminous and rich theoretical and clinical literature—based primarily on but not limited to the single subject case study method may attest to the effectiveness of psychoanalysis and psychodynamic psychotherapy for MDD (201,202).

Psychodynamic practitioners have traditionally been ambivalent about other methods of empirical research that focus more narrowly on symptoms and behaviors given the inherent complexity of unconscious mental processes, which are the specialized focus of psychodynamic treatments (203). The exigencies of managed care and the pressure of the empirically supported treatments (ESTs) movement (i.e., CT, IPT), however, pose a significant challenge to tradition. Psychodynamically oriented researchers have responded by proposing multiple methods for psychotherapy research and developing dynamically sensitive process and outcome measures (204–206). They have also critiqued the underlying assumptions of ESTs and have challenged research diagnostic series as a valid and reliable basis for research on depression (207–210).

Two large-scale MDD studies are particularly noteworthy in terms of demonstrating comparable effectiveness by virtue of large numbers of subjects, randomization, quality of implementation, specificity of interventions, and range of assessment measures. In the Sheffield Psychotherapy Project, subjects who met criteria for MDD ($n = 169$) were randomized to CBT or short-term psychodynamic psychotherapy (STPP) (211). Both treatments were equally effective when assessed at 16 sessions. The Helsinki Psychotherapy Study ($n = 381$) compared a new problem-solving, solution-focused therapy to short- and long-term psychodynamic psychotherapy for mood disorders in a randomized clinical trial (212). No significant differences between the treatment groups were observed on a wide range of measures of depression and anxiety. Smaller scale studies have also been conducted. Another RCT ($n = 30$) compared brief dynamic therapy, supportive therapy, and a waiting-list control condition in the treatment of minor depressive disorders (213). Assessment at baseline, termination, and 9-, 18-, and 60-month follow-ups showed that patients improved significantly in both psychotherapeutic treatments when compared to controls but that brief dynamic therapy was more effective at six-month follow-up. An additional randomized control trial ($n = 193$) compared nondirective counseling, CBT, and psychodynamic therapy with a control condition of routine primary care in the treatment of women with postpartum depression (214). All three treatments demonstrated significant impact at 4.5 months, but only psychodynamic therapy produced a reduction of depression superior to control. Treatment benefits, however, were not apparent at nine months postpartum and treatment did not reduce subsequent episodes of postpartum depression.

An RCT ($n = 74$) compared a combination of clomipramine and psychodynamic psychotherapy and clomipramine alone for MDD to investigate the cost effectiveness of combined treatment (215). Combined treatment as compared to medication alone demonstrated less treatment failure, better work adjustment at 10 weeks, better global functioning, fewer lost workdays, and lower hospitalization. These findings support the cost effectiveness of providing supplemental psychodynamic psychotherapy for patients with MDD on antidepressant medication.

Naturalistic clinical trials have replicated earlier studies of STPP for depression. Hilsenroth et al. examined process and outcome in a hybrid effectiveness/efficacy study ($n = 21$), which followed guidelines in four treatment manuals (216). Duration of treatment was determined by clinical judgment, patient decision, progress in treatment, and life changes. This study is the first to rate treatment credibility, fidelity, and satisfaction, which were high, demonstrating that changes in depressive symptoms were related to techniques derived from the models utilized. This approach and findings are comparable to those utilized by CT and IPT. All areas of functioning demonstrated large statistical effects and clinically significant improvements in depressive symptoms.

In another study, patients with chronic and recurrent depressive, anxiety, and/or personality disorders ($n = 53$) were followed in a naturalistic study of long-term psychodynamic psychotherapy (217). Subjects demonstrated significant improvement on measures of defenses, symptoms, global functioning, and the Hamilton Depression Rating Scale over the course of three to five years.

A sample of patients ($n = 59$) with a range of depressive conditions was gathered from an archival database at the University of Pennsylvania Center for Psychotherapy Research to test the hypothesis that explanatory style changed in a manualized supportive–expressive (SE) dynamic therapy (218). Data originally came from four separate and independent open trials conducted on chronic or double depression, generalized anxiety disorder, and avoidant and obsessive–compulsive disorder. Analyses of data demonstrated that patients' explanatory style became more positive during SE dynamic therapy and that this change was associated with an improvement in mood, a finding usually associated with CBT.

Meta-analytic reviews have also consistently shown that different therapy modalities are comparably effective for depression (219). Leichsenring critiqued and addressed the restrictions and distortions of previous meta-analyses in his review of the efficacy of STPP for depression as compared to CBT or BT (220). Six studies met inclusion criteria: target symptoms (depression), general level of psychiatric symptoms, and social functioning were assessed. No statistically significant difference between STPP and CBT was detected in 58 of 60 comparisons performed on the six studies and their follow-ups. Leichsenring considers these findings preliminary due to the small number of studies reviewed and recommends further studies in controlled and naturalistic settings to determine the effects of specific forms of STPP and CBT.

Researchers have questioned the validity of conclusions drawn from both efficacy and effectiveness studies on the basis that efficacy studies bear little resemblance to treatment delivered in the community, and effectiveness studies, while less restrictive, are difficult to assess in terms of causal connections between treatment and outcome. Ablon and Jones studied psychotherapy process in the NIMH TDCRP using the Psychotherapy Process Q-Set to investigate the basic premise underlying RCTs, i.e., the interventions compared were separate and distinct treatments (221,222). The study showed that there was considerable overlap between CBT and IPT that was correlated with change but was not detected in adherence checks.

While the evidence base for psychodynamic psychotherapy of depression is less robust than for other treatment modalities, findings from RCTs, open trials, hybrid effectiveness/efficacy studies, naturalistic studies, and meta-analyses provide preliminary and reasonable support for its comparable effectiveness in the treatment of MDD in adults.

Combined Psychotherapy and Antidepressant Treatment

Given that both a wide range of antidepressant medications and two depression-focused psychotherapies—CBT and IPT—have been found efficacious in the acute-phase treatment of depression, it makes sense that efforts have been made to combine the two. The rationale for this strategy includes the hope that the combined treatment increases the overall level of symptom relief (degree of response), increases the breadth of response, and increases acceptability of either treatment for the patient (e.g., receiving psychotherapy increases the likelihood of a patient starting and complying with needed antidepressant treatment) (223). A positive effect in one or more of the above areas would justify the decision to use combined treatment.

Many of the early studies that examined the combination of antidepressant medication and CBT found no advantage for this treatment combination when compared with either treatment as monotherapy (109,224). Subsequent meta- and mega-analyses (225,226), addressing the problem of small sample sizes in these earlier studies, concluded that the combination treatment does provide an advantage over either monotherapy. This was especially true for more severely depressed and more chronic patients (227,228). The most recent study to examine combined treatment (229), using nefazodone as a medication treatment and the Cognitive-Behavioral Analysis System of Psychotherapy (CBASP) as the study talk therapy, demonstrated that the combination of nefazodone and CBASP was significantly superior to either treatment alone in a large sample of chronically depressed patients. The difference in response rate, for study completers, between the combined treatment group and either monotherapy group was greater than 25%.

In summary, more severely and/or more chronically depressed patients will likely benefit from a treatment that combines antidepressant medication with psychotherapy. However, more research is needed to definitely determine if these or other patient characteristics (e.g., axis II comorbidity) predict which patients benefit most from the combined treatment. Finally, other methods for combining treatments (e.g., sequencing antidepressants and psychotherapy) that focus on resolution of residual symptoms and relapse prevention show great promise and are discussed in later chapters of this book.

CONCLUSIONS

The depression-focused psychotherapies, as exemplified by IPT, several models of BT, and Beck's CT are practical and effective outpatient treatments of mild to moderately severe MDD. Each therapy assesses the depressed patient's current state and problem areas, provides psychoeducation, explicitly instills hope, and guides patients through specific strategies to help them resolve the depressive episode. These principles though less manualized and structured exist in the dynamic therapies as well. No one form of psychotherapy has emerged as superior to the others. Similar to the antidepressants globally offering no distinct advantage over one another, the psychotherapies may also show subtle differences as noted above. Again, in any individual patient, response rates to specific psychotherapies may emerge. It also remains to be seen if an eclectic model of psychotherapy for depression will emerge, fusing the more clinically germane aspects of IPT, CT, and dynamics (120,157,195).

The depression-focused psychotherapies probably do best alone, without concomitant pharmacotherapy, for more acutely depressed patients with higher levels of premorbid functioning and adequate social support (100,230,231). This indication should not be trivialized as a nonspecific response because these psychotherapies have been consistently shown to be superior to waiting-list or low-contact control conditions.

The depression-focused psychotherapies should be conducted by appropriately trained clinicians and, ideally, should be preferentially recommended for patients who are motivated to participate in this style of treatment. When used as the primary treatment of MDD, clinicians should follow the AHCPR's (5) suggestion to re-evaluate the need for pharmacotherapy after several months of therapy if only partial response occurs with this modality. Unfortunately, this is not always done. A survey by Kendall et al. (170) indicated that nonmedical psychotherapists typically wait between 6 and 14 months before concluding that patients are not progressing in therapy. In such cases, months of unproductive suffering might have been circumvented by the more timely use of antidepressant medication. For example, one group found that more than 70% of IPT nonresponders responded to a sequential trial of imipramine or fluoxetine (232). One reason for this lag in time to initiate pharmacotherapy could be the relative lack of use of adequate rating scales in clinical practice. Ratings scales would more quickly alert a clinician to inadequate responses.

Finally, it is clear that both psychotherapy and pharmacotherapy are useful tools in the treatment of MDD. The reader should be cautioned that most of the clinical studies above allow relatively noncomorbid patients to enter. Given this, response rates in the usually comorbid psychiatric patient population may differ. The goal of treatment, regardless of modality, is complete symptom remission, and combining medications and psychotherapies is generally considered the standard of care in the MDD population.

REFERENCES

1. Thase ME, Kupfer DJ. Recent developments in the pharmacotherapy of mood disorders. J Consult Clin Psychol 1996; 64:646–659.
2. Stahl SM. J Clin Psychiat 2003; 64(11):1282–1283.
3. Morris JB, Beck AT. The efficacy of antidepressant drugs: a review of research (1958–1972). Arch Gen Psychiat 1974; 30:667–674.
4. Klein DF, Gittelman R, Quitkin F, Rifkin A. Diagnosis and Drug Treatment of Psychiatric Disorders: Adult and Children. 2d ed. Baltimore, MD: Williams & Wilkins, 1980.
5. Depression Guideline Panel. Depression in Primary Care. Treatment of Major Depression. Vol. 2. Rockville, MD: US Depart of Health and Human Services Agency for Health Care Policy and Research, 1993. Clinical Practice Guideline Number 5. AHCPR publication 93–0551.
6. American Psychiatric Association. Practice guideline for the treatment of patients with major depressive disorder (revision). Am J Psychiat 2000; 157(suppl 4):1–45.
7. Thase ME. Studying new antidepressants: if there was a light at the end of the tunnel could we see it? J Clin Psychiat 2002; 63(suppl 2):24–28.
8. Thase ME. Comparing the methods used to compare antidepressants. Psychopharmacol Bull 2002; 36(suppl 1):4–17.
9. Hamilton M. A rating scale for depression. J Neurol Neurosurg Psychiat 1960; 23:56–62.
10. Montgomery SA, Åsberg M. A new depression scale designed to be sensitive to change. Br J Psychiat 1979; 134:382–389.
11. Cohen J. Statistical Power Analysis for the Behavioral Sciences. New York: Academic Press, 1977.
12. Kirsch I, Moore TJ, Scoboria A, Nicholls SS. The emperor's new drugs: an analysis of antidepressant medication data submitted to the U.S. Food and Drug Administration. Prevention Treatment 2002; 5 (Article 23) (http://journals.apa.org/prevention/volume5/pre0050023a.html).
13. Walsh BT, Seidman SN, Sysko R, Gould M. Placebo response in studies of major depression: variable, substantial, and growing. JAMA 2002; 287:1840–1847.
14. Khan A, Warner HA, Brown WA. Symptom reduction and suicide risk in patients treated with placebo in antidepressant clinical trials: an analysis of the Food and Drug Administration database. Arch Gen Psychiat 2000; 57:311–317.
15. Stahl SM, Entsuah R, Rudolph RL. Comparative efficacy between venlafaxine and SSRIs: a pooled analysis of patients with depression. Biol Psychiat 2002; 52:1166–1174.

16. Frank E, Prien RF, Jarrett RB, et al. Conceptualization and rationale for consensus definitions of terms in major depressive disorder. Remission, recovery, relapse, and recurrence. Arch Gen Psychiat 1991; 48:851–855.

17. Thase ME, Sloan DM, Kornstein S. Remission as the critical outcome of depression treatment. Psychopharmacol Bull 2002; 36(suppl 3):12–25.

18. Zimmerman M, Posternak MA, Chelminski I. Implications of using different cut-offs on symptom severity scales to define remission from depression. Int Clin Psychopharmacol 2004; 19:215–220.

19. Paykel ES, Ramana R, Cooper Z, Hayhurst H, Kerr J, Barocka A. Residual symptoms after partial remission: an important outcome in depression. Psychol Med 1995; 25:1171–1180.

20. Thase ME, Simons AD, McGeary J, et al. Relapse after cognitive BT of depression: potential implications for longer courses of treatment? Am J Psychiat 1992; 149:1046–1052.

21. Miller IW, Keitner GI, Schatzberg AF, et al. The treatment of chronic depression. Part 3: Psychosocial functioning before and after treatment with sertraline and imipramine. J Clin Psychiat 1998; 59:608–619.

22. Thase ME, Trivedi MH, Rush AJ. MAOIs in the contemporary treatment of depression. Neuropsychopharmacology 1995; 12:185–219.

23. Stewart JS, McGrath PJ, Rabkin JG, Quitkin FM. A typical depression: a valid clinical entity? Psychiat Clin North Am 1993; 16(3):479–495.

24. Buckley NA, McManus PR. Fatal toxicity of serotoninergic and other antidepressant drugs: analysis of UK mortality data. BMJ 2002; 325:1332–1333.

25. Buckley NA, Faunce TA. 'Atypical' antidepressants in overdose: clinical considerations with respect to safety. Drug Saf 2003; 26:539–551.

26. Song F, Freemantle N, Sheldon TA, et al. Selective serotonin reuptake inhibitors: meta-analysis of efficacy and acceptability. BMJ 1993; 306:683–687.

27. Anderson IM, Tomenson BM. The efficacy of selective serotonin re-uptake inhibitors in depression: a meta-analysis of studies against tricyclic antidepressants. J Psychopharmacol 1994; 8:238–249.

28. Anderson IM. Selective serotonin reuptake inhibitors versus tricyclic antidepressants: a meta-analysis of efficacy and tolerability. J Affect Disord 2000; 58:19–36.

29. Freemantle N, Anderson IM, Young P. Predictive value of pharmacological activity for the relative efficacy of antidepressant drugs. Br J Psychiat 2000; 177:292–302.

30. Barbui C, Hotopf M. Amitriptyline v. the rest: still the leading antidepressant after 40 years of randomised controlled trials. Br J Psychiat 2001; 178:129–144.

31. Montgomery SA, Henry J, McDonald G, et al. Selective serotonin reuptake inhibitors: meta-analysis of discontinuation rates. Int Clin Psychopharmacol 1994; 9:47–53.

32. Roose SP, Laghrissi-Thode F, Kennedy JS, et al. Comparison of paroxetine and nortriptyline in depressed patients with ischemic heart disease. JAMA 1998; 279:287–291.

33. Kornstein SG, Schatzberg AF, Thase ME, et al. Gender differences in treatment response to sertraline versus imipramine in chronic depression. Am J Psychiat 2000; 157(9):1445–1452.

34. Anderson IM. SSRIS versus tricyclic antidepressants in depressed inpatients: a meta-analysis of efficacy and tolerability. Depress Anxiety 1998; 7(suppl 1): 11–17.
35. Edwards JG, Anderson I. Systematic review and guide to selection of selective serotonin reuptake inhibitors. Drugs 1999; 57:507–533. [Erratum appears in Drugs 1999; 58(6):1207–1209].
36. Anderson IM. Meta-analytical studies on new antidepressants. Br Med Bull 2001; 57:161–178.
37. Gorman JM, Korotzer A, Su G. Efficacy comparison of escitalopram and citalopram in the treatment of major depressive disorder: pooled analysis of placebo-controlled trials. CNS Spectrums 2002; 7(suppl 1):40–44.
38. Svensson S, Mansfield PR. Escitalopram: superior to citalopram or chiral chimera? Psychother Psychosomat 2004; 73:10–16.
39. Stórustovu SI, Sánchez C, Pörzgen P, et al. R-citalopram functionally antagonizes escitalopram in vivo and in vitro: evidence for kinetic interaction at the serotonin transporter. Br J Pharmacol 2004; 142:172–180.
40. Baron BM, Ogden A, Siegel BW, Stegeman J, Ursillo RC, Dudley MW. Rapid down regulation of β adrenoceptors by co-administration of desipramine and fluoxetine. Eur J Pharmacol 1988; 154:125–134.
41. Clerc GE, Ruimy P, Verdeau PJ. A double-blind comparison of venlafaxine and fluoxetine in patients hospitalised for major depression and melancholia. Int Clin Psychopharmacol 1994; 9:139–143.
42. Dierick M, Ravizza L, Realini R, Martin A. A double-blind comparison of venlafaxine and fluoxetine for treatment of major depression in outpatients. Prog Neuropsychopharmacol Biol Psychiat 1996; 20:57–71.
43. Bolden-Watson C, Richelson E. Blockade by newly-developed antidepressants of biogenic amine uptake into rat brain synaptosomes. Life Sci 1993; 52: 1023–1029.
44. Thase ME. Effects of venlafaxine on blood pressure: a meta-analysis of original data from 3744 depressed patients. J Clin Psychiat 1998; 59(10):502–508.
45. Harvey AT, Rudolph RL, Preskorn SH. Evidence of the dual action of venlafaxine. Arch Gen Psychiat 2000; 57:503–509.
46. Olver JS, Burrrows GD, Norman TR. The treatment of depression with different formulations of venlafaxine: a comparative analysis. Hum Psychopharmacol 2004; 19:9–16.
47. Thase ME, Friedman ES, Howland RH. Venlafaxine and treatment-resistant depression. Depress Anxiety 2000; 12(suppl 1):55–62.
48. Kelsey JE. Dose-response relationship with venlafaxine. J Clin Psychopharmacol 1996; 16:21S–26S.
49. Khan A, Upton GV, Rudolph RL, Entsuah R, Leventer SM. The use of venlafaxine in the treatment of major depression and major depression associated with anxiety: a dose-response study. J Clin Psychopharmacol 1998; 18:19–25.
50. Einarson TR, Arikian SR, Casciano J, Doyle JJ. Comparison of extended-release venlafaxine, selective serotonin reuptake inhibitors, and tricyclic antidepressants in the treatment of depression: a meta-analysis of randomized controlled trials. Clin Ther 1999; 21:296–308.

51. Smith D, Dempster C, Glanville J, Freemantle N, Anderson I. Efficacy and tolerability of venlafaxine compared with selective serotonin reuptake inhibitors and other antidepressants: a meta-analysis. Br J Psychiat 2002; 180:396–404.

52. Thase ME, Entsuah AR, Rudolph RI. Remission rates during treatment with venlafaxine or selective serotonin reuptake inhibitors. Br J Psychiat 2001; 178:234–241.

53. Nemeroff CB, Entsuah AR, Willard L, Demitrack M, Thase M. Venlafaxine and SSRIs: pooled remission analysis. Eur Neuropsychopharmacol 2003; 13(suppl 4):S255.

54. Nemeroff C. Poster Presented at 2003 American Psychiatric Association Annual Meeting, San Francisco.

54a. Thase ME, Entsuah P, Cantillon M, Kornstein SG. Relative antidepressant efficacy of venlafaxine and SSRIs: sex-age interactions. J Women's Health 2005; 14(7):609–616.

54b. Shelton C, Entsuah P, Padmanabhan SK, Vinall PE. Venlafaxine XR demonstrates higher rates of sustained remission compared to fluoxetine, paroxemine or placebo. Int Clin Psychopharm 2005; 20(4):233–238.

55. Shelton RC, Haman K, Kiev A, et al. NR380 sertraline versus venlafaxine extended release in depressed outpatients. Poster presented at American Psychiatric Association Annual Meeting 2004, New York.

56. Bielski RJ, Ventura D, Chang CC. A double-blind comparison of escitalopram and venlafaxine extended release in the treatment of major depressive disorder. J Clin Psychiat 2004.

57. Poirier M-F, Boyer P. Venlafaxine and paroxetine in treatment-resistant depression: double-blind, randomised comparison. Br J Psychiat 1999; 175:12–16.

58. Spencer CM, Wilde MI. Milnacipran. A review of its use in depression. Drugs 1998; 56:405–427.

59. Vaishnavi SN, Nemeroff CB, Plott SJ, Rao SG, Kranzler J, Owens MJ. Milnacipran: a comparative analysis of human monoamine uptake and transporter binding affinity. Biol Psychiat 2004; 55:320–322.

60. Puech A, Montgomery S, Prost JF, Solles A, Briley M. Milnacipran, a new serotonin and noradrenaline reuptake: an overview of its antidepressant effects and clinical tolerability. Int Clin Psychopharmacol 1997; 12:99–108.

61. Fukuchi T, Kanemoto K. Differential effects of milnacipran and fluvoxamine, especially in patients with severe depression and agitated depression: a case-control study. Int Clin Psychopharmacol 2002; 17:53–58.

62. Guelfi JD, Ansseau M, Corruble E, et al. A double-blind comparison of the efficacy and safety of milnacipran and fluoxetine in depressed patients. Int Clin Psychopharmacol 1998; 13:121–128.

63. Clerc G. Milnacipran/fluvoxamine study group. Antidepressant efficacy and tolerability of milnacipran a dual serotonin and noradrenaline reuptake inhibitor: a comparison with fluvoxamine. Int Clin Psychopharmacol 2001; 16:145–151.

64. Morishita S, Aritz S. Differential period of onset of action of fluvoxamine, paroxetine and milnacipran for depression. Hum Psychopharmacol 2003; 18:479–482.

65. Ansseau M, von Frenckell R, Gerard M-A, et al. Interest of a loading dose of milnacipran in endogenous depressive inpatients. Comparison with the standard regimen and with fluvoxamine. Eur Neuropsychopharmacol 1991; 1:113–121.

66. Ansseau M, Papart P, Troisfontaines B, et al. Controlled comparison of milnacipran and fluoxetine in major depression. Psychopharmacology 1994; 114:131–137.

67. Nemeroff CB, Schatzberg AF, Goldstein DJ, et al. Duloxetine for the treatment of major depressive disorder. Psychopharmacol Bull 2002; 36:106–132.

68. Thase ME, Tran PV, Wiltse C, Pangallo BA, Mallinckrodt C, Detke MJ. Cardiovascular profile of duloxetine, a dual reuptake inhibitor of serotonin and norepinephrine. J Clin Psychopharmacol 2005; 25:132–140.

69. Thase M, Schutte AJ, Van der flier S, Heukels A. Remission with mirtazapine versus SSRIs: a meta analysis on data of more than 2500 depressed patients treated in randomized controlled trials. J Affect Disord 2004; 78(suppl 1):S136.

70. Khan A, Leventhal RM, Khan SR, Brown WA. Severity of depression and response to antidepressants and placebo: an analysis of the Food and Drug Administration database. J Clin Psychopharmacol 2002; 22:40–45.

71. Rush AJ, Armitage R, Gillin JC, et al. Comparative effects of nefazodone and fluoxetine on sleep in outpatients with major depressive disorder. Biol Psychiat 1998; 44:3–14.

72. Feiger AD, Bielski RJ, Bremner J, et al. Double-blind, placebo-substitution study of nefazodone in the prevention of relapse during continuation treatment of outpatients with major depression. Int Clin Psychopharmacol 1999; 14:19–28.

73. Ferguson JM, Shrivastava RK, Stahl SM, et al. Reemergence of sexual dysfunction in patients with major depressive disorder: double blind comparison of nefazodone and sertraline. J Clin Psychiat 2001; 62:24–29.

74. Quitkin FM, Taylor BP, Kremer C. Does mirtazapine have a more rapid onset than SSRIs? J Clin Psychiat 2001; 62:358–361.

75. Thase ME, Howland RH, Friedman ES. Onset of action of selective and multi-action antidepressants. In: den Boer JA, Westenberg HGM, eds. Antidepressants: Selectivity or Multiplicity? Benecke, NI: Amsterdam, The Netherlands, 2001:101–116.

76. Guelfi JD, Ansseau M, Timmerman L, Kørsgaard S. Mirtazapine-venlafaxine study group. Mirtazapine versus venlafaxine in hospitalized severely depressed patients with melancholic features. J Clin Psychopharmacol 2001; 21:425–431.

77. Ferster CB. A functional analysis of depression. Am Psychol 1973; 28: 857–870.

78. Liberman RP, Raskin DE. Depression. A behavioral formulation. Arch Gen Psychiat 1971; 24:515–523.

79. Rush AT. Psychotherapy of the affective psychoses. Am J Psychoanal 1980; 40:99–123.

80. Weissman MM. The psychological treatment of depression: research evidence for the efficacy of psychotherapy alone, in comparison and in combination with pharmacotherapy. Arch Gen Psychiat 1979; 36:1261–1269.

81. Arieti S. Affective disorders: manic-depressive psychosis and psychotic depression: manifest symptomatology, psychodynamics, sociological factors

and psychotherapy. In: Arieti S, ed. American Handbook of Psychiatry. Basic Books. New York: Basic Books, 1976.

82. Jacobson E. Depression. New York: International Universities Press, 1964.

83. Mohl PC, Lomax J, Tasman A, et al. Psychotherapy training for the psychiatrist of the future. Am J Psychiat 1990; 147:7–13.

84. Olfson M, Klerman GL, Pincus HA. The roles of psychiatrists in organized outpatient mental health settings. Am J Psychiat 1993; 150:625–631.

85. Windle C, Poppen PJ, Thompson JW, Marvelle K. Types of patients served by various providers of outpatient care in CMHCs. Am J Psychiat 1988; 145: 457–463.

86. Scott J. Social and community approaches. In: Paykel ES, ed. Handbook of Affective Disorders. New York: The Guilford Press, 1992.

87. Wolpe J. Psychotherapy by Reciprocal Inhibition. Stanford, California: Stanford University Press, 1958.

88. Beck AT. Cognitive Therapy and the Emotional Disorders. New York: International Universities Press, 1976.

89. Klerman GL, Weissman MM, Rounsaville BJ, Chevron RS. Interpersonal Psychotherapy of Depression. New York: Basic Books, 1984.

90. Agency for Health Care Policy and Research, U.S. Public Health Service. Clinical Practice Guideline Number 5. Depression in Primary Care. Treatment of Major Depression. Vol. 2. Rockville, Maryland, 1993; American Psychiatric Association: practice guideline for major depressive disorder in adults. Am J Psychiat 1993; 150(suppl).

91. Dobson KS. A meta-analysis of the efficacy of cognitive therapy for depression. J Consult Clin Psychol 1989; 57:414–419.

92. Robinson LA, Berman JS, Neimeyer RA. Psychotherapy for the treatment of depression: a comprehensive review of controlled outcome research. Psychol Bull 1990; 108(1):30–49.

93. Gloaguen V, Cottraux J, Cucherat M, et al. A meta-analysis of the effects of cognitive therapy in depressed patients. J Affect Disord 1998; 49:59–72.

94. Elkin I, Shea MT, Watkins JT, et al. National Institute of Mental Health Treatment of Depression Collaborative Research Program: general effectiveness of treatments. Arch Gen Psychiat 1989; 46:971–982.

95. Jarrett RB, Schaffer M, McIntire D, et al. Treatment of atypical depression with cognitive therapy or phenelzine. A double-blind, placebo-controlled trial. Arch Gen Psychiat 1999; 56:431–437.

96. Beach SR, O'Leary KD. Treating depression in the context of marital discord: outcome and predictors of response of marital therapy versus cognitive therapy. Behav Ther 1992; 23:428–507.

97. Neimeyer RA, Robinson LA, Berman JS, et al. Clinical outcome of group therapies for depression. Group Anal 1989; 22:73–86.

98. Propst LR, Ostrom R, Watkins P, et al. Comparative efficacy of religious and nonreligious cognitive-behavioral therapy for the treatment of clinical depression in religious individuals. J Consult Clin Psychol 1992; 60:94–103.

99. Ross M, Scott M. An evaluation of the effectiveness of individual and group cognitive therapy in the treatment of depressed patients in an inner city health centre. J Roy College Gen Pract 1985; 35:239–242.

100. Rude SS. Relative benefits of assertion or cognitive self-control treatment for depression as a function of proficiency in each domain. J Consult Clin Psychiat 1986; 54:390–394.

101. Scott MJ, Stradling SG. Group cognitive therapy for depression produces clinically significant reliable change in community-based settings. Behav Psychother 1990; 18:1–19.

102. Selmi PM, Klein MH, Greist JH, et al. Computer-administered cognitive-behavioral therapy for depression. Am J Psychiat 1990; 147:51–56.

103. Thompson LW, Gallagher D, Breckenridge JS. Comparative effectiveness of psychotherapies for depressed elders. J Consult Clin Psychol 1987; 55:385–390.

104. Stewart JW, Garfinkel R, Nunes EV, et al. Atypical features and treatment response in the National Institute of Mental Health Treatment of Depression Collaborative Research Program. J Clin Psychopharmacol 1998; 18:429–434.

105. Blackburn IM, Bishop S, Glen AIM, et al. The efficacy of cognitive therapy in depression: a treatment trial using cognitive therapy and pharmacotherapy, each alone and in combination. Br J Psychiat 1981; 139:181–189.

106. Scott C, Tacchi MJ, Jones R, et al. Acute and one-year outcome of a randomised controlled trial of brief cognitive therapy for major depressive disorder in primary care. Br J Psychiat 1997; 171:131–134.

107. Teasdale JD, Fennell MJV, Hibbert GA, et al. Cognitive therapy for major depressive disorder in primary care. Br J Psychiat 1984; 144:400–406.

108. Blackburn IM, Moore RG. Controlled acute and follow-up trial of cognitive therapy and pharmacotherapy in out-patients with recurrent depression. Br J Psychiat 1997; 171:328–334.

109. Hollon SD, DeRubeis RJ, Evans MD, et al. Cognitive-therapy and pharmacotherapy for depression: singly and in combination. Arch Gen Psychiat 1992; 49:774–781.

110. McKnight DL, Nelson-Gray RO, Barnhill J. Dexamethasone suppression test and response to cognitive therapy and antidepressant medication. Behav Ther 1992; 1:99–111.

111. Murphy GE, Simons AD, Wetzel RD, et al. Cognitive therapy and pharmacotherapy. Arch Gen Psychiat 1984; 41:33–41.

112. Rush AJ, Beck AT, Kovacs M, et al. Comparative efficacy of cognitive therapy and pharmacotherapy in the treatment of depressed outpatients. Cogn Ther Res 1977; 1:17–38.

113. Murphy GE, Carney RM, Knesevich MA, et al. Cognitive behaviour therapy, relaxation training, and tricyclic antidepressant medication in the treatment of depression. Psychol Rep 1995; 45:403–420.

114. Markowitz JC, Kocsis JH, Fishman B, et al. Treatment of depressive symptoms in human immunodeficiency virus-positive patients. Arch Gen Psychiat 1988; 55:452–457.

115. Elkin I, Gibbons RD, Shea MT, et al. Initial severity and differential treatment outcome in the National Institute of Mental Health Treatment of Depression Collaborative Research Program. J Consult Clin Psychol 1995; 63:841–847.

116. Watkins JT, Leber WR, Imber SD, et al. Temporal course of change of depression. J Consult Clin Psychol 1993; 61:858–864.

117. Gibbons RD, Hedeker D, Elkin I, et al. Some conceptual and statistical issues in analysis of longitudinal psychiatric data. Arch Gen Psychiat 1993; 50: 739–750.

118. Kocsis JH, Rush AJ, Markowitz JC, et al. Continuation treatment of chronic depression: a comparison of nefazodone, cognitive behavioral analysis system of psychotherapy, and their combination. Psychopharmacol Bull 2003; 37(4):73–87.

119. McCullough JP. Cognitive Behavioral Analysis System of Psychotherapy: Treatment of Chronic Depression. New York, NY: Guilford Press, 1999.

120. Jacobson NS, Dobson K, Fruzzetti AE, et al. Marital therapy as a treatment for depression. J Consult Clin Psychol 1991; 59:547–557.

121. Gallagher DE, Thompson LW. Treatment of major depressive disorder in older adult outpatients with brief psychotherapies. Psychotherapy 1982; 19:482–490.

122. Jacobson NS, Dobson KS, Truax PA, et al. A component analysis of cognitive-behavioral treatment for depression. J Consult Clin Psychol 1996; 64:295–304.

123. Shapiro DA, Barkham M, Rees A, et al. Effects of treatment duration and severity of depression on the effectiveness of cognitive-behavioral and psychodynamic-interpersonal psychotherapy. J Consult Clin Psychol 1994; 62: 522–534.

124. Barkham M, Rees A, Shapiro DA, et al. Outcomes of time-limited psychotherapy in applied settings: replicating the second Sheffield Psychotherapy Project. J Consult Clin Psychol 1996; 64:1079–1085.

125. Hogg JA, Deffenbacher JL. A comparison of cognitive and interpersonal-process group therapies in the treatment of depression among college students. J Consult Clin Psychol 1998; 35:304–310.

126. Rush AJ, Watkins JT. Group versus individual cognitive therapy: a pilot study. Cogn Ther Res 1981; 5:95–103.

127. Beutler LE, Scogin F, Kirkish P, et al. Group cognitive therapy and alprazolam in the treatment of depression in older adults. J Consult Clin Psychol 1987; 55:550–556.

128. Covi L, Lipman RS. Cognitive-behavioral group psychotherapy combined with imipramine in major depression. Psychopharmacol Bull 1987; 23: 173–177.

129. Ravindran AV, Anisman H, Merali Z, et al. Treatment of primary dysthymia with group cognitive therapy and pharmacotherapy: clinical symptoms and functional impairments. Am J Psychiat 1999; 156:1608–1617.

130. Stuart S, Simons AD, Thase ME, et al. Are personality assessments valid in acute major depression? J Affect Disord 1992; 24:281–290.

131. Wright J, Thase M, Beck A, et al. Cognitive therapy with inpatients. Depression 1993; 1:329–330.

132. Shaw BF. Cognitive therapy with an inpatient population. In: Emery G, Hollon SD, Bedrosian RC, eds. New Directions in Cognitive Therapy. New York: Guilford Press, 1981:29–49.

133. Scott J. Cognitive therapy with depressed inpatients. In: Dryden W, Trower P, eds. Developments in Cognitive Psychotherapy. London: Sage Publications, 1988:177–189.

134. DeJong R, Treiber R, Henrich G. Effectiveness of two psychological treatments for inpatients with severe and chronic depressions. Cogn Ther Res 1986; 10:645–663.

135. Thase ME, Dub S, Bowler K, et al. Hypothalamic-pituitary-adrenocortical activity and response to cognitive behavior therapy in unmedicated, hospitalized depressed patients. Am J Psychiat 1996; 153:886–891.

136. Thase ME, Howland RH. Refractory depression: relevance of psychosocial factors and therapies. Psych Ann 1994; 24:232–240.

137. Thase ME, Howland R. Biological processes in depression: updated review and integration. In: Beckham EE, Leber WR, eds. Handbook of Depression. New York, NY: Guilford Press, 1995:213–279.

138. Bowers WA. Treatment of depressed inpatients. Cognitive therapy plus medication, relaxation plus medication, and medication alone. Br J Psychiat 1990; 156:73–78.

139. Miller IW, Norman WH, Keitner GI, et al. Cognitive-behavioral treatment of depressed inpatients. Behav Ther 1989; 20:25–47.

140. Weissman MM, Klerman GL, eds. New Applications of Interpersonal Psychotherapy. Washington, D.C.: American Psychiatric Press, 1993.

141. Barber JP, Muenz LR. The role of avoidance and obsessiveness in matching patients to cognitive and interpersonal psychotherapy: empirical findings from the treatment for depression collaborative research program. J Consult Clin Psychol 1996; 64:951–958.

142. Jarrett RB, Eaves GG, Grannenmann BD, et al. Clinical, cognitive, and demographic predictors of response to cognitive therapy for depression: a preliminary report. Psychiat Res 1991; 37:245–260.

143. Simons AD, Gordon JS, Monroe SM. Toward an integration of psychologic, social, and biologic factors in depression: effects on outcome and course of cognitive therapy. J Consult Clin Psychol 1995; 63:369–377.

144. Thase ME, Reynolds CF III, Frank E, et al. Do depressed men and women respond similarly to cognitive behavior therapy? Am J Psychiat 1994; 151:500–505.

145. Shea MT, Pilkonis PA, Beckham E, et al. Personality disorders and treatment outcome in the NIMH treatment of depression collaborative research program. Am J Psychiat 1990; 147:711–718.

146. Persons JB, Burns DD, Perloff JM. Predictors of dropout and outcome in cognitive therapy for depression in a private practice setting. Cogn Ther Res 1988; 12:557–575.

147. Burns DD, Nolen-Hoeksema S. Therapeutic empathy and recovery from depression in cognitive-behavioral therapy: a structural equation model. J Consult Clin Psychol 1992; 60:441–449.

148. Simons AD, Epstein LH, McGowan CR, et al. Exercise as a treatment for depression: an update. Clin Psychol Rev 1985; 5:553–568.

149. Kavanaugh DJ, Wilson PH. Prediction of outcome with group cognitive therapy for depression. Behav Res Ther 1989; 27:333–343.

150. Seligman MEP, Castellon C, Cacciola J, et al. Explanatory style change during cognitive therapy for unipolar depression. J Abnorm Psychol 1988; 97:13–18.

151. Fennell MJV, Teasdale JD, Jones S, et al. Distraction in neurotic and endogenous depression: an investigation of negative thinking in major depressive disorder. Psychol Med 1987; 17:441–452.

152. Bryant MJ, Simons AD, Thase ME. Therapist skill and patient variables in homework compliance: controlling an uncontrolled variable in cognitive therapy outcome research. Cogn Ther Res 1999; 23:381–399.

153. Beckham EE. Improvement after evaluation in psychotherapy of depression: evidence of a placebo effect? J Clin Psychol 1989; 45:945–950.

154. Burns DD, Sayers SL, Moras K. Intimate relationships and depression: Is there a causal connection? J Consult Clin Psychol 1994; 62(5):1033–1043.

155. DeRubeis RJ, Feeley M. Determinants of change in cognitive therapy for depression. Cogn Ther Res 1990; 14:469–482.

156. DeRubeis RJ, Evans MD, Hollon SD, et al. How does cognitive therapy work? Cognitive change and symptom change in cognitive therapy and pharmacotherapy for depression. J Consult Clin Psychol 1990; 58:862–869.

157. Jacobson NS, Hollon SD. Prospects for future comparisons between drugs and psychotherapy: lessons from the CBT-versus pharmacotherapy exchange. J Consult Clin Psychol 1996; 64:104–108.

158. Reynolds CF III, Miller MD, Pasternak RE, et al. Treatment of bereavement-related major depressive episodes in later life: a controlled study of acute and continuation treatment with nortriptyline and interpersonal psychotherapy. Am J Psychiat 1999; 156:202–208.

159. Schneider LS, Sloane RB, Staples FR, et al. Pretreatment orthostatic hypotension as a predictor of response to nortriptyline in geriatric depression. J Clin Psychopharmacol 1986; 6:172–176.

160. DiMascio A, Weissman MM, Prusoff BA, et al. Differential symptom reduction by drugs and psychotherapy in acute depression. Arch Gen Psychiat 1979; 36:1450–1456.

161. Sloane RB, Staples FR, Schneider LR. Interpersonal therapy versus nortriptyline for depression in the elderly. In: Burrows G, Norman TR, Dennerstein L, eds. Clinical and Pharmacological Studies in Psychiatric Disorders. London: John Libbey, 1985:344–346.

162. Sotsky SM, Glass DR, Shea MT, et al. Patient predictors of response to psychotherapy and pharmacotherapy: findings in the NIMH Treatment of Depression Collaborative Research Program. Am J Psychiat 1991; 148:997–1008.

163. Brown C, Schulberg HC, Madonia MJ, et al. Treatment outcomes for primary care patients with major depression and lifetime anxiety disorders. Am J Psychiat 1996; 153:1293–1300.

164. Feske U, Frank E, Kupfer DJ, et al. Anxiety as a predictor of response to interpersonal psychotherapy for recurrent major depression: an exploratory investigation. Depression Anxiety 1998; 8:135–141.

165. Schulberg HC, Block MR, Madonia M, et al. Treating major depression in primary care practice. Eight-month clinical outcomes. Arch Gen Psychiat 1996; 53:913–919.

166. Lave JR, Frank RG, Schulberg HC, et al. Cost-effectiveness of treatments for major depression in primary care patients. Arch Gen Psychiat 1998; 55: 645–651.

167. Prusoff BA, Weissman MM, Klerman GL, et al. Research Diagnostic Criteria subtypes of depression: their role as predictors of differential response to psychotherapy and drug treatment. Arch Gen Psychiat 1980; 37:796–803.

168. Elkin I, Gibbons RD, Shea MT, et al. Science is not a trial (but it can sometimes be a tribulation). J Consult Clin Psychol 1996; 64:92–103.

169. Buysse D, Kupfer DJ, Frank E, et al. Electroencephalographic sleep studies in depressed patients treated with psychotherapy—I. Baseline studies in responders and nonresponders. Psychiat Res 1992; 42:13–26.

170. Kendall PC, Kipnis D, Otto-Salaj L. When clients don't progress: influences on and explanations for lack of therapeutic progress. Cogn Ther Res 1992; 16:269–281.

171. Weissman MM, Klerman GL, Prusoff BA, et al. Depressed outpatients: results one year after treatment with drugs and/or interpersonal psychotherapy. Arch Gen Psychiat 1981; 38:51–55.

172. Imber SD, Pilkonis PA, Sotsky SM, et al. Mode-specific effects among three treatments for depression. J Consult Clin Psychol 1990; 58:352–359.

173. Klerman GL, DiMascio A, Weissman M, et al. Treatment of depression by drugs and psychotherapy. Am J Psychiat 1974; 131:186–191.

174. Frank E, Kupfer DJ, Perel JM, et al. Three-year outcomes for maintenance therapies in recurrent depression. Arch Gen Psychiat 1990; 47:1093–1099.

175. Mufson L, Dorta KP, Wickramaratne P, Nomura Y, Olfson M, Weissman MM. A randomized effectiveness trial of interpersonal psychotherapy for depressed adolescents [see comment]. Arch Gen Psychiat 2004; 61(6):577–584.

176. Bleiberg KL, Markowitz JC. A pilot study of interpersonal psychotherapy for posttraumatic stress disorder. Am J Psychiat 2005; 162(1):181–183.

177. O'Hara MW, Stuart S, Gorman LL, Wenzel A. Efficacy of interpersonal psychotherapy for postpartum depression. Arch Gen Psychiat 2000; 57(11): 1039–1045.

178. Zlotnick C, Johnson SL, Miller IW, Pearlstein T, Howard M. Postpartum depression in women receiving public assistance: pilot study of an interpersonal-therapy-oriented group intervention. Am J Psychiat 2001; 158(4):638–640.

179. Spinelli MG, Endicott J. Controlled clinical trial of interpersonal psychotherapy versus parenting education program for depressed pregnant women. Am J Psychiat 2003; 160(3):555–562.

180. Wilfley DE, Welch RR, Stein RI, et al. A randomized comparison of group cognitive-behavioral therapy and group interpersonal psychotherapy for the treatment of overweight individuals with binge-eating disorder [see comment]. Arch Gen Psychiat 2002; 59(8):713–721.

181. Hoberman H, Lewinsohn PM. Behavioral approaches to the treatment of unipolar depression. In: Klerman GL, ed. Treatment of Psychiatric Disorders. Vol. 3. Washington, D.C.: American Psychiatric Association, 1989:1846–1862.

182. Crits-Christoph. The efficacy of brief dynamic psychotherapy: a meta-analysis. Am J Psychiat 1992; 149:151–158.

183. Meterissian GB, Bradwejn J. Comparative studies on the efficacy of psychotherapy, pharmacotherapy, and their combination in depression: was adequate pharmacotherapy provided? J Clin Psychopharmacol 1989; 9:334–339.

184. Hersen M, Bellack AS, Himmelhoch JM, et al. Effects of social skill training, amitriptyline, and psychotherapy in unipolar depressed women. Behav Ther 1984; 15:21–40.

185. McLean PD, Hakstian AR. Clinical depression: comparative efficacy of outpatient treatments. J Consult Clin Psychol 1979; 47:818–836.

186. Bellack AS, Hersen M, Himmelhoch JM. A comparison of social-skills training, pharmacotherapy, and psychotherapy for depression. Behav Res Ther 1983; 2:101–107.

187. Brown RA, Lewinsohn PM. A psychoeducational approach to the treatment of depression: comparison of group, individual, and minimal contact procedures. J Consult Clin Psychol 1984; 52:774–783.

188. Lerner MS, Clum GA. Treatment of suicide ideators: a problem-solving approach. Behav Ther 1990; 21:403–411.

189. Nezu AM. Efficacy of a social problem-solving therapy approach for unipolar depression. J Consult Clin Psychol 1986; 54:196–202.

190. Arean PA, Perri MG, Nezu Am, et al. Comparative effectiveness of social problem-solving therapy and reminiscence therapy as treatments for depression in older adults. J Consult Clin Psychol 1993; 61:1003–1010.

191. Fuchs CZ, Rehm LP. A self-control BT program for depression. J Consult Clin Psychol 1977; 45:206–215.

192. Kornblith SJ, Rehm LP, O'Hara MW, et al. The contribution of self-reinforcement training and behavioral assignments to the efficacy of self-control therapy for depression. Cogn Ther Res 1983; 7:499–528.

193. Rehm LP, Fuchs CZ, Roth DM, et al. A comparison of self-control and assertion skills treatment of depression. Behav Ther 1979; 10:429–442.

194. Rehm LP, Kornblith SJ, O'Hara MW, et al. An evaluation of major components in a self-control therapy program for depression. Behav Mod 1981; 5:459–489.

195. Rehm LP, Kaslow NJ, Rabin AS. Cognitive and behavioral targets in a self-control therapy program for depression. J Consult Clin Psychol 1987; 55: 60–67.

196. Lewinsohn PM, Antonuccio DA, Steinmetz J, et al. The Coping with Depression Course: A Psychoeducational Intervention for Unipolar Depression. Eugene, Oregon: Castalia Press, 1984.

197. Mynors-Wallis LM, Gath DH, Lloyd-Thoms AR, et al. Randomised controlled trial comparing problem solving treatment with amitriptyline and placebo for major depression in primary care. Gen Pract 1995; 310: 441–445.

198. Gabbard GO. Psychodynamic Psychiatry in Clinical Practice. In: Psychodynamic Psychiatry in Clinical Practice. 3rd. Washington, D.C.: American Psychiatric Press, 2004.

199. Gabbard GO. Long-Term Psychodynamic Psychotherapy: A Basic Text. Washington, D.C.: American Psychiatric Publishing, 2004.

200. Groves JE, ed. Essential Papers on Short-Term Dynamic Therapy. New York: New York University Press, 1996.
201. Coynes JC, ed. Essential Papers on Depression. New York, NY: University Press, 1986.
202. Busch FN, Rudden M, Shapiro T. Psychodynamic Treatment of Depression. D.C.: American Psychiatric Publishing, Inc., 2004.
203. Levy R, Ablon JS. Psychoanalytic research: progress and process. Psychoanal Psychol 2000; 23:23–25.
204. Fonagy P, ed. Open Door Review of Outcome Studies in Psychoanalysis. 2d ed. London: International Psychoanalytical Association, 2002.
205. Wallerstein RS. Outcome research. In: Person ES, Cooper AM, Gabbard, GO, eds. American Psychiatric Publishing Textbook of Psychoanalysis, 2005: 301–315.
206. Bucci W. Process research. In: Person ES, Cooper AM, Gabbard GO, eds. American Psychiatric Publishing Textbook of Psychoanalysis, 2005:317–333.
207. Westen D, Novotny C, Thompson-Brenner H. The empirical status of empirically-supported psychotherapies: assumptions, findings, and reporting in clinical trials. Psychol Bull 2004; 130(4):631–663.
208. Westen D, Novotny C, Thompson-Brenner H. The new generation of psychotherapy research: reply to Ablon and Marci (2004), Goldfried and Eubanks-Carter (2004), and Haaga (2004). Psychol Bull 2004; 130(4):677–683.
209. Westen D, Novotny C, Thompson-Brenner H. EBP $\neq$ EST: reply to Crits-Cristoph et al. (2005) and Weiz et al. (2005). Psychol Bull 2005; 131(3): 427–433.
210. Blatt SJ, Levy KN. A psychodynamic approach to the diagnosis of psychopathology. In: Barron JW, ed. Making Diagnosis Meaningful 73–109. Washington, D.C.: American Psychological Association Press, 1998.
211. Barkham M, Rees A, Stiles Shapiro DA, Hardy GE, Reynolds S. Dose-effect relations in time-limited psychotherapy for depression. J Clin Consult Psychol 1996; 64(5):927–935.
212. Knedt P, Lindfors O, eds. A Randomized Trial of the Effects of Four Forms of Psychotherapy on Depression and Anxiety Disorders: Design Methods and Results on the Effectiveness of Short-Term Psychodynamic Psychotherapy and Solution-Focused Therapy During a 1-Year Follow-Up. Vol. 77. Helsinki: Social Insurance Institution, 2004.
213. Maina G, Forner F, Bogetto F. Randomized controlled trial comparing brief dynamic and supportive therapy with waiting list control in minor depressive disorders. Psychother Psychosomat 2005; 74(1):43–50.
214. Copper L, Cooper P, Wilson A, Romaniuk H. Controlled trial of the short- and long-term effect of psychological treatment of post-partum depression: impact on the mother-child relationship and child outcome. Br J Psychiat 2003; 182(5):420–427.
215. Burnand Y. Psychodynamic psychotherapy and clomipramine in the treatment of major depression. Psychiat Serv 2002; 53(5):585–590.
216. Hilsenroth MJ, Ackerman SJ, Blagys MD, Baity MR, Mooney MA. Short-term psychodynamic psychotherapy for depression: an examination of

statistical, clinically significant, and technique-specific change. J Nerv Mental Dis 2003; 191(6):349–357.

217. Bond M, Perry CJ. Long-term changes in defense styles with psychodynamic psychotherapy for depressive, anxiety, and personality disorders. Am J Psychiat 2004; 161:1665–1671.

218. Barber J, Abrams MJ, Connolly-Gibbons MB, et al. J Clin Psychol 2005; 16(3):257–268.

219. Wampold B. The Great Psychotherapy Debate. Mahwah, NJ: Lawrence Erlbaum, 2001.

220. Leichsenring F. Comparative effects of short-term psychodynamic psychotherapy and cognitive-behavioral therapy in depression: a meta-analytic approach. Clin Psychol Rev 2001; 21(3):401–419.

221. Fisher S, Greenberg R. Freud Scientifically Reappraised: Testing the Theories and the Therapies. New York: Wiley and Sons, 1996.

222. Ablon JS, Jones EE. Validity of controlled clinical trials of psychotherapy: findings from the NIMH collaborative study of depression. Am J Psychiat 2002; 159:775–783.

223. Hollon SD, Jarrett RB, Nierenberg AA, Thase ME, Trivedi M, Rush AJ. Psychotherapy and medication in the treatment of adult and geriatric depression: which monotherapy or combined treatment? J Clin Psychiat 2005; 66: 455–468.

224. Murphy GE, Simons AD, Wetzel RD, et al. Cognitive therapy and pharmacotherapy, singly and together, in the treatment of depression. Arch Gen Psychiat 1984; 41:33–41.

225. Conte HR, Plutchik R, Wild KV, et al. Combined psychotherapy and pharmacotherapy for depression. Arch Gen Psychiat 1986; 43:471–479.

226. Thase ME, Greenhouse JB, Frank E, et al. Treatment of major depression with psychotherapy-pharmacotherapy combinations. Arch Gen Psychiat 1997; 54:1009–1015.

227. Friedman MA, Detweiler-Bedell JB, Leventhal HE, et al. Combined psychotherapy and pharmacotherapy for the treatment of major depressive disorder. Clin Psychol Sci Pract 2004; 11:47–68.

228. Pampallona S, Bollini P, Tiabaldi G, et al. Combined pharmacotherapy and psychological treatment for depression: a systematic review. Arch Gen Psychiat 2004; 61:714–719.

229. Keller MB, McCullough JP, Klein DN, et al. A comparison of nefazodone, the cognitive behavioral-analysis system of psychotherapy, and their combination for the treatment of chronic depression. N Engl J Med 2000; 342:1462–1470.

230. Klerman GL, Weissman MM. Interpersonal psychotherapy: theory and research. In: Rush AJ, ed. Short-Term Psychotherapies for Depression. New York: Guilford Press, 1982:88–106.

231. Safran JD, Segal ZV, Vallis TM, et al. Assessing patient suitability for short-term cognitive therapy with an interpersonal focus. Cogn Ther Res 1993; 17:23–28.

232. Thase ME, Buysse DJ, Frank E, et al. Which depressed patients will respond to interpersonal psychotherapy? The role of abnormal electroencephalographic sleep profiles. Am J Psychiat 1997; 154:502–509.

5

Depression: Treatment Outcomes with Long-Term Maintenance

I. Pharmacotherapy

Richard C. Shelton

Department of Psychiatry, Vanderbilt University School of Medicine, Nashville, Tennessee, U.S.A.

II. Psychotherapy

Chiara Ruini and Giovanni A. Fava

Department of Psychology, University of Bologna, Bologna, Italy and Department of Psychiatry, State University of New York at Buffalo, Buffalo, New York, U.S.A.

I. PHARMACOTHERAPY
Richard C. Shelton

Depression is often treated as a short-term, self-limiting condition, and some patients do experience the illness in this manner. However, this is the exception rather than the rule (1). Most unipolar depressive conditions are either chronic or recurring in 80% or more of patients (2–4). The long-term nature of the condition tends to result in sustained or recurrent impairment, making unipolar depression possibly the single most disabling of all medical conditions (5). Nonetheless, the condition remains under-recognized and under-treated, particularly in considering long-term management (6). Although acute management is important, the management of depression should focus primarily on the improvement of long-term outcome, in the same manner as other chronic medical conditions.

Alternatively, even pharmacotherapeutic or psychotherapeutic management can leave much to be desired with both short- and long-term outcome. For example, with any given antidepressant trial, one-third or more of patients remain ill. In fact, the overall outcome in clinical practice appears to be even poorer, given more clinical comorbidity. One study of depression treatment outcomes in a primary care practice setting suggested that half or less of patients achieved remission, regardless of whether they were treated with a tricyclic antidepressant (TCA) or serotonin selective reuptake inhibitor (SSRI) (7). This implies that the gains in side effect burden achieved by post-TCA development may not translate into better outcomes in treatment. This is a public health crisis given the potential for negative outcome, including social impairment or suicide.

Alternatively, the capacity for a more positive outcome appears relatively high. Based on data from the NIMH Collaborative Depression Study and others, more than 90% of patients achieve recovery over periods of a decade or more (8,9). Even patients who have remain depressed for at least five years continue to remit; nearly 40% will recover over the subsequent five-year period (10). These data suggest a troublesome aspect of the treatment of depression: Most patients can recover, but many do not. Further, relapse [typically defined as the return of depression within the first year after initiating treatment (11)] or recurrence [the occurrence of a wholly new episode (11)] is common, even with ongoing treatment (12,13). Therefore, the overall outcome of depression tends to be relatively poor. Ideally, treatment will achieve full therapeutic remission in the first place, and maintain that remission indefinitely.

This chapter will at first look at some of the predictors of poor prognosis in regard to major depressive disorder (MDD), and will then discuss management issues and outcomes from a long-term or "maintenance of euthymia" point of view.

PREDICTORS OF CHRONICITY, RELAPSE, AND RECURRENCE (TABLE 1)

A number of factors appear to be associated with a poorer overall outcome, including incomplete initial response and subsequent relapse or recurrence. Incomplete initial effect is associated with both treatment- and patient-specific factors. Treatment variables include inadequate dose or duration of antidepressant; premature discontinuation, which is often associated with intractable side effects (especially sexual side effects); or incorrect diagnosis (14). Patient variables reported in some studies that impact acute outcome include both medical and psychiatric comorbidities, including substance abuse (15–18), pretreatment severity and chronicity (18,19), history of severe emotional trauma (20), and poor psychosocial support (16,19). Early relapse or recurrence can be associated with similar factors [e.g., baseline severity (21,22), comorbidity (18,23–25), trauma history (26), or poor interpersonal support (27,28)], and also early onset of illness (29), a high frequency of

Table 1 Patients-specific Factors That May Be Associated with Relapse or Recurrence

Chronic depression or dysthymia
Comorbidities (medical and psychiatric)
Family history of mood disorders
Later onset of first episode
Multiple prior episodes (prior recurrence)
Poor psychosocial support
Recurring on ongoing psychosocial stressors
Residual functional impairment
Residual symptoms
Temperamental characteristics (high neuroticism, low extroversion)
Trauma history

Source: From Ref. 1.

recurrence (12,24,30), prior chronicity (31), recurring or ongoing psychosocial stressors (25,26,32,33), ongoing functional impairment (even in the face of apparent symptomatic recovery) (34) or poorer quality of life (22,35), and temperamental qualities including high neuroticism and low extraversion (25,36,37).

One of the principal predictors of poorer outcome is incomplete acute phase treatment to full response or remission (22,38). For example, Judd et al. (38) found that residual but subclinical depressive symptoms were significantly associated with both a reduced time to recurrence and frequency of recurrence in first episode major depression. Paykel et al. showed that patients with significant residual symptoms had a 76% rate of recurrence by 15 months, in contrast to 25% of patients who had full symptomatic recovery. Aggressive pharmacotherapy seems to be associated with better short- and long-term outcomes, in spite of baseline severity of illness (22,39). Therefore, clinician variables, which include the ability of the clinician to persistently engage the patient in long-term treatment, particularly in the absence of early response, may be very important determinants of clinical outcome. Also, the aggressiveness of the intervention strategies, which may reflect personal practice style, knowledge base, availability of office time for patient visits, availability of multiple antidepressants, etc. may substantially influence the outcome.

DRUG DISCONTINUATION

Some patients do not have the characteristics that predict poorer outcome, and others may prefer to discontinue medication management despite having these features. A limited amount of data suggests that slow tapering is superior to abrupt discontinuation (9), and this is now considered standard practice. This is particularly important with regard to drugs that are particularly prone to discontinuation effects, especially the short half-life SSRIs and SNRIs, including paroxetine and venlafaxine (40,41). Although these drugs appear to be particularly prone to more severe discontinuation effects, such reactions have been reported even with drugs with longer half-lives (42). In these latter agents, the withdrawal symptoms appear to be less severe and delayed over time postdiscontinuation. Typical discontinuation effects include anxiety, crying, dizziness, headache, increased dreaming, insomnia, irritability, myoclonus, nausea, paresthesias (including "electrical sensations"), and tremor (43). These effects are usually mitigated by tapering; however, some patients appear to be particularly prone to these effects and may require a short-term addition of a long-acting SSRI such as fluoxetine, or even complete conversion to the longer-acting drug followed by another slow tapering. Clearly, making the patient aware of the discontinuation effects should be a part of the informed consent process. If possible, patients with known poor compliance should preferentially avoid SSRI/ SNRI, known to have great discontinuation effects.

Other situations may pose problems in long-term treatment. For example, even with ongoing continuation or maintenance pharmacotherapy, patients can miss doses intermittently that may cause discontinuation effects (including apparent relapse or recurrence) and that may be incorrectly attributed to a loss of therapeutic effect of the drug. Increasing dosage or switching medications may not solve this problem. Intermittently missing doses can be problematic even with longer half-life drugs. A regular pattern of missed doses may result in a lower plasma level of drugs such as fluoxetine or sertraline leading to a loss of biological and ultimately therapeutic effect. Similar effects may also be seen when patients surreptitiously reduce or discontinue treatment. Therefore, the patient should be carefully queried about the possibility of missed doses if there is a loss of therapeutic effect, and certainly whenever discontinuation-like effects occur.

The possibility of a pregnancy during ongoing medication management poses another set of potential problems. For example, the SSRI discontinuation–like syndrome has been observed in neonates exposed to maternal use of antidepressant particularly shorter-acting antidepressants such as paroxetine during pregnancy (44,45). Therefore, pre- and perinatal exposure to antidepressants must be considered a potential outcome of treating any woman of reproductive potential.

Several other more "common sense" issues relate to termination of treatment. For example, it seems unwise to discontinue treatment in a person who is undergoing significant stressors or who anticipates new onset of stressors in the near future. Similarly, significant residual symptoms or impairment of functioning suggests an ongoing disease process that is likely to result in early relapse or recurrence. Finally, we are not aware of any data to support a relationship between the season in which a drug is discontinued and relapse or recurrence; however, given the potential impact of season on mood, it seems prudent to avoid discontinuation between late fall and the end of winter.

MAINTENANCE PHARMACOTHERAPY (TABLE 2)

Ongoing pharmacotherapy can be conceptually divided into continuation treatment, which reflects management during the original episode of illness (typically thought of as the first 6–12 months after initiation) or maintenance, reflecting prevention of a wholly new episode (beyond the continuation period). Continuation treatment has long been known to improve outcome. For example, as early as the 1970s, Prien et al. (48,49) showed that ongoing treatment after initial response reduced the frequency of relapse. In a now classic study, Prien and Kupfer (50) demonstrated that discontinuation of treatment at less than 16 weeks resulted in a much higher rate of relapse than did discontinuation of longer treatment. These studies served as the basis for the common recommendation that treatment be continued for at least six to nine months after initial full response (51).

By contrast, the concept that treatment should be continued indefinitely in some patients is a relatively more recent development. This is based on the observation that the rate of recurrence after the initial year or so of treatment is very high (21). For example, one large-scale long-term follow-up study found that 85% of 350 patients who achieved therapeutic remission eventually had a recurrence, including 58% of those who had maintained remission for five years (13). Ongoing treatment with antidepressants generally reduces the likelihood of a recurrence (1,6,46). Taking into consideration factors associated with increased likelihood of relapse or recurrence, people with any of a number of characteristics—marked lethality, recurrence, comorbidity, medication or psychotherapy resistance, etc.—may benefit from indefinite maintenance treatment.

The typical method for assessing continuation or maintenance prophylaxis against relapse or recurrence is double-blind randomization into active drug or placebo treatment after initial response is achieved for a given time period (1). Virtually all studies of continuation or maintenance prophylaxis of this type have shown beneficial effects of continuing pharmacotherapy (1,6,9). However, rates of relapse or recurrence with ongoing pharmacotherapy are not trivial. Relapse rates in continuation pharmacotherapy studies have ranged from about 10% to 50%, with a roughly 15% to 40% differential

Table 2 Factors Commending Maintenance Treatment

Chronicity (≥ 2 years of symptoms) or dysthymia
Early age of onset for first episode
Family history of mood disorder (especially recurrent depression)
Frequent recurrence ($\geq$ prior episodes)
Older age of onset of first episode
Residual functional impairment
Residual symptoms

Source: From Refs. 1, 9, 46, 47.

between placebo and drug (1,9). For example, a recent study by Hollon et al. (52) randomly assigned patients who had experienced an initial response to paroxetine (with or without augmentation) after 16 weeks to blinded continuation pharmacotherapy or placebo. The latter placebo group had a 76% rate of relapse over the first year of treatment; however ongoing medication was associated with a relapse rate of only 31%.

If pharmacotherapy is to be sustained over long periods, then dosing becomes a key issue. One study that directly addresses this issue is that of Frank et al. (53), in which patients who had experienced an initial response to imipramine were randomly assigned to continuation of the same dose versus one half of the dose that produced the initial effect, and followed over three years. The continuation of full dose was superior to that of half-dose in terms of both the likelihood of experiencing relapse [70% vs. 30% (9)] and the time to relapse. Although there are no data to address the question of SSRIs, SNRIs, or other novel antidepressant medications, the general recommendation has been to continue the dose that produced the optimum clinical antidepressant effect into the continuation and maintenance periods. This concept assumes that there are no ongoing, dose-limiting side effects in which tapering to a lower dose, using combination therapies (e.g., reduced dose SSRI plus bupropion), or using a different drug would be indicated.

In conclusion, there are some maintenance regulatory approvals and some guidelines for long-term antidepressant use, and there are very few, if any, "head-to-head" comparative studies between antidepressants to show superiority of one agent over another (47,54–61).

Sertraline, paroxetine, venlafaxine, and fluoxetine have the best evidence base, but comparative studies are limited. There is a paucity of long-term data regarding the use of trazodone, nefazodone, bupropion, mirtazapine, and duloxetine. The available long-term studies are not comparative in nature and often proceed from 26 to 52 weeks. Unlike in the previous chapter, where there was a reasonable database of comparative data and hence the ability to perform secondary meta-analyses, here we are unable to obtain the data regarding the maintenance phase of treating depression. We must rely on the survival analysis studies of these few specific antidepressants and on naturalistic data noted above which suggest that antidepressant therapy must be continued for longer periods of time at adequate doses given the chronicity of depression as an illness. The following paragraphs will extensively detail the available literature in this area.

STUDIES OF LONG-TERM PHARMACOTHERAPY

Long-Term Course of Depression: Observational Studies

Observational studies often show a worse long-term prognosis for MDD patients than do controlled trials. As part of the NIMH Collaborative

Program on the Psychobiology of Depression, Lavori et al. (62) followed 359 patients. These patients had recovered from their index episode of depression for at least eight weeks and were then followed for up to five years. Of those patients who continued to take high levels of somatic treatment, over 20% became depressed again within the first six months. Thereafter, patients who had continued to feel well up until that time relapsed at the same rate regardless of treatment status. Overall, 88% of the entire cohort had a relapse or recurrence by the end of five years.

Mueller et al. (13) in another analysis examined 15 years of naturalistic follow-up data for 380 patients who recovered from the index episode of MDD. In addition, the authors identified 105 of these patients who had remained well for at least five years after recovery. Baseline demographic and clinical characteristics were also examined as predictors of recurrence. A cumulative proportion of 85% of the 380 recovered patients experienced a recurrence, as did 58% of those who remained well for at least five years. Female patients with a longer index episode, more prior episodes, and never marrying were significant predictors of recurrence in the larger group, but not for the patients who remained well for at least five years. Naturalistic treatment was characterized by lower than recommended doses for all phases of treatment.

In another observational study, Ramana et al. (63) followed 70 patients (53 in- and 17 out-patients) for up to 15 months: 80% remitted by 15 months; of those who remitted, Kaplan–Meier survival analysis (64) showed that 40% experienced at least one depressive relapse within 10 months of remission. Relapsers and nonrelapsers had the same levels of long-term antidepressant treatment, again consistent with the findings of Lavori et al. (62).

Montgomery et al. (65) followed a group of 217 patients who had remitted to three different six-week acute phase treatments—mirtazapine, amitriptyline, or placebo—and then continued on the same treatments during a two-year follow-up phase. Dosing during follow-up was flexible but maximum permitted dosages were 35 mg/day, mirtazapine; 280 mg/day, amitriptyline; and 7 capsules/day, placebo. Survival analysis indicated that patients treated with mirtazapine had a significantly longer time to relapse than recipients of amitriptyline or placebo, and amitriptyline-treated patients showed a significantly longer time to relapse than recipients of placebo. At study endpoint, survival analysis indicated that patients treated with mirtazapine or amitriptyline had a significantly longer time to relapse than did recipients of placebo. Relapse rates during the first 20 weeks of follow-up were 4.1%, 7.0%, and 28.0% for the mirtazapine, amitriptyline, and placebo groups, respectively. At study endpoint, relapse rates were 4.1%, 11.6%, and 28.1%. Tolerability was lower to amitriptyline than to mirtazapine or placebo.

Claxton et al. (66) utilized the U.K. Primary Care Database to identify 7293 patients treated for depression with an SSRI. The authors then examined rates of relapse and recurrence during an 18-month follow-up period. Four cohorts were identified: patients who had less than 120 days of any antidepressant treatment (73% of sample); patients who had at least 120 days of treatment, but who switched agents or added a second antidepressant (4% of sample); patients who maintained treatment on the original SSRI for at least 120 days, but had their dosage titrated upward during the six-month treatment period (2% of sample); and patients who used the index SSRI at a stable dosage throughout the treatment period (21% of sample). The authors found that the stable use cohort experienced a somewhat lower rate of relapse or recurrence (20%) than the other three groups—23%, 29%, and 24%. Younger age, increased psychiatric comorbidity, and anxiolytic use during the index episode were associated with higher rates of relapse and recurrence. Primary limitations of this study were a small effect size for risk between groups and heterogeneity within definitions of relapse and recurrence. Moreover, inferences regarding causality are limited by the nonrandomized design.

Controlled Studies of Continuation Treatment

Sackheim et al. (67) randomized 84 patients (stratified by medication resistance) who had remitted to acute phase electroconvulsive therapy (ECT) to three continuation treatment groups: nortriptyline (NT), NT and lithium (NT + Li), or placebo. By the end of this 24-week continuation phase, relapse rates were 60%, 39%, and 84% for the NT, NT + Li, and placebo groups, respectively. NT + Li combination therapy had a marked advantage in time to relapse, superior to both placebo and NT alone. All but one instance of relapse with NT + Li occurred within five weeks of ECT termination, while relapse continued throughout treatment with placebo or NT alone. Medication-resistant patients, female patients, and those with more severe depressive symptoms following ECT had more rapid relapse.

Versiani et al. (68) treated 283 patients with recurrent depression during a six-week open trial of reboxetine. Responders went on to be randomized to continuation reboxetine versus placebo for a 46-week period. During this time period, 22% of patients receiving reboxetine and 56% of patients receiving placebo relapsed. Confirming previous work that indicates the importance of treating patients acutely to full remission, Versiani et al. found that patients in full remission at the end of acute treatment had even lower relapse rates: 16% and 48% for the reboxetine and placebo groups, respectively.

Feiger et al. (69) conducted a trial in which patients were treated acutely with open nefazodone. One hundred and thirty-one remitters were then randomized to continuation nefazodone versus placebo. Rates of relapse during the 36-week continuation treatment phase were 1.8% and 18.3% for the nefazodone and placebo groups, respectively. Rates of discontinuation due to lack of efficacy were 17.3% and 32.8% for the same two groups.

Several other studies have examined the effectiveness of continuation of active treatments versus placebo in patients having demonstrated partial and/or full acute phase response. In a pooled analysis from four randomized controlled trials, Entsuah et al. (70) found that relapse rates (after six months of continuation treatment) between acute phase responders treated with continuation placebo versus venlafaxine were 23% and 11%, respectively. Thase et al. (71) treated 410 patients, diagnosed with moderate to severely recurrent or chronic major depression, with open mirtazapine. One hundred and fifty-six fully remitted patients were randomized to mirtazapine or placebo for a 40-week continuation phase. Relapse rates during continuation treatment were 19.7% for the mirtazapine group and 43.8% for the placebo group. Rates of discontinuation due to adverse events were 11.8% and 2.5% for these groups. Ferreri et al. (72) used 200 mg of open label amineptine to treat 458 patients with depression during a three-month acute trial. The authors report an acute phase response rate of 66%. These responders ($N = 284$) were then randomized to continuation amineptine or placebo during a nine-month continuation phase. Relapse rates were found to be 6.6% for the medication group and 18.7% for the placebo group. Of note is that patients in this protocol met criteria for MDD or dysthymia.

Some more recent work has evaluated a switch to weekly fluoxetine for those patients who responded acutely to an SSRI. Miner et al. (73) found that responders to paroxetine, citalopram, or sertraline demonstrated a 9.3% relapse or discontinuation rate over a 12-week continuation treatment phase. Schmidt et al. (74) randomized acute phase fluoxetine responders to fluoxetine, 20 mg/day, fluoxetine, 90 mg weekly, and placebo, and found no difference in efficacy between the two active drug groups.

Doogan and Caillard (75) followed depressed patients who responded to an eight-week trial of sertraline. After patients responded, they were randomized to either continue on the sertraline ($N = 184$) or be switched to placebo ($N = 105$). Thirteen percent of the sertraline-treated patients and over 45% of the placebo-substituted patients had another episode of major depression within 44 weeks. Note that if a depression reappeared, the dose of sertraline could be increased to up to 200 mg daily (mean daily dose ranged between 69.3 and 82.1 mg). The authors do not specify if patients who had another depressive episode, and then responded to an increase in dose, were considered to have a relapse or recurrence. No mention is made of how many patients required, and then responded to an increase in dose. Furthermore, although about 75% of the original group had recurrent depression, information that describes the number of prior episodes is missing. For these reasons, the investigators' finding that 13% of patients relapsed during long-term sertraline treatment may be an underestimate of the true relapse rate.

Montgomery and Dunbar (76) treated 172 depressed patients who had a history of recurrences with open paroxetine (20–40 mg/day) for eight weeks.

Patients who responded were randomized to either continue on paroxetine (20–30 mg/day; $N = 68$) or placebo ($N = 67$) for the next 52 weeks. Three percent of the patients who took paroxetine had depressive relapses as compared to 19% of the placebo group. Similarly, Claghorn and Feighner (77) followed patients for 52 weeks and found relapse rates of 25% among 32 patients who had responded to placebo initially, 15% among 60 paroxetine-treated patients, and 4% among imipramine-treated patients. The dose of long-term medication used in Montgomery's study could be maintained, decreased, or increased at the discretion of the physician. The mean dose of paroxetine that patients responded to was 40 mg during the acute trial and 38 mg during the extension phase. The dose of the SSRI in this study, therefore, was stable during continuation and maintenance treatment. As with the studies noted above, no information is provided about subsequent treatment of those patients who had breakthrough depressions while on active medications.

Quitkin et al. (78) have proposed that the loss of efficacy within six weeks after an acute response may reflect the loss of an initial placebo response to an antidepressant rather than a true drug effect. They reported the results of a 12-week double-blind trial of imipramine ($N = 174$), phenelzine ($N = 169$), and placebo ($N = 164$) for patients with atypical depression. Of the group that responded by six weeks, the proportions of patients that had a relapse were 11.8% (imipramine), 8.8% (phenelzine), and 31.3% (placebo). The authors' hypothesis is that between 36% and 100% of relapsers initially had a placebo response to medication and then lost it. Given the parallel design used in this study, such inference may be tentative because, after all, the majority of the placebo responders still remained well during continuation treatment. Nevertheless, it is not an uncommon clinical observation that early (less than two weeks into treatment) dramatic responses to antidepressants are suspect; the ebbing of these responses with time seems likely to reflect heterogeneous influences including loss of placebo response, mood cycling in individuals who have undiagnosed bipolar disorder, or, for some, perhaps, a nonspecific regression to the mean.

Uncontrolled Studies of Maintenance Antidepressant Treatment

Peselow et al. (79) studied 217 patients with unipolar depression who responded to TCAs (mean imipramine-equivalence dose: 159.6 mg daily), were stable for at least six months, and then followed for up to five years. They compared patients who stayed on medication with a group of 28 patients who were stable for six months and then discontinued medication. Relapse rates were 30%, 50%, and 60%, at one, two, and three years, respectively, while on active drug versus 51%, 74%, and 83% on no treatment. Overall, 87 of 217 patients on active drug (40.1%) were observed to have suffered a depressive relapse over the five-year course.

Controlled Studies of Maintenance Antidepressant Treatment

Controlled studies suggest that imipramine therapy, either alone or with Li, is more effective in preventing recurrence than therapy with Li alone. Prien et al. (80) compared strategies for maintenance treatment for 150 unipolar depressed patients. These patients were treated initially for their index depressive episode with a variety of antidepressants (usually imipramine), antidepressants +Li, Li alone, neuroleptics, or ECT and then stabilized for two months with a combination of imipramine +Li. After stabilization, patients were randomized to take imipramine alone (mean daily dose: 137 mg), Li alone (mean blood level: 0.66 ng/mL), the combination of imipramine +Li, or placebo. Over the next 27 months, 33% of the imipramine group, 26% of the combination group, 57% of the Li group, and 65% of the placebo group had a recurrence. Although imipramine prevented recurrences in a substantially higher proportion of patients than either placebo or Li alone, a third of these patients experienced a depressive recurrence while taking maintenance imipramine. Greenhouse et al. (81) suggest that the reappearance of the depressive syndrome in patients treated with Li alone may have been due to discontinuation of the imipramine rather than to a loss of efficacy of this agent. This explanation, however, does not apply to those who became depressed again while they continued imipramine therapy.

Frank et al. (82) demonstrated the advantages of taking full doses of imipramine for three years after an acute response to imipramine plus interpersonal therapy in those patients who had at least their third episode of depression; only about 20% of patients had a recurrence while taking imipramine at the acute effective dose [with and without interpersonal psychotherapy (IPT)] as compared to about 80% of those who were switched over to placebo alone. Prior studies that examined the usefulness of lower doses of maintenance antidepressants tend to have recurrence rates of about 50% to 70% (80). Even though Frank et al.'s (82) data are encouraging when compared with previous reports, note that (i) these patients had been treated with IPT during the acute treatment phase and might have been more able to cope with stressors and less likely to suffer from recurrences, and (ii) 20% of the patients who took full antidepressant doses for maintenance became depressed again. No mention is made of how these patients were subsequently treated.

In a follow-up study of those patients who experienced a recurrence when treated with IPT, Frank et al. (53) restabilized these patients on a full dose of imipramine plus interpersonal therapy. They were then randomized to continue on full or half-dose imipramine ($N = 10$ each group). Thirty percent of the full dose group and 70% of the half-dose group had a recurrence. Note that although the full dose group had a lower recurrence rate as compared with the half-dose group, the 30% recurrence rate of the full dose group is substantial.

Rouillon et al. (83) examined patients who had remitted to acute phase milnacipran treatment and maintained remission throughout the 18-week continuation treatment phase. These patients were randomized to maintenance phase milnacipran versus placebo. Recurrence rates were significantly different between groups—23.6% for placebo and 16.3% for active drug. Gilaberte et al. (47), in another placebo-controlled maintenance phase trial, randomized patients who had maintained a total of 32 weeks of response to fluoxetine to the same dose of fluoxetine or placebo. The authors found recurrence rates (20% fluoxetine and 40% placebo) as well as time to recurrence to significantly differ between groups. Adverse events did not significantly differ between groups.

In a study of geriatric patients, Klysner et al. (84) randomized 121 patients (who had maintained response to 20–40 mg of citalopram throughout acute and continuation treatment phases) to same dose of citalopram or placebo. He found recurrence rates of 32% for citalopram and 66% for placebo. Using a similar study design, Terra and Montgomery (85) followed 204 patients who maintained response to fluvoxamine for both six weeks of acute treatment and 18 weeks of continuation treatment. These patients were randomized to continuing on active drug or placebo. Significantly fewer recurrences were observed in the active drug group when compared with the placebo group.

Robinson et al. (86) studied the long-term efficacy of maintenance phenelzine in 47 depressed patients. Patients were first treated with phenelzine at a dose of 1 mg/kg for 6 to 13 weeks. Responders were stabilized for 16 weeks after acute recovery and then randomized to phenelzine, 60 mg daily ($N = 19$), phenelzine, 45 mg daily ($N = 12$), or placebo ($N = 16$) for two years. Although maintenance phenelzine at both doses was superior to placebo, after 12 months a substantial proportion of patients relapsed while taking the active drug (total proportions of patients who had either a relapse or recurrence were phenelzine 60 mg = 26%; phenelzine 45 mg = 33%; and placebo = 81%). One problem with these data is that only eight patients were able to complete the entire two-year maintenance phase.

Montgomery et al. (87) compared fluoxetine ($N = 88$) with placebo ($N = 94$) to prevent recurrences in unipolar depressed patients who had responded to an open trial of fluoxetine (40–80 mg daily). Subjects were stable for six months on fluoxetine 40 mg/day prior to randomization to either staying on the same dose of fluoxetine 40 mg or switching to placebo. At the end of one year, 26% of subjects who took prophylactic fluoxetine and 57% who took placebo had a recurrence. As with the studies of Frank et al. (11) and Kupfer et al. (88), Montgomery et al. (87) demonstrated that active antidepressant maintenance therapy is superior to placebo, but that a substantial proportion (26%) of patients experience a depressive recurrence despite active treatment.

Stewart et al. (89) applied pattern analysis to distinguish between "true drug response," which was delayed and sustained, and "placebo response," which was early or nonpersistent, among 428 responders to 12 weeks of open treatment with fluoxetine 20 mg/day. Among the 392 subjects willing to be randomized to fluoxetine versus placebo over the next 12 months, those identified as true drug responders showed a significant drug–placebo difference in relapse/recurrence rates during continuation/maintenance while those with an initial placebo response pattern had an equivalent outcome regardless of whether they were maintained on fluoxetine or not. In addition, placebo pattern responders were significantly more likely to experience depressive breakthrough on drug compared with those who had shown a true drug response.

One study of the long-term treatment of depression with paroxetine differentiated continuation and maintenance prophylaxis (76). Paroxetine was superior to placebo, but 14% of patients experienced a recurrence during active long-term paroxetine treatment.

Montgomery et al. (90) randomized 147 patients who had responded to either citalopram 20 mg ($N = 68$) or 40 mg ($N = 79$) during a six-week acute treatment trial to receive the same dose or placebo over a 24-week period. Relapse rates were significantly lower on citalopram (8% on 20 mg and 12% on 40 mg) than placebo (31%). In a similar study, 226 responders to citalopram, flexibly dosed between 20 and 60 mg over eight weeks were randomized 2:1 to citalopram or placebo (91). Citalopram-treated subjects continued on the dose to which they had responded acutely. Relapse rates were 13.8% on citalopram compared with 24.3% on placebo. In an active comparator study among 297 depressed patients treated in general practice, there was no significant difference in depression severity at 22 weeks between patients randomized to one of two levels of citalopram (10–30 or 20–60 mg) versus imipramine (50–150 mg), although relapse rates were not reported (92).

Franchini et al. (93) reported a high recurrence rate (50%) among 32 patients with recurrent major depression who had maintained response to citalopram 40 mg/day over a four-month period and were then treated with 20 mg/day over 24 months. Although the absence of a comparison group treated with 40 mg/day hinders any definitive conclusions, the high rate of depressive breakthrough on the lower dose would tend to support the premise that full dose maintenance treatment of this SSRI is required for adequate prophylaxis among patients at risk for recurrence. In an extension of this work, Franchini et al. (59) examined 32 patients who had maintained response through acute and continuation phases of treatment at citalopram 40 mg/day, and continued on the same dosage during maintenance phase treatment. The authors report a 34% recurrence rate for patients on the maintenance citalopram dose of 40 mg/day. Hochstrasser et al. (60) also examined citalopram as a maintenance phase treatment, but in a placebo-controlled manner. Time to recurrence was found to be significantly longer in the maintenance phase citalopram-treated group versus placebo. All of these patients ($N = 269$) had demonstrated response to flexible citalopram dosing (20–60 mg) throughout the acute and continuation phases of treatment.

Overall, controlled trials show that, within one to three years of long-term antidepressant treatment after an acute response, at least 14% to 30% of patients have a recurrence of depression. In contrast to controlled trials, observational studies show that, within five years of acute response, 40% to 80% of patients have depressive breakthrough.

Meta-Analyses of Relapse Prevention

Geddes et al. (94) recently published a comprehensive meta-analysis of randomized trials of continuing treatment with antidepressants in patients with depressive disorders who have responded to acute treatment. The authors pooled data from 31 randomized trials (a total of 4410 patients) and found that continued antidepressant treatment (following acute phase response) reduced the odds of relapse by 70% compared with treatment discontinuation (placebo). The average rate of relapse on placebo was 41% compared with 18% on active treatment. The modal length of follow-up after randomization for these trials was 12 months, with a range of 6 to 36 months. Rates of relapse did not differ between types of antidepressant or treatment duration before randomization. This latter fact, as suggested by the authors, challenges the validity of clear demarcation of continuation and maintenance treatment phases. In addition, the proportional risk reduction was found to be similar in patients with short (six months) and long (36 months) follow-up periods, suggesting no increased or decreased risk with increasing time since response. As acknowledged by these researchers, one limitation of this meta-analysis is that patients were mainly drawn from secondary care settings, where patients may have a higher risk for relapse. Nevertheless, these findings confirm the clear benefit of continued antidepressant treatment in terms of reduction of relapse risk.

II. PSYCHOTHERAPY
Chiara Ruini and Giovanni A. Fava

The combination of psychotherapy and pharmacotherapy in the treatment of depressive and anxiety disorders has attracted considerable attention during the past two decades (95). However, it has obtained limited support from controlled trials (96,97). Indeed, a detrimental effect (exposure and alprazolam in panic disorder) has also been reported (98). The underlying assumption of the integrated approach was that of an additive model of interaction between pharmacotherapy and psychotherapy, which could take place on the basis of specific changes to be induced by specific treatments. Further, the simultaneous administration of pharmacotherapy and psychotherapy is based on a cross-sectional, flat view of the disorders that ignores their longitudinal development (99). An alternative way of integrating pharmacotherapy and psychotherapy involves their sequential administration according to the stages of the disorder.

Administration of treatments in sequential order is a common practice in other medical specialties when a treatment fails. If the physician prescribes the antibiotic A to eradicate an infection and the ensuing response is judged to be unsatisfactory, he or she switches to the antibiotic B, hoping to get a better outcome. The process is by approximation, applies only if treatment fails, and can be potentially avoided by appropriate pretreatment tests (e.g., in vitro determination of the susceptibility of bacteria to antimicrobial drugs). In clinical psychiatry, administration of treatment in sequential order has been mainly limited to instances of treatment resistance and has involved different types of drugs, such as in drug-refractory depression (100). However, cognitive-behavioral strategies have been successful in the management of drug-resistant MDDs (101), to the same extent that imipramine was found to be effective after unsuccessful cognitive therapy (CT) of depression (102). Similar results have been obtained in other disorders, such as panic disorder (103).

Within psychotherapeutic approaches, Emmelkamp et al. (104) suggested the feasibility of applying different therapies consecutively instead of in combination and the need to compare the two approaches in controlled studies. A first attempt to demonstrate the effectiveness of the sequential approach (involving exposure in vivo followed by CT) compared to a strategy where the two approaches were integrated from the start did not yield significant differences in the treatment outcome for social phobia (105). Similarly disappointing results were obtained with application of CT to panic disorder patients who failed to respond to exposure in vivo (106).

This type of sequential approach, however, was not targeted to stages of illness (99), or to residual symptoms (107). The arbitrary nature of the clinical and research decision along a response continuum that may range from treatment-resistant disorder to full remission via partial remission is not frequently acknowledged. In particular, treatment of depression by pharmacological means is likely to leave a substantial amount of residual symptomatology in most patients (108). The presence of residual symptoms after completion of drug or psychotherapeutic treatment has been correlated with poor long-term outcome (108). Further, some residual symptoms of MDD may progress to prodromal symptoms of relapse (109). This has led to the development of a sequential strategy based on the use of pharmacotherapy in the acute phase of depression and CT in its residual phase (110–114).

In this chapter, we will outline clinically significant findings concerned with residual symptoms of unipolar depression, provide an overview of the use of psychotherapy in later stages of treatment, describe the studies upon which the development of a sequential approach is based, and describe how this approach can be implemented in clinical practice.

RESIDUAL SYMPTOMS OF UNIPOLAR DEPRESSION

In 1973, Paykel and Weissman found social and interpersonal maladjustments in fully recovered depressed patients compared to controls, despite considerable improvement in social adjustment upon treatment. Submissive dependency and family attachment improved almost completely, whereas two other personal dysfunctions, interpersonal friction and inhibited communication, showed little change and greatest residual impairment (115). Residual social maladjustment was subsequently reported by other investigators (116–118) and was found to correlate with poorer long-term outcome (118). Similarly, dysfunctional attitudes and attributions were found to persist after recovery, despite clinical and cognitive improvement (119–121). These cognitive patterns were positively correlated with vulnerability to persistent depression or relapse (120,122,123). Social maladjustments and dysfunctional attitudes may overlap with characterological traits assessed after clinical recovery (124–127) or premorbid personality features (128). In any case, there appears to be a residual attributional interpersonal component that is refractory to otherwise successful treatment of depression. Such a component may have considerable predictive value for long-term illness course.

The notion that the majority of depressed patients experience mild but chronic residual symptoms or recurrence of symptoms after complete remission that was well delineated in the 1970s (129) did not receive the attention it deserved in subsequent years. This phenomenon was emphasized, in fact, mainly in its etiological role in dysthymia. Akiskal (130) subdivided chronic depression into primary depression (usually of late onset and occurring as a sequela to one or more syndromal episodes of primary MDD), chronic secondary dysphoria (having a variable onset age and occurring in the setting of pre-existing and incapacitating nonaffective disorders), and characterologic depression (with insidious and early developmental onset and fluctuating course). Hirschfeld et al. (131) suggested that chronicity in depression either results from an illness of a minor nature with insidious onset in early adult life or is a function of an unresolved MDD. However, the presence of residual symptoms after completion of drug treatment (48,132–135) or cognitive behavior therapy (CBT) (136,137) of depression has been correlated with poor long-term outcome. Methodological problems in the assessment of residual symptoms, however, emerge. There are few psychometric studies addressing the phenomenology of depressed patients after benefiting from treatment. Recovered depressed patients displayed significantly more depression and anxiety than did control subjects in one study (138), but not in another (139). Differences in the sensitivity of the rating scales that were employed (140,141) may account for such discrepant results. In a study using an observer-rated scale, Paykel's Clinical Interview for Depression (142)—that was found to be a suitable and sensitive instrument for detecting subclinical symptomatology (141)—only six (12%) of 49 patients with MDD successfully treated with antidepressant drugs and judged to be fully remitted had no residual symptoms (110). The majority of residual symptoms were present also in the prodromal phase of illness. The most frequently reported symptoms involved anxiety and irritability. This was consistent with previous studies on prodromal symptoms of depression (143,144) and overlapped with findings concerned with interpersonal friction (115) and trait anxiety (126).

PSYCHOTHERAPY DURING CONTINUATION AND MAINTENANCE PHASES OF TREATMENT

A limited number of controlled studies have examined the use of psychotherapy during the continuation and maintenance phases of treatment for depression. The goal of using psychotherapy during these treatment phases is twofold—to resolve any residual symptoms and prevent relapse or recurrence. The best-studied therapies for this purpose are IPT and CT. IPT was, in fact, first developed and tested as a continuation phase treatment for patients who had responded acutely to amitriptyline (145). Two important findings emerged from this early study. The first was that the combination of IPT with antidepressant treatment produced the best outcomes and, secondly, receiving IPT was associated with more significantly improved social functioning. In the most pivotal long-term IPT study (82,146), patients who responded to acute phase antidepressant treatment and remained remitted on the same treatment during continuation phase treatment were assigned to one of five maintenance treatment arms of three years' duration—(i) high-dose antidepressant, (ii) high-dose antidepressant plus monthly IPT sessions, (iii) monthly IPT sessions only, (iv) monthly IPT sessions plus placebo pill, or (v) placebo pill plus clinical management visits. The primary finding was that continued high-dose antidepressant treatment had the greatest prophylactic effect, and while not as effective, monthly IPT sessions as a continuation phase monotherapy were clearly superior to placebo. These findings were quite similar to a later study conducted by Reynolds et al. (147) involving a sample of depressed geriatric patients. In this study, patients who attained recovery from depression were assigned to one of four maintenance treatment arms. When comparing this study to Frank et al.'s earlier investigation, the missing treatment assignment was IPT monthly sessions alone as a monotherapy. The IPT delivered in Reynolds' study also differed because it was adapted for the unique needs of this geriatric patient group (e.g., fear of death, etc.). Results indicated that patients receiving the combination of IPT and NT experienced the lowest rates of recurrence (20%). Patients receiving either monotherapy (IPT or NT) experienced similar recurrence rates (64% vs. 43%) while those assigned to placebo experienced a 90% recurrence rate. In both the Frank and Reynolds studies, IPT was delivered in a once-per-month format. It is unknown what differences in results may have been seen if the frequency of sessions had been increased. Taken together, these studies suggest that IPT may be effective in prevention of depressive relapse and recurrence, and may be associated with more improvement in social functioning when compared with antidepressants taken as a continuation or maintenance treatment monotherapy.

CBTs have also been investigated as continuation and maintenance treatments in several recent studies. Jarrett et al. (148,149) conducted two studies in which patients who achieved remission following acute phase CT did or did not receive continuation phase CT. The earlier of these studies was nonrandomized while the latter was a true randomized trial. Both studies suggested that patients who continue CT past the point of remission attainment fare better in the long run (reduced relapse rates) than those patients who terminated CT at the end of acute phase treatment. In an earlier study of recurrently depressed patients, Blackburn and Moore (150) found maintenance phase CT to be as efficacious as maintenance antidepressant treatment in the prevention of recurrence. A series of studies also suggest that the preventive effects of receiving CT are more enduring than those of receiving antidepressant medication alone. Most recently, Hollon et al. (52) found that severely depressed outpatients receiving acute phase CT fared better (30.8% relapse rate) in one year of no treatment follow-up than patients receiving acute phase antidepressant medication (76.2% relapse rate). Even when antidepressant medication was continued for those patients who had responded acutely to antidepressant treatment, relapse rates were higher (47.2%) when compared with the acute phase CT only group.

Fava et al. (112) randomly assigned recovered depressed patients to either discontinuation of antidepressant treatment or discontinuation of antidepressant treatment and 10 sessions of CBT modified to enhance well-being. Over a six-year follow-up period, patients who received the cognitive-behavioral intervention experienced significantly lower rates of relapse and recurrence. Continuing with the theme of adapting cognitive therapies for later stages of depression treatment, Teasdale et al. (151) found that mindfulness-based CT (MBCT), when added to continuation antidepressant therapy (a group-based treatment), reduced relapse occurrence more than continuation medications alone. However, this finding was only true for patients with more recurrent forms of depression.

As can be seen, there are potentially significant benefits in using IPT or CBT—either alone or in combination with antidepressant medications—during later stages of treatment for depression. It is possible that use of these psychotherapies during the continuation and/or maintenance phases of treatment may confer a better long-term illness course. In addition, focus on this area of research has led to the development of some exciting modifications to address the unique needs of a patient who has already received acute phase treatment.

EFFICACY OF THE SEQUENTIAL APPROACH IN TREATING RESIDUAL SYMPTOMS

In a controlled therapeutic trial (110) previously mentioned, 40 patients with a MDD who had been successfully treated with antidepressant drugs were randomly assigned to either CBT or clinical management of residual symptoms. In both groups, antidepressant drugs were tapered and discontinued. The group that received CBT treatment had a significantly lower level of residual symptoms after drug discontinuation in comparison with the clinical management group. CBT also resulted in a lower rate of relapse, with achievement of statistical significance at a four-year follow-up (111). These differences faded at a six-year follow-up (112). However, when multiple relapses were considered, patients in the CBT group had a significantly lower number of depressive episodes than those in the standard clinical management group (112). The aim of this approach was to use CBT resources when they are most likely to make a unique and separate contribution to patient well-being and to achieve a more pervasive recovery. This sequential approach was applied also to 40 patients with recurrent major depression by the same group of investigators (113). These patients met the criteria outlined by Frank et al. (82), that is, three or more episodes of unipolar depression (with the immediately preceding episode being no more than 2.5 years before the onset of the present episode). Patients were randomly assigned to either CBT of residual symptoms—supplemented by lifestyle modification and well-being therapy (152,153)—or clinical management. In both groups, antidepressant drugs were tapered and discontinued. At a two-year follow-up, CBT resulted in a significantly lower relapse rate (25%) than did clinical management (80%). The differential relapse rate was found to be significantly related to the abatement of residual symptoms (114). At a six-year follow-up, CBT still resulted in a significantly lower relapse rate (40%) than clinical management (90%) (154).

Other groups of investigators lent support to the sequential use of pharmacotherapy and psychotherapy for relapse prevention in unipolar depression. Paykel et al. (155) randomized 158 patients with recent major depression, partially remitted with antidepressant treatment but with residual symptoms, to clinical management or clinical management associated with CT. Patients received continuation and maintenance antidepressants during a one-year follow-up. CBT reduced relapse rate from 47% in the clinical management group to 29% with CBT. At a six-year follow-up (156), effects in prevention of relapse and recurrence were found to persist up to 3.5 years after the end of CBT. A relationship between degree of improvement in residual symptoms and outcome was not found, unlike in previous studies (110,114), suggesting that the mechanism of action in CBT may be the change in coping skills rather than to ameliorate all depressive symptoms (157).

Similar results were obtained with MBCT. Teasdale et al. (151) randomized 145 patients in remission or recovery from major depression to treatment as usual (TAU) or TAU supplemented by MBCT. For patients with three or more previous episodes of depression, who constituted 77% of the sample, relapse rates were 66% for the TAU controls, and 37% for the patients also receiving MBCT (151). Because MBCT was administered in groups, this study provided the first demonstration that the sequential model may yield beneficial results also in the group format. There were no significant differences in outcome, however, for patients with only two previous episodes of depression. The favorable results concerned with MBCT were replicated in a subsequent study (158), involving 75 patients in remission or recovery from major depression.

Bockting et al. (159) recently reported the outcome of a randomized controlled trial of cognitive group therapy to prevent relapse in a group of high-risk patients diagnosed with recurrent depression. One hundred and eighty-seven patients were randomized to TAU, including continuation of pharmacotherapy, or to TAU associated with group CT. During a two-year follow-up, CT resulted in a significant protective effect, which increased with the previous number of depressive episodes experienced.

One study, however, has failed to substantiate the clinical advantages of the sequential model (160). One hundred and thirty-two patients with major depression who achieved remission with fluoxetine were randomized to receive CBT and medication or medication management alone and were followed for up to 28 weeks. Relapse rates did not differ between the two groups, even though the addition of CBT was associated with attributional style gains (161). Major limitations of this study were, however, the duration of follow-up (in previous studies maximal gains tended to occur at a later point) and that maintenance CBT was not directly comparable to the sequential use of therapeutic tools performed by Fava et al. (110,154) and Paykel et al. (155,156).

The results of the randomized controlled trials lend support, therefore, to the use of a sequential treatment model (pharmacotherapy followed by psychotherapy) for preventing relapse in unipolar depression. This approach appears to be particularly important in recurrent depression. However, because incomplete recovery from the first lifetime major depressive episode was found to predict a chronic course of illness during a 12-year prospective naturalistic follow-up (38), this sequential approach may be indicated whenever substantial residual symptomatology is present.

The advantages of continuing medication during psychotherapy versus tapering and discontinuation have not been directly compared in a controlled study. Some inferential indications may come from a study by Blackburn and Moore (150). Seventy-five outpatients with recurrent major depression were allocated to three groups: short-term and maintenance (two years) treatment with antidepressant drugs, CBT in the short-term and maintenance phases, and antidepressant use in the short-term phase and CBT for maintenance. CBT displayed a similar prophylactic effect to maintenance medication. There were no significant differences among treatments.

A novel indication for the sequential model has been provided by a pilot study, which concerned 10 patients with recurrent depression who relapsed while taking maintenance antidepressant drugs (162). They were randomly assigned to dose increase and clinical management or to CBT and maintenance of the antidepressant drug at the same dose. Four of five patients responded to a larger dose, but all relapsed again at the higher dose by a one-year follow-up. Four of five patients responded to CBT, but only one relapsed during follow-up. The data of this pilot study (162) and of a case report (163) suggest that the application of a sequential model is feasible when there is a loss of clinical effects during long-term antidepressant treatment (164) and may carry long-term benefits. The results, however, need to be confirmed with large-scale controlled studies.

STANDARD FORMAT OF SEQUENTIAL TREATMENT SESSIONS

Suitability and Motivation for Treatment

Before undergoing sequential treatment, patients should have displayed a satisfactory response to antidepressant drug treatment. They should thus have undergone at least three months of drug treatment and no longer present with depressed mood. During pharmacological treatment and clinical management it is, however, essential to introduce the subsequent part of treatment.

One helpful example (113) is the following:

"When we first saw you, you were very depressed. You went off the road. We gave you antidepressant drugs and these put you back on the road. Things are much better now. However, if you keep on driving the way you did, you will go off the road again, sooner or later."

The example outlines the need for lifestyle modification and introduces a sense of control to the patient about his or her depressive illness. This psychological preparation paves the way for subsequent psychotherapeutic approaches.

Standard Format

Psychotherapeutic intervention extends over 10 sessions, of 30 to 45 minutes each, every other week. The first session is mainly concerned with assessment and introduction of the psychotherapeutic treatment by the therapist, rehearsing the example provided before formal initiation of treatment. Sessions two through six are concerned with cognitive-behavioral treatment of residual symptoms and lifestyle modification. The last four sessions involve well-being therapy.

Table 3   Example of the Assessment Diary

Situation	Distress (0–100)	Thoughts
I am watching TV, when the telephone rings	40	Something has certainly happened to...

Assessment

It is most important to reassess the remitted patient as if he or she is a new patient. This means to go through symptoms developed in the most recent weeks in a careful way. Exploration should not only concern symptoms, which characterize the diagnosis of MDD, but also those which characterize anxiety disturbances (including phobic and obsessive-compulsive symptoms) and irritability. In the original studies (110,113) a modified version of Paykel's Clinical Interview for Depression (142) was employed, but other semistructured interviews may be used as long as these are sufficiently comprehensive as to anxiety and irritability. This is the first step in recognizing residual symptomatology.

The second step deals with self-observation of the patient. He or she is instructed to report in a diary (Table 3) all episodes of distress, which may ensue in the following two weeks. It is important to emphasize that distress (which is left unspecified) does not need to be prolonged, but may also be short lived. Patients are also instructed to build a list of situations that elicit distress and/or tend to induce avoidance. Each situation should be rated on a 0 to 100 point scale (0 = no problem; 100 = panic). Patients are instructed to bring the diary to the following visit.

COGNITIVE-BEHAVIORAL TREATMENT OF RESIDUAL SYMPTOMS

After patient's assessment and reading the diary brought by the patient, a cognitive-behavioral package is formulated. This may encompass both exposure and cognitive restructuring. Exposure consists of homework exposure only. An exposure strategy is planned with the patient, based on the list of situations outlined in the diary. The therapist writes an assignment per day in the diary, following a graded exposure (165). The patient assigns a score from 0 to 100 for each homework assignment. At the following visit, the therapist reassesses the homework done and discusses the next steps, and/or problems in compliance that may have ensued.

Cognitive restructuring follows the classic format of Beck et al. (166,167) and is based on introduction of the concept of automatic thoughts (second session) and of observer's interpretation (third session and on). The problems that may be the object of cognitive restructuring strictly depend on the material offered by the patient. They may encompass insomnia (sleep hygiene instructions are added), hypersomnia, diminished energy and concentration, residual hopelessness, re-entry problems (diminished functioning at work, avoidance, and procrastination), lack of assertiveness and self-care, perfectionism, and unrealistic self-expectations.

WELL-BEING THERAPY

At the seventh session well-being therapy is introduced (152). Well-being therapy is a short-term psychotherapeutic strategy, with sessions that may take place every week or every other week. The duration of each session may range from 30 to 50 minutes. It is a technique that emphasizes self-observation (168), with the use of a structured diary, and interaction between patients and therapists. Well-being therapy is based on Ryff's cognitive model of psychological well-being (169). This model was selected on the basis of its easy applicability to clinical populations (170,171). Well-being therapy is structured, directive, problem oriented, and based on an educational model. The development of sessions is given below.

Seventh session. It is simply concerned with identifying episodes of well-being and setting them into a situational context, no matter how short lived they were. Patients are asked to report in a structured diary the circumstances surrounding their episodes of well-being, rated on a 0 to 100 scale, with 0 being absence of well-being and 100 the most intense well-being that could be experienced (Table 4). When patients are assigned this homework, they often reply that they will bring a blank diary, because they never feel well. It is helpful to reply that these moments do exist but tend to pass unnoticed. Patients should therefore monitor them anyway.

Meehl (172) described "how people with low hedonic capacity should pay greater attention to the 'hedonic book keeping' of their activities than would be necessary for people located midway or high on the hedonic capacity continuum. That is, it matters more to someone cursed with an inborn hedonic defect whether he is efficient and sagacious in selecting friends, jobs, cities, tasks, hobbies, and activities in general" (p. 305).

Eighth session. Once the instances of well-being are properly recognized, the patient is encouraged to identify thoughts and beliefs leading to premature interruption of well-being. For instance, in the example reported

Table 4 Self-Observation of Episodes of Well-Being

Situation	Feeling of well-being	Intensity (0–100)
I went to visit my nephews and they greeted me with great enthusiasm and joy	They like me and care for me	40

in Table 4, the patients added "it is just because I brought two presents." The similarities between the search for irrational, tension-evoking thoughts in Ellis and Becker's rational-emotive therapy (173) and automatic thoughts in CT (166) are obvious. The trigger for self-observation is, however, different, being based on well-being instead of distress.

This phase is crucial, because it allows the therapist to identify areas of psychological well-being which are unaffected by irrational or automatic thoughts and which are saturated with them. The therapist may challenge these thoughts with appropriate questions, such as "what is the evidence for or against this idea?" or "are you thinking in all or none terms?" (166). The therapist may also reinforce and encourage activities that are likely to elicit well-being (for instance, assigning the task of undertaking particular pleasurable activities for a certain time each day). Such reinforcement may also result in graded task assignments (166). However, the focus of this phase of well-being therapy is always on self-monitoring of moments and feelings of well-being. The therapist refrains from suggesting conceptual and technical alternatives, unless a satisfactory degree of self-observation (including irrational or automatic thoughts) has been achieved.

Ninth session. Monitoring the course of episodes of well-being allows the therapist to realize specific impairments in well-being dimensions according to Ryff's conceptual framework. Ryff's six dimensions of psychological well-being are progressively introduced to the patients, if the material recorded is appropriate. Errors in thinking and alternative interpretations are then discussed.

Cognitive restructuring in well-being therapy follows Ryff's conceptual framework (174). The goal of the therapist is to lead the patient from an impaired level to an optimal level in the six dimensions of psychological well-being.

Environmental mastery (Table 5): This is the most frequent impairment that emerges. It was expressed by a patient as follows: "I have got a filter that nullifies any positive achievement (I was just lucky) and amplifies any negative outcome, no matter how much expected (this once more confirms I am a failure)." This lack of sense of control leads the patient to miss surrounding opportunities, with the possibility of subsequent regret over them.

Personal growth (Table 5): Patients often tend to emphasize their distance from expected goals much more than the progress that has been made toward goal achievement. A basic impairment that emerges is the inability to identify the similarities between events and situations that were handled successfully in the past and those that are about to come (transfer of experiences). Impairments in perception of personal growth and environmental mastery thus tend to interact in a dysfunctional way. A university student who is unable to realize the common contents and methodological similarities between the exams he or she successfully passed and the ones that

Table 5 Modification of the Six Dimensions of Psychological Well-Being According to Ryff's Model

Dimensions	Impaired level	Optimal level
Environmental mastery	The subject has or feels difficulties in managing everyday affairs; feels unable to change or improve surrounding context; is unaware of surrounding opportunities; lacks sense of control over external world	The subject has a sense of mastery and competence in managing the environment; controls external activities; makes effective use of surrounding opportunities; able to create or choose contexts suitable to personal needs and values
Personal growth	The subject has a sense of personal stagnation; lacks sense of improvement or expansion over time; feels bored and uninterested with life; feels unable to develop new attitudes or behaviors	The subject has a feeling of continued development; sees self as growing and expanding; is open to new experiences; has sense of realizing own potential; sees improvement in self and behavior over time
Purpose in life	The subject lacks a sense of meaning in life; has few goals or aims, lacks sense of direction, does not see purpose in past life; has no outlooks or beliefs that give life meaning	The subject has goals in life and a sense of directedness; feels there is meaning to present and past life; holds beliefs that give life purpose; has aims and objectives for living
Autonomy	The subject is overconcerned with the expectations and evaluation of others; relies on judgment of others to make important decisions; conforms to social pressures to think or act in certain ways	The subject is self-determining and independent; able to resist to social pressures; regulates behavior from within; evaluates self by personal standards
Self-acceptance	The subject feels dissatisfied with self; is disappointed with what has occurred in past life; is troubled about certain personal qualities; wishes to be different than what he or she is	The subject has a positive attitude toward the self; accepts his/her good and bad qualities; feels positive about past life

(Continued)

Table 5 Modification of the Six Dimensions of Psychological Well-Being According to Ryff's Model (*Continued*)

Dimensions	Impaired level	Optimal level
Positive relations with others	The subject has few close, trusting relationships with others; finds difficult to be open and is isolated and frustrated in interpersonal relationship; not willing to make compromises to sustain important ties with others	The subject has warm and trusting relationships with others; is concerned about the welfare of others; capable of strong empathy affection, and intimacy; understands give and take of human relationships

Source: From Ref. 72.

are to be given shows impairments in both environmental mastery and personal growth.

Purpose in life (Table 5): An underlying assumption of psychological therapies (whether pharmacological or psychotherapeutic) is to restore pre-morbid functioning. In case of treatments that emphasize self-help such as cognitive behavioral, therapy itself offers a sense of direction and hence a short-term goal. However, this does not persist when acute symptoms abate and/or premorbid functioning is suboptimal. Patients may perceive a lack of sense of direction and may devalue their function in life. This particularly occurs when environmental mastery and sense of personal growth are impaired.

Autonomy (Table 5): It is a frequent clinical observation that patients may exhibit a pattern whereby a perceived lack of self-worth leads to unassertive behavior. For instance, patients may hide their opinions or preferences, go along with a situation that is not in their best interests, or consistently put their needs behind the needs of others. This pattern undermines environmental mastery and purpose in life, and these, in turn, may affect autonomy, because these dimensions are highly correlated in clinical populations. Such attitudes may not be obvious to the patients, who hide their considerable need for social approval. A patient who tries to please everyone is likely to fail to achieve this goal, and the unavoidable conflicts that may ensue result in chronic dissatisfaction and frustration.

Self-acceptance (Table 5): Patients may maintain unrealistically high standards and expectations, driven by perfectionistic attitudes (that reflect lack of self-acceptance) and/or endorsement of external instead of personal standards (that reflect lack of autonomy). As a result, any instance of well-being is neutralized by a chronic dissatisfaction with oneself. A person may set unrealistic standards for their performance. For instance, it is a frequent clinical observation that patients with social phobia tend to aspire to outstanding social performances (being sharp, humorous, etc.) and are not satisfied with average performances (despite the fact that these latter would not put them under the spotlights, which could be seen as their apparent goal).

Positive relations with others (Table 5): Interpersonal relationships may be influenced by strongly held attitudes of which the patient may be unaware and that may be dysfunctional. For instance, a young woman who recently got married may have set unrealistic standards for her marital relationship and find herself frequently disappointed. At the same time she may avoid pursuing social plans that involve other people and may lack sources of comparison. Impairments in self-acceptance (with the resulting belief of being rejectable and unlovable) may also undermine positive relations with others.

LIFESTYLE MODIFICATION

One of the aims of therapy is making the patient aware of allostatic loads (i.e., chronic and often subtle life stresses that exert harmful consequences on the individual over a certain amount of time). Examples may be excessive work loads, being unaware that an increasing age requires a longer time to recover from demanding days, inability to protect oneself from requests that exceed the potential of the individual, and inappropriate sleeping habits.

Such awareness (and the resulting lifestyle implementation) is pursued in all phases of psychotherapy, but particularly with well-being therapy. Patients are given instructions in the diary as to this implementation.

DRUG TAPERING AND DISCONTINUATION

Sequential treatment offers a unique opportunity for antidepressant drug tapering and discontinuation. It offers the opportunity to monitor the patient in one of the most delicate aspects of treatment. In the original studies (110,113) antidepressant drugs were mainly tricyclics and were decreased at the rate of 25 mg of amitriptyline or its equivalent every other week. When SSRI are involved, the more the gradual tapering is, the better the result.

It is important to warn the patient that he or she should not perceive "steps" (as one patient defined them) in this tapering (i.e., patients should not perceive substantial differences in their sleep, energy, mood, and appetite from 200 mg of amitriptyline per day to 175 mg). If they do, the appropriateness of tapering the antidepressant drug should be questioned. Indeed, in the original studies, drug discontinuation could not take place in a few patients.

The sequential format offers an ideal opportunity to support psychologically the patient when withdrawal syndromes (despite slow tapering, particularly with SSRI) do occur.

At times patients are fearful of drug discontinuation. It is then helpful to emphasize that a drug-free status is a step forward in therapy and may be associated with an increased quality of life. It is thus a sign of progress. Antidepressant drugs may be prescribed again if they are needed, at the prodromal symptoms of mood deterioration, and patients should be reassured about this possibility that is always available.

CONCLUSIONS

This sequential model that was developed for preventing relapse in depression (16) may potentially apply to any type of psychiatric disorder (107) or when psychotherapy is associated with medical illness. Marks (175) suggested that current prevailing therapeutic mechanisms for explaining therapeutic effectiveness in psychotherapy are about to change. Foa and Kozak (176) wondered whether the slowing advance of cognitive behavior may be the result of an alienation from psychopathology. The sequential model introduces a conceptual shift in psychotherapy research and practice. The target of psychotherapeutic efforts is not predetermined and therapy driven (e.g., cognitive triad), but depends on the type and intensity of residual symptomatology (110,113) or the specific impairments in psychological well-being (113,152). The cognitive-behavioral approach that is entailed by the sequential model is thus pragmatic, realistic instead of idealistic, with a strictly evidence-based appraisal of its ingredients (177). There is limited awareness that current techniques of treating affective disorders are geared to acute situations more than residual phases of illness (108) and neglect psychological well-being (174). The model may be frustrating to the purist, in its blurring of clear-cut interpretative instruments. However, it is more in keeping with the complexity of the balance of positive and negative affects (178) in health and disease and the clinical needs of patients with affective disorders.

ACKNOWLEDGMENTS

The work described in this paper was supported in part by grants from the Mental Health Project (Istituto Superiore di Sanità, Roma), from the Outcome Evaluation Project (Istituto Superiore di Sanità, Roma), and the Ministero dell'Università e della Ricerca Scientifica e Tecnologica (Roma) to Dr. Fava.

REFERENCES

1. Nierenberg AA, Petersen TJ, Alpert JE. Prevention of relapse and recurrence in depression: the role of long-term pharmacotherapy and psychotherapy. J Clin Psychiat 2003; 64(suppl 15):13–17.

2. Robins LN, Helzer JE, Weissman MM, et al. Lifetime prevalence of specific psychiatric disorders in three sites. Arch Gen Psychiat 1984; 41:949–958.

3. Kessler RC, McGonagle KA, Zhao S, et al. Lifetime and 12-month prevalence of DSM-III-R psychiatric disorders in the United States. Results from the National Comorbidity Survey. Arch Gen Psychiat 1994; 51:8–19.

4. Keller MB. Long-term treatment of recurrent and chronic depression. J Clin Psychiat 2001; 62(suppl 24):3–5.

5. Murray CJ, Lopez AD. Alternative projections of mortality and disability by cause 1990–2020: Global Burden of Disease Study. Lancet 1997; 349:1498–1504.

6. Keller MB. The long-term treatment of depression. J Clin Psychiat 1999; 60(suppl 17):41–45.

7. Simon GE, VonKorff M, Heiligenstein JH, et al. Initial antidepressant choice in primary care. Effectiveness and cost of fluoxetine vs. tricyclic antidepressants. JAMA 1996; 275:1897–1902.

8. Solomon DA, Keller MB, Leon AC, et al. Recovery from major depression. A 10-year prospective follow-up across multiple episodes. Arch Gen Psychiat 1997; 54:1001–1006.

9. Keller MB, Boland RJ. Implications of failing to achieve successful long-term maintenance treatment of recurrent unipolar major depression. Biol Psychiat 1998; 44:348–360.

10. Mueller TI, Keller MB, Leon AC, et al. Recovery after 5 years of unremitting major depressive disorder. Arch Gen Psychiat 1996; 53:794–799.

11. Frank E, Prien RF, Jarrett RB, et al. Conceptualization and rationale for consensus definitions of terms in major depressive disorder. Remission, recovery, relapse, and recurrence. Arch Gen Psychiat 1991; 48:851–855.

12. Solomon DA, Keller MB, Leon AC, et al. Multiple recurrences of major depressive disorder. Am J Psychiat 2000; 157:229–233.

13. Mueller TI, Leon AC, Keller MB, et al. Recurrence after recovery from major depressive disorder during 15 years of observational follow-up. Am J Psychiat 1999; 156:1000–1006.

14. Shelton RC. Treatment options for refractory depression. J Clin Psychiat 1999; 60(suppl 4):57–61.

15. Zubenko GS, Zubenko WN, Spiker DG, Giles DE, Kaplan BB. Malignancy of recurrent, early-onset major depression: a family study. Am J Med Genet 2001; 105:690–699.

16. Mueller TI, Kohn R, Leventhal N, et al. The course of depression in elderly patients. Am J Geriatr Psychiat 2004; 12:22–29.

17. Ezquiaga E, Garcia-Lopez A, de Dios C, Leiva A, Bravo M, Montejo J. Clinical and psychosocial factors associated with the outcome of unipolar major depression: a one year prospective study. J Affect Disord 2004; 79:63–70.

18. Melartin TK, Rytsala HJ, Leskela US, Lestela-Mielonen PS, Sokero TP, Isometsa ET. Severity and comorbidity predict episode duration and recurrence of DSM-IV major depressive disorder. J Clin Psychiat 2004; 65:810–819.

19. Spijker J, de Graaf R, Bijl RV, Beekman AT, Ormel J, Nolen WA. Determinants of persistence of major depressive episodes in the general population

Results from the Netherlands Mental Health Survey and Incidence Study (NEMESIS). J Affect Disord 2004; 81:231–240.

20. Barbe RP, Bridge JA, Birmaher B, Kolko DJ, Brent DA. Lifetime history of sexual abuse, clinical presentation, and outcome in a clinical trial for adolescent depression. J Clin Psychiat 2004; 65:77–83.

21. Kennedy N, Abbott R, Paykel ES. Remission and recurrence of depression in the maintenance era: long-term outcome in a Cambridge cohort. Psychol Med 2003; 33:827–838.

22. Paykel ES, Ramana R, Cooper Z, Hayhurst H, Kerr J, Barocka A. Residual symptoms after partial remission: an important outcome in depression. Psychol Med 1995; 25:1171–1180.

23. Lewinsohn PM, Rohde P, Seeley JR, Klein DN, Gotlib IH. Natural course of adolescent major depressive disorder in a community sample: predictors of recurrence in young adults. Am J Psychiat 2000; 157:1584–1591.

24. Hart AB, Craighead WE, Craighead LW. Predicting recurrence of major depressive disorder in young adults: a prospective study. J Abnorm Psychol 2001; 110:633–643.

25. Oldehinkel AJ, Van DB, Bouhuys AL, Ormel J. Do depressive episodes lead to accumulation of vulnerability in the elderly? Depress Anxiety 2003; 18:67–75.

26. Daley SE, Hammen C, Rao U. Predictors of first onset and recurrence of major depression in young women during the 5 years following high school graduation. J Abnorm Psychol 2000; 109:525–533.

27. Paykel ES, Cooper Z, Ramana R, Hayhurst H. Life events, social support and marital relationships in the outcome of severe depression. Psychol Med 1996; 26:121–133.

28. Hayhurst H, Cooper Z, Paykel ES, Vearnals S, Ramana R. Expressed emotion and depression A longitudinal study. Br J Psychiat 1997; 171:439–443.

29. Klein DN, Schatzberg AF, McCullough JP, et al. Age of onset in chronic major depression: relation to demographic and clinical variables, family history, and treatment response. J Affect Disord 1999; 55:149–157.

30. Kessing LV, Hansen MG, Andersen PK, Angst J. The predictive effect of episodes on the risk of recurrence in depressive and bipolar disorders—a life-long perspective. Acta Psychiat Scand 2004; 109:339–344.

31. McGrath PJ, Stewart JW, Petkova E, et al. Predictors of relapse during fluoxetine continuation or maintenance treatment of major depression. J Clin Psychiat 2000; 61:518–524.

32. Paykel ES, Tanner J. Life events, depressive relapse and maintenance treatment. Psychol Med 1976; 6:481–485.

33. Paykel ES. Life events and affective disorders. Acta Psychiat Scand Suppl 2003:61–66.

34. Solomon DA, Leon AC, Endicott J, et al. Psychosocial impairment and recurrence of major depression. Compr Psychiat 2004; 45:423–430.

35. Wells K, Sherbourne C, Schoenbaum M, et al. Five-year impact of quality improvement for depression: results of a group-level randomized controlled trial. Arch Gen Psychiat 2004; 61:378–386.

36. Ormel J, Oldehinkel AJ, Brilman EI. The interplay and etiological continuity of neuroticism, difficulties, and life events in the etiology of major and subsyndromal, first and recurrent depressive episodes in later life. Am J Psychiat 2001; 158:885–891.

37. Oldehinkel AJ, Bouhuys AL, Brilman EI, Ormel J. Functional disability and neuroticism as predictors of late-life depression. Am J Geriatr Psychiat 2001; 9:241–248.

38. Judd LL, Paulus MJ, Schettler PJ, et al. Does incomplete recovery from first lifetime major depressive episode herald a chronic course of illness? Am J Psychiat 2000; 157:1501–1504.

39. Leon AC, Solomon DA, Mueller TI, et al. A 20-year longitudinal observational study of somatic antidepressant treatment effectiveness. Am J Psychiat 2003; 160(suppl 4):727–733.

40. Lejoyeux M, Ades J. Antidepressant discontinuation: a review of the literature. J Clin Psychiat 1997; 58(suppl 7):11–15.

41. Haddad PM. Antidepressant discontinuation syndromes. Drug Saf 2001; 24:183–197.

42. Black K, Shea C, Dursun S, Kutcher S. Selective serotonin reuptake inhibitor discontinuation syndrome: proposed diagnostic criteria. J Psychiat Neurosci 2000; 25:255–261.

43. Schatzberg AF, Haddad P, Kaplan EM, et al. Serotonin reuptake inhibitor discontinuation syndrome: a hypothetical definition. Discontinuation Consensus panel. J Clin Psychiat 1997; 58(suppl 7):5–10.

44. Costei AM, Kozer E, Ho T, Ito S, Koren G. Perinatal outcome following third trimester exposure to paroxetine. Arch Pediatr Adolesc Med 2002; 156:1129–1132.

45. Sanz EJ, Las-Cuevas C, Kiuru A, Bate A, Edwards R. Selective serotonin reuptake inhibitors in pregnant women and neonatal withdrawal syndrome: a database analysis. Lancet 2005; 365:482–487.

46. Nierenberg AA. Long-term management of chronic depression. J Clin Psychiat 2001; 62(suppl 6):17–21.

47. Gilaberte I, Montejo AL, de la Gandara J, et al. Fluoxetine Long-Term Study Group. Fluoxetine in the prevention of depressive recurrences: a doubleblind study [Clinical Trial. Journal Article. Multicenter Study. Randomized Controlled Trial]. J Clin Psychopharmacol 2001; 21(suppl 4):417–424.

48. Prien RF, Klett CJ, Caffey EM Jr. Lithium carbonate and imipramine in prevention of affective episodes. A comparison in recurrent affective illness. Arch Gen Psychiat 1973; 29:420–425.

49. Prien RF, Caffey EM Jr. Long-term maintenance drug therapy in recurrent affective illness: current status and issues. Dis Nerv Syst 1977; 38:981–992.

50. Prien RF, Kupfer DJ. Continuation drug therapy for major depressive episodes: how long should it be maintained? Am J Psychiat 1986; 143:18–23.

51. Clinton JJ. From the Agency for Health Care Policy and Research. JAMA 1993; 270(suppl 2):172.

52. Hollon SD, DeRubeis RJ, Shelton RC, et al. Prevention of relapse following cognitive therapy versus medications in moderate to severe depression. Arch Gen Psychiat 2005; 58(suppl 4):381–388.

53. Frank E, Kupfer DJ, Perel JM, et al. Comparison of full-dose versus half-dose pharmacotherapy in the maintenance treatment of recurrent depression. J Affect Disord 1993; 27:139–145.

54. Lepine JP, Caillard V, Bisserbe JC, Troy S, Hotton JM, Boyer P. A randomized, placebo controlled trial of sertraline for prophylactic treatment of highly recurrent major depressive disorder [Erratum appears in Am J Psychiat 2004; 161(suppl 7):1320] [Clinical Trial. Journal Article. Randomized Controlled Trial]. Am J Psychiat 2004; 161(suppl 5):836–842.

55. Mavissakalian MR. Imiprmaine versus sertraline in panic disorder: 24-week treatment completers [Clinical Trial. Journal Article. Randomized Controlled Trial]. Ann Clin Psychiat 2003; 15(suppl 3, 4):171–180.

56. Mauri MC, Fiorentini A, Cerveri G, et al. Long-term efficacy and therapeutic drug monitoring of sertraline in major depression [Clinical Trial. Journal Article]. Hum Psychopharmacol 2003; 18(suppl 5):385–388.

57. Kocsis JH, Schatzberg A, Rush AJ, et al. Psychosocial outcomes following long-term, double-blind treatment of chronic depression with sertraline vs placebo [see comment] [Clinical Trial. Journal Article. Randomized Controlled Trial]. Arch Gen Psychiat 2002; 59(suppl 8):723–728.

58. Bump GM, Mulsant BH, Pollock BG, et al. Paroxetine versus nortriptyline in the continuation and maintenance treatment of depression in the elderly [Clinical Trial. Journal Article. Randomized Controlled Trial]. Depress Anxiety 2001; 13(suppl 1):38–44.

59. Franchini L, Spagnolo C, Rampoldi R, Zanardi R, Smeraldi E. Long-term treatment with citalopram in patients with highly recurrent forms of unipolar depression [Journal Article]. Psychiat Res 2001; 105(suppl 1, 2):129–133.

60. Hochstrasser B, Isaksen PM, Koponen H, et al. Prophylactic effect of citalopram in unipolar, recurrent depression: placebo-controlled study of maintenance therapy [see comment] [Clinical Trial. Journal Article. Multicenter Study. Randomized Controlled Trial]. Br J Psychiat 2001; 178:304–310.

61. Montgomery SA, Entsuah R, Hackett D, Kunz NR, Rudolph RL. Venlafaxine 335 Study Group. Venlafaxine versus placebo in the preventive treatment of recurrent major depression [Clinical Trial. Journal Article. Multicenter Study. Randomized Controlled Trial]. J Clin Psychiat 2004; 65(suppl 3): 328–336.

62. Lavori PW, Keller MB, Scheftner W, et al. Recurrence after recovery in unipolar MDD: an observational follow-up study of clinical predictors and somatic treatment as a mediating factor. Int J Meth Psychiat Res 1994; 4:211–220.

63. Ramana R, Paykel E, Cooper Z. Remission and relapse in major depression: a two-year prospective follow-up study. Psychol Med 1995; 25:1161–1170.

64. Kaplan E, Meier P. Nonparametric estimation from incomplete observations. J Am Stat Assoc 1958; 58:690–700.

65. Montgomery SA, Reimitz PE, Zivkov M. Mirtazapine versus amitriptyline in the long-term treatment of depression: a double-blind placebo-controlled study. Int Clin Psychopharmacol 1998; 13(suppl 2):63–73.

66. Claxton AJ, Li Z, McKendrick J. Selective serotonin reuptake inhibitor treatment in the UK: risk of relapse or recurrence of depression. Br J Psychiat 2000; 177:163–168.

67. Sackheim HA, Haskett RE, Mulsant BH, et al. Continuation pharmacotherapy in the prevention of relapse following electroconvulsive therapy: a randomized controlled trial. JAMA 2001; 285(suppl 10):1299–1307.

68. Versiani M, Mehilane L, Gaszner P, Arnaud-Castiglioni R. Reboxetine, a unique selective NRI, prevents relapse and recurrence in long-term treatment of major depressive disorder. J Clin Psychiat 1999; 60(suppl 6):400–406.

69. Feiger AD, Bielski RJ, Bremner J, et al. Double-blind, placebo-substitution study of nefazodone in the prevention of relapse during continuation treatment of outpatients with major depression. Int Clin Psychopharmacol 1999; 14(suppl 1):19–28.

70. Entsuah AR, Rudolph RL, Hackett D, Miska S. Efficacy of venlafaxine and placebo during long-term treatment of depression: a pooled analysis of relapse rates. Int Clin Psychopharmacol 1996; 11(suppl 2):137–147.

71. Thase ME, Nierenberg AA, Keller MB, Panagides J. The relapse prevention study group: efficacy of mirtazapine for prevention of depressive relapse: a placebo controlled double-blind trial of recently remitted high-risk patients. J Clin Psychiat 2001; 62(suppl 10):782–788.

72. Ferreri M, Colonna L, Leger JM. Efficacy of amineptine in the prevention of relapse in unipolar depression. Int Clin Psychopharmacol 1997; 12(suppl 3): 39–45.

73. Miner CM, Brown EB, Gonzales JS, Munir R. Switching patients from daily citalopram, paroxetine, or sertraline to once-weekly fluoxetine in the maintenance of response for depression. J Clin Psychiat 2002; 63(suppl 3):232–240.

74. Schmidt ME, Fava M, Robinson JM, Judge R. The efficacy and safety of a new enteric-coated formulation of fluoxetine given once weekly during the continuation treatment of major depressive disorder. J Clin Psychiat 2000; 61(suppl 11):851–857.

75. Doogan DP, Caillard V. Sertraline in the prevention of depression. Br J Psychiat 1992; 160:217–222.

76. Montgomery SA, Dunbar G. Paroxetine is better than placebo in relapse prevention and prophylaxis of recurrent depression. Int Clin Psychopharmacol 1993; 8:181–195.

77. Claghorn JL, Feighner JP. A double-blind comparison of paroxetine with imipramine in the long term treatment of depression. J Clin Psychopharmacol 1993; 13(suppl 2, 6):23–27.

78. Quitkin FM, Stewart JW, McGrath PJ. Loss of drug effects during continuation therapy. Am J Psychiat 1993; 150:562–565.

79. Peselow ED, Dunner DL, Fieve RR, et al. The prophylactic efficacy of tricyclic antidepressants—a five year followup. Prog Neuropsychopharmacol Biol Psychiat 1991; 15:71–82.

80. Prien RF, Kupfer DJ, Mansky PA. Drug therapy in the prevention of recurrences in unipolar and bipolar affective disorders: a report of the NIMH

Collaborative Study Group comparing lithium carbonate, imipramine, and a lithium carbonate-imipramine combination. Arch Gen Psychiat 1984; 41:1096–1104.

81. Greenhouse JB, Stangl D, Kupfer DJ, et al. Methodologic issues in maintenance therapy clinical trials. Arch Gen Psychiat 1991; 48:313–318.

82. Frank E, Kupfer DJ, Perel JM. Three-year outcomes for maintenance therapies in recurrent depression. Arch Gen Psychiat 1990; 47:1093–1099.

83. Rouillon F, Warner B, Pezous N, Bisserbe JC. Milnacipran efficacy in the prevention of recurrent depression: a 12-month placebo-controlled study. Int Clin Psychopharmacol 2000; 15(suppl 3):133–140.

84. Klysner R, Bent-Hansen J, Hansen HL, et al. Efficacy of citalopram in the prevention of recurrent depression in elderly patients: placebo-controlled study of maintenance therapy. Br J Psychiat 2002; 181:29–35.

85. Terra JL, Montgomery SA. Fluvoxamine prevents recurrence of depression: results of long-term, double-blind, placebo-controlled study. Int Clin Psychopharmacol 1998; 13(suppl 2):55–62.

86. Robinson DS, Lerfald SC, Bennett B, et al. Continuation and maintenance treatment of major depression with the monoamine oxidase inhibitor phenelzine: a double-blind placebo-controlled discontinuation study. Psychopharmacol Bull 1991; 27:31–39.

87. Montgomery SA, Dufour H, Brion S. The prophylactic efficacy of fluoxetine in unipolar depression. Br J Psychiat 1988; 153(suppl 3):69–73.

88. Kupfer DJ, Frank E, Perel JM, et al. Five year outcome for maintenance therapies in recurrent depression. Arch Gen Psychiat 1992; 49:769–773.

89. Stewart J, Quitkin F, McGrath PJ, et al. Use of pattern analysis to predict differential relapse of remitted patients with major depression during 1 year of treatment with fluoxetine or placebo. Arch Gen Psychiat 1998; 55:334–343.

90. Montgomery SA, Rasmussen JGC, Tanghoj P. A 24-week study of 20 mg citalopram, 40 mg citalopram, and placebo in the prevention of relapse of major depression. Int Clin Psychopharmacol 1993; 8:181–188.

91. Robert PH, Montgomery SA. Citalopram in doses of 20–60 mg is effective in depression relapse prevention: a placebo-controlled 6 month study. Int Clin Psychopharmacol 1995; 10(suppl 1):29–35.

92. Rosenberg et al. 1994.

93. Franchini L, Zanardi R, Gasperini M, et al. Two-year maintenance treatment with citalopram, 20 mg, in unipolar subjects with high recurrence rate. J Clin Psychiat 1999; 60:861–865.

94. Geddes JR, Carney SM, Davies C, et al. Relapse prevention with antidepressant drug treatment in depressive disorders: a systematic review. Lancet 2003; 361(9358):653–661.

95. Fava GA. Conceptual obstacles to research progress in affective disorders. Psychother Psychosom 1997; 66:283–285.

96. Wexler BE, Nelson JC. The treatment of depressive disorders. Int J Mental Health 1993; 22:7–41.

97. Gelder MG. Treatment of the neuroses. Int J Mental Health 1993; 21:3–42.

98. Basoglu M. Pharmacological and behavioral treatment of panic disorder. Psychother Psychosom 1992; 58:57–59.

99. Fava GA, Kellner R. Staging: a neglected dimension in psychiatric classification. Acta Psychiat Scand 1993; 87:225–230.
100. Ananth J. Treatment-resistant depression. Psychother Psychosom 1998; 67:61–70.
101. Fava GA, Savron G, Grandi S, et al. Cognitive-behavioral management of drug-resistant major depression disorder. J Clin Psychiat 1997; 58: 278–282.
102. Stewart JW, Mercier MA, Agosti V, et al. Imipramine is effective after unsuccessful cognitive therapy. J Clin Psychopharmacol 1993; 13:114–119.
103. Pollack MH, Otto MW, Rosenbaum JF. Challenges in Clinical Practice. New York: Guilford, 1996.
104. Emmelkamp PMG, Bouman TK, Scholing A. Anxiety Disorders. Chichester: Wiley, 1993.
105. Scholing A, Emmelkamp PMG. Cognitive and behavioral treatments of fear of blushing, sweating or trembling. Behav Res Ther 1993; 31:155–170.
106. Fava GA, Savron G, Zielezny M, et al. Overcoming resistance to exposure in panic disorder with agoraphobia. Acta Psychiat Scand 1997; 95:306–312.
107. Fava GA. The concept of recovery in affective disorders. Psychother Psychosom 1996; 65:2–13.
108. Fava GA. Subclinical symptoms in mood disorders. Pathophysiological and therapeutic implications. Psychol Med 1999; 29:47–61.
109. Fava GA, Kellner R. Prodromal symptoms in affective disorders. Am J Psychiat 1991; 48:823–830.
110. Fava GA, Grandi S, Zielezny M, et al. Cognitive behavioral treatment of residual symptoms in primary major depressive disorder. Am J Psychiat 1994; 151:1295–1299.
111. Fava GA, Grandi S, Zielezny M, et al. Four year outcome for cognitive behavioral treatment of residual symptoms in major depression. Am J Psychiat 1996; 153:945–947.
112. Fava GA, Rafanelli C, Grandi S, et al. Six-year outcome for cognitive behavioral treatment of residual symptoms in major depression. Am J Psychiat 1998; 155:1443–1445.
113. Fava GA, Rafanelli C, Grandi S, et al. Prevention of recurrent depression with cognitive behavioral therapy. Arch Gen Psychiat 1998; 55:816–820.
114. Fava GA, Rafanelli C, Grandi S, et al. The role of residual subthreshold symptoms in early episode relapse in unipolar depressive disorder [Letter to the editor]. Arch Gen Psychiat 1999; 56:765.
115. Paykel ES, Weissman MM. Social adjustment and depression. Arch Gen Psychiat 1973; 28:659–664.
116. Coryell W, Scheftner W, Keller MB, et al. The enduring psychosocial consequences of mania and depression. Am J Psychiat 1993; 150:720–727.
117. Bauwens F, Tray A, Pardoen D, et al. Social adjustment of remitted bipolar and unipolar out-patients. Br J Psychiat 1991; 159:239–244.
118. Goering PN, Lancee WJ, Freeman SJJ. Marital support and recovery from depression. Br J Psychiat 1992; 160:76–82.
119. Eaves G, Rush AJ. Cognitive patterns in symptomatic and remitted unipolar major depression. J Abnorm Psychol 1984; 93:31–40.

120. Williams JMG, Healy D, Teasdale JD, et al. Dysfunctional attitudes and vulnerability to persistent depression. Psychol Med 1990; 20:375–381.
121. Brown GW, Bifulco A, Andrews B. Self-esteem and depression. Soc Psychiat Psychiat Epidemiol 1990; 25:244–249.
122. Power MJ, Duggan CF, Lee AS, et al. Dysfunctional attitudes in depressed and recovered depressed patients and their first degree-relatives. Psychol Med 1995; 25:97–93.
123. Scott J, Eccleston D, Boys R. Can we predict the persistence of depression? Br J Psychiat 1992; 161:633–637.
124. Peselow ED, Sanfilipo MP, Fieve RR, et al. Personality traits during depression and after clinical recovery. Br J Psychiat 1994; 164:349–354.
125. Fava M, Bouffides E, Pava JA, et al. Personality disorder comorbidity with major depression and response to fluoxetine treatment. Psychother Psychosom 1994; 62:160–167.
126. Murray LO, Blackburn IM. Personality differences in patients with depressive illness and anxiety neurosis. Acta Psychiat Scand 1974; 50:183–191.
127. Perris C, Eisemann M, von Knorring L, et al. Personality traits in former depression patients and in healthy subjects without past history of depression. Psychopathology 1984; 17:178–186.
128. Clayton PJ, Ernst C, Angst J. Premorbid personality traits of men who develop unipolar or bipolar disorder. Eur Arch Psychiat Clin Neurosci 1994; 243:340–346.
129. Weissman MM, Kasl SV, Klerman GL. Follow-up of depressed women after maintenance treatment. Am J Psychiat 1976; 133:757–760.
130. Akiskal HS. Dysthymic disorder. Am J Psychiat 1983; 140:11–20.
131. Hirschfeld RMA, Klerman GL, Andreasen NC, et al. Psychosocial predictors of chronicity in depressed patients. Br J Psychiat 1986; 148:648–654.
132. Mindham RH, Howland C, Shepherd M. An evaluation of continuation therapy with tricyclic antidepressants in depressive illness. Psychol Med 1973; 3:5–17.
133. Faravelli C, Ambonetti A, Pallanti S, et al. Depressive relapses and incomplete recovery from index episode. Am J Psychiat 1986; 143:888–891.
134. Georgotas A, McCue RE. Relapse of depressed patients after effective continuation therapy. J Affect Disord 1989; 17:159–164.
135. Maj M, Veltro F, Pirozzi R, et al. Pattern of recurrence of illness after recovery from an episode of major depression. Am J Psychiat 1992; 149:795–800.
136. Simons AD, Murphy GE, Levine JL, et al. Cognitive therapy and pharmacotherapy of depression. Arch Gen Psychiat 1986; 43:43–50.
137. Thase ME, Simons AD, McGeary J, et al. Relapse after cognitive behavior therapy of depression. Am J Psychiat 1992; 149:1046–1052.
138. Fava GA, Kellner R, Lisansky J, et al. Rating depression in normals and depressives. J Affect Disord 1986; 11:29–33.
139. Agosti V, Stewart JW, Quitkin FM, et al. How symptomatic do depressed patients remain after benefiting from medication treatment? Comp Psychiat 1993; 34:182–186.
140. Kellner R. The development of sensitive scales for research in therapeutics. In: Fava M, Rosenbaum JF, eds. Research Design and Methods in Psychiatry. Amsterdam: Elsevier, 1992.

141. Fava GA. Measurement of prodromal and subclinical symptoms. In: Fava M, Rosenbaum JF, eds. Research Design and Methods in Psychiatry. Amsterdam: Elsevier, 1992:223–230.
142. Paykel ES. The clinical interview for depression. J Affect Disord 1985; 9:85–96.
143. Fava GA, Grandi S, Canestrari R, et al. Prodromal symptoms in primary major depressive disorder. J Affect Disord 1990; 19:149–152.
144. van Praag HM. About the centrality of mood disorders. Eur Neuropsychopharmacol 1992; 2:393–404.
145. Klerman GL, DiMascio A, Weissman M, Prusoff B, Paykel ES. Treatment of depression by drugs and psychotherapy. Am J Psychiat 1974; 131:186–191.
146. Frank E, Kupfer DJ, Wagner EF, McEachran AB, Cornes C. Efficacy of interpersonal psychotherapy as a maintenance treatment of recurrent depression. Arch Gen Psychiat 1991; 48:851–855.
147. Reynolds CF III, Frank E, Perel JM, et al. Nortriptyline and interpersonal psychotherapy as maintenance therapies for recurrent major depression: a randomized controlled trial in patients older than 59 years. JAMA 1999; 281: 39–45.
148. Jarrett RB, Basco MR, Risser R, et al. Is there a role for continuation phase cognitive therapy for depressed outpatients? J Consult Clin Psychol 1998; 66:1036–1040.
149. Jarrett RB, Kraft D, Doyle J, Foster BM, Eaves GG, Silver PC. Preventing recurrent depression using cognitive therapy with and without a continuation phase: a randomized clinical trial. Arch Gen Psychiat 2001; 58:381–388.
150. Blackburn IM, Moore RG. Controlled acute and follow-up trial of cognitive therapy in outpatients with recurrent depression. Br J Psychiat 1997; 171: 328–334.
151. Teasdale JD, Segal ZV, Williams JMG, et al. Prevention of relapse/recurrence in major depression by mindfulness-based cognitive therapy. J Consult Clin Psychol 2000; 68:615–623.
152. Fava GA, Ruini C. Development and characteristics of a well-being enhancing psychotherapeutic strategy: well-being therapy. J Behav Ther Exp Psychiat 2003; 34:45–63.
153. Fava GA, Ruini C. The sequential approach to relapse prevention in unipolar depression. World Psychiat 2002; 1:10–15.
154. Fava GA, Ruini C, Rafanelli C, et al. Six-year outcome of cognitive behavior therapy for prevention of recurrent depression. Am J Psychiat 2004; 161:1872–1876.
155. Paykel ES, Scott J, Teasdale JD, et al. Prevention of relapse in residual depression by cognitive therapy. Arch Gen Psychiat 1999; 56:829–835.
156. Paykel ES, Scott J, Cornwall PL, et al. Duration of relapse prevention after cognitive therapy in residual depression: follow-up of controlled trial. Psychol Med 2005; 35:59–68.
157. Scott J, Teasdale JD, Paykel ES, et al. Effects of cognitive therapy on psychological symptoms and social functioning in residual depression. Br J Psychiat 2004; 177:440–446.
158. Ma SH, Teasdale JD. Mindfulness-based cognitive therapy for depression. J Consult Clin Psychol 2004; 72:31–40.

159. Bockting CLH, Schene AH, Spinhoven P, et al. Preventing relapse/recurrence in recurrent depression using cognitive therapy. J Consult Clin Psychol 2005; 73:647–657.

160. Perlis RH, Nierenberg AA, Alpert JE, et al. Effects of adding cognitive therapy to fluoxetine dose increase on risk of relapse and residual depressive symptoms in continuation treatment of major depressive disorder. J Clin Psychopharmacol 2002; 22:474–480.

161. Petersen T, Harley R, Papakostas G, et al. Continuation cognitive behavioral therapy maintains attributional style improvement in depressed patients responding acutely to fluoxetine. Psychol Med 2004; 34:555–561.

162. Fava GA, Ruini C, Rafanelli C, et al. Cognitive behavior approach to loss of clinical effect during long-term antidepressant treatment. Am J Psychiat 2002; 159:2094–2095.

163. Fabbri S. Family intervention approach to loss of clinical effect during antidepressant treatment. Psychother Psychosom 2004; 73:124.

164. Fava GA. Can long-term treatment with antidepressant drugs worsen the course of depression? J Clin Psychiat 2003; 64:123–133.

165. Marks IM. Fears, Phobias, and Rituals: Panic, Anxiety and Their Disorders. New York: Oxford University Press, 1987.

166. Beck AT, Rush AJ, Shaw BF, et al. Cognitive Therapy of Depression. New York: Guilford Press, 1979.

167. Beck AT, Emery G. Anxiety Disorders and Phobias. New York: Basic Books, 1985.

168. Emmelkamp PMG. Self-observation versus flooding in the treatment of agoraphobia. Behav Res Ther 1974; 12:229–237.

169. Ryff CD. Happiness is everything, or is it? Explorations on the meaning of psychological well-being. J Pers Soc Psychol 1989; 57:1069–1081.

170. Rafanelli C, Park SK, Ruini C, et al. Rating well-being and distress. Stress Med 2000; 16:55–61.

171. Fava GA, Rafanelli C, Ottolini F, et al. Psychological well-being and residual symptoms in remitted patients with panic disorder and agoraphobia. J Affect Disord 2001; 65:185–190.

172. Meehl PE. Hedonic capacity: some conjectures. Bull Menninger Clin 1975; 39:295–307.

173. Ellis A, Becker I. A Guide to Personal Happiness. Hollywood, CA: Melvin Powers Wilshire Book Company, 1982.

174. Ryff CD, Singer B. Psychological well-being: meaning, measurement, and implications for psychotherapy research. Psychother Psychosom 1996; 65:14–23.

175. Marks I. Is a paradigm shift occurring in brief psychological treatments? Psychother Psychosom 1999; 68:169.

176. Foa EB, Kozak MJ. Beyond the efficacy ceiling? Cognitive behavior therapy in search of theory. Behav Ther 1997; 28:601–611.

177. Fava GA. Cognitive behavioral therapy. In: Fink M, ed. Encyclopedia of Stress. San Diego, CA: Academic Press, 2000:484–487.

178. Ryff CD, Singer B. The contours of positive human health. Psychol Inquiry 1998; 9:1–28.

6

Combining Medications to Achieve Remission

John M. Zajecka and Corey Goldstein

Department of Psychiatry, Rush University Medical Center, Chicago, Illinois, U.S.A.

Jeremy Barowski

Department of Psychiatry, SUNY Upstate Medical Univeristy, Syracuse, New York, U.S.A.

INTRODUCTION

Depression is currently among the most treatable illnesses that we see in medicine. Similar to any other medical illness, depression should be treated to full remission and, ultimately, to recovery. Remission has now become the standard of treatment for treating individuals with major depression, and should be the goal of treatment for the patient who partially responds in the first episode, or the patient who may have failed to respond to multiple treatments. Unfortunately, up to 50% of patients who "respond" to their antidepressant treatment fail to fully "remit." (1) Residual emotional or physical symptoms of depression jeopardize achieving remission for any individual patient and can also significantly increase the risk of relapse and recurrence (2). There are several possible consequences of failing to achieve remission, including higher rates of relapse and recurrence, continued psychosocial impairments, increased use of medical services, potential worsening of prognosis of any comorbid medical/psychiatric illnesses, ongoing risk of suicide, and at least the theoretical possibility of the patient becoming "treatment resistant" (3,4).

In the last several decades, an abundance of pharmacological, psychological, and other somatic treatment options for the effective treatment of depression have been introduced. There is also growing literature on both the acute and long-term efficacy of these treatments used either alone or in combination with each other. These findings have been extensively discussed in previous chapters. One of the more common themes that has emerged in the last several years is the importance of treating the index episode of depression as aggressively as possible to achieve remission and avoid any potential negative outcomes. Remission remains among the strongest variables that predict whether a patient will do well in the long term (4). In clinical research, one of the accepted definitions of remission is a Hamilton Depression Rating Scale (HAMD-17) score of 7 or less (5–7). This is in contrast to "response," which has been defined as having a minimum of a 50% decrease from baseline in the total HAMD-17 score (5–7). It is not uncommon for patients to respond by having a drop in their baseline HAMD-17 score of more than 50%, but fail then to achieve a remission HAMD-17 score of ≤ 7. In clinical practice, patients are said to be in remission when they are virtually asymptomatic, and over time, have a return of psychosocial functioning to that of their premorbid state (5–7). Remission is still a significant unmet target in the treatment of depression, and clinical expectations are moving toward defining more specific strategies to get depressed patients into full remission and subsequent recovery.

Strategies to Achieve and Sustain Remission

Major depressive disorder (MDD) carries significant morbidity and mortality if not treated or if inadequately treated, the latter being defined as a condition in which a patient may be responding to treatment, but continues to have residual depressive symptoms. The clinician must always consider the risk/benefit ratio of specific treatment strategies that should be tailored to the individual patient. Doing so will provide an optimal acute and long-term response and avoid the risks associated with inadequate response. Educating patients that the goal of treatment is complete symptom resolution is vital, in addition to confirmation of diagnosis and comorbidities. It is also important to ensure adequate dosage and duration of each specific treatment when assessing its success or failure. Inadequate dosing or duration of a "therapeutic dose" is a common error made in what may otherwise appear to be treatment failure. Maximizing the dose of a primary antidepressant should always be considered even for those antidepressants that have not been proven to show a dose–response effect. As discussed in Chapter 4, many of the monotherapy-controlled studies are not adequately powered to reveal these anecdotally reported dose–response findings. Medications such as tricyclics (TCA), monoamine oxidase inhibitors (MAOIs), and ven-lafaxine [a serotonin norepinephrine reuptake inhibitor (SNRI)] are examples of medications that may have a dose–response effect in some patients, and maximizing the dose of a particular antidepressant should be considered as long as it is not at the risk of development of significant tolerability and/or compromising on safety issues. Antidepressant dosages in some patients may be safely increased to the equivalent of 500 mg/day of imipramine (8–10). In such cases, monitoring of the blood levels of the antidepressant or even an electrocardiogram to ensure cardiac safety in such doses may be recommended. While some patients may respond to a treatment within the first two to three weeks of the use of antidepressant, others may not show a response for 12 to 16 weeks, and full response may not be evident until the latter time. Tolerability and safety issues are paramount in treating all depressed patients whether using monotherapy or combination treatments, the clinician needs to remain cognizant of these issues over time because patients may develop comorbid medical illnesses or other factors that may affect the safety and tolerability of a particular treatment. Additionally, clinicians should always remain cognizant of problems with adherence to treatment because it is among the more common causes for failure to achieve and sustain a remission.

If monotherapy with a particular treatment is not effective, the clinician should then consider one of several strategies, including switching the antidepressant, combining antidepressants, or augmenting the antidepressant with another somatic/pharmacological treatment. Additional considerations include psychotherapeutic interventions and other somatic treatments including electroconvulsive therapy (ECT), vagus nerve stimulation, phototherapy, and even "investigational treatments." It is also important for clinicians to remember that symptoms and treatments may change over time to sustain a remission, and the specific strategies should always be tailored to the individual patient.

Treatment-Resistant Depression

Despite the increasing literature on treatment-resistant depression, this population remains poorly defined. This chapter addresses the use of combination treatments in a "treatment-resistant patient"; however, this can describe a patient who is showing a partial response to the first antidepressant, or a patient who has potentially failed to show any response to multiple antidepressant treatment strategies. The various clinical presentations of a treatment-resistant patient include (1) the patient who shows a partial response, yet has residual symptoms of depression; (2) the patient who shows a response or remission and subsequently relapses or suffers a recurrence later in the course of treatment; or (3) the patient who completely fails to respond to treatment. Before making a decision regarding the treatment for any of these patient subtypes, clinicians should always attempt to identify any potentially "modifiable" factors that account for the lack of an acute or long-term remission; these factors include an accurate diagnosis, failure to achieve remission of the index episode, an inadequate trial of the treatment (dose and/or duration), problems with adherence, intolerance to treatment, inaccurate assessment of response, and psychosocial factors that prevent a full remission. Managing any of these modifiable factors should always be considered when facing a patient who appears to be resistant to treatment, whether it is the first treatment or a failure to respond to multiple treatment trials.

Managing these patients also includes confirming the presence or absence of all potential diagnoses, especially other Axis I disorders that may be contributing to what may otherwise appear to be depressive symptoms or loss of an initial response. Examples include the discovery of a patient with a bipolar disorder, psychosis, substance use disorder, anxiety disorder, or eating disorder. It is important to consider the role of Axis II disorders in contributing to a lack of achieving an optimal antidepressant response, and clinicians should be encouraged to treat the Axis I disorder aggressively. Axis II traits can improve when the underlying mood disorder is improved, particularly for those patients with chronic or recurrent mood disorders. It is also important that clinicians keep reasonable expectations about overt Axis II pathology that may improve the outcome of a psychosocial management strategy. Additionally, Axis III disorders, considering the role of ongoing or new medical illnesses that may complicate an underlying depression, are part of the acute and long-term management strategies for any clinician who treats depression.

MAKING THE DECISION TO SWITCH, COMBINE, OR AUGMENT AN ANTIDEPRESSANT

When a patient is failing to respond optimally to a particular antidepressant treatment, the clinician is faced with making a decision to either switch to another antidepressant, combine the existing antidepressant with another, or sometimes, "bridge" one antidepressant with another with the intention of stopping the first antidepressant. While there is a growing literature in regard to providing guidelines for clinical practice based upon clinical research, it is still important for the clinician to tailor their decision to an individual patient's needs. Before making a decision to switch, combine, or augment, it is imperative to ensure that the dose of the antidepressant has been maximized for an adequate duration of time, the latter at least four to six weeks of an adequate dose, although other factors such as suicidality, psychotic symptoms, persistant anxiety or severity of the underlying depression are examples of situations where combining or augmenting may need to occur at an earlier time. The quality of published reports on combining or augmenting antidepressants to achieve optimal responses has improved over the last several years; however, there are still significant methodological flaws with many of the studies. The assessment of baseline severity and comorbidity before the initiation of the primary antidepressant, the variety of patient subtypes including severity, chronicity, and history of treatment resistance of the depressive subtypes, and also whether the study is placebo controlled or is based on open-label or case reports are factors that can impact what we extrapolate from the clinical research literature. There is an apparent gap in the evidence base where polypharmacy of MDD is concerned. In short, the clinician should remain on top of the current literature in regard to combining or augmenting antidepressants in specific patient populations and must keep in mind the methodology of published studies in terms of extrapolating the use of such strategies in their own clinical practice. It is always helpful to be able to refer to published literature when using specific strategies, especially when documenting this in the patient's chart as well as when obtaining informed consent from the patient. The clinician may feel more comfortable utilizing a strategy that has been well-substantiated in the literature with double-blind, placebo-controlled trials that demonstrate both safety and efficacy compared to an open series of case reports that suggests efficacy and may be limited in describing safety and tolerability limits.

In addition to staying informed on the evidence in the literature in regard to safety and efficacy, some other factors that clinicians must take into account when deciding what to do when the initial antidepressant fails to provide remission include the cost of treatment, the potential for drug interactions, adherence, the rapidity of response, the type of symptoms that the patient continues to present with, family history, previous past history, and the degree of symptomology. When the clinician is faced with the choice of either augmenting or combining an antidepressant, there are some very basic guidelines that may help make that decision. Our group finds that, if a patient has less than 25% efficacy after an adequate dose and duration, we may be more likely to consider switching the antidepressant, rather than augmenting with a pharmacological agent that alone may not have inherent antidepressant effects. In this process, the clinician can consider combining two antidepressants as long as there are no issues with safety or tolerability. If the patient remits in the process of the switch during this "bridging" of antidepressants, they may choose to continue the patient on the combination. For the patient who shows a greater than 50% effect to a particular antidepressant, the clinician may err toward augmenting that antidepressant with another pharmacological strategy to "enhance" the primary antidepressant effect, rather than risk switching to an antidepressant that may not provide the same degree of improvement as the initial treatment. Finally, for those patients who fall between 25% to 50% improvement, switching versus augmenting the primary antidepressant needs to take into account the factors mentioned above, including questions such as: Is this the first treatment the patient failed, or is it the tenth treatment of a totally different class of antidepressants?

There are a number of practical issues to consider when augmenting or combining antidepressants. It is important to tailor the choice of the treatment to the symptoms. It is also important to consider "synergistic" pharmacological profiles. For example, if the individual is on a selective serotonin reuptake inhibitor (SSRI), adding a noradrenergic or dopaminergic agent may be warranted (atomoxetine, stimulants, bupropion). For depressed patients who have comorbid illnesses that contribute to the underlying residual symptomology, using pharmacological strategies to target those symptoms may be warranted, examples of which include: for attention deficit disorder, adding a stimulant, modafinil, or atomoxetine; for obsessive-compulsive symptoms, premenstrual dysphoric disorder symptoms, or eating disorders, the use of an SSRI may be warranted; for anxiety disorders, using buspirone, benzodiazepines, or even atypical antipsychotics may be considered; and for bipolar disorders, the use of lithium, lamotrigine, carbamazepine, or atypical antipsychotics may be considered. Morever, side effects from the primary antidepressant may guide a clinician to choose a particular pharmacological strategy. For example, a patient who may be suffering sexual side effects and continues to have depressive symptoms may benefit from adding bupropion or a stimulant. Another example is the patient who may be showing a partial antidepressant response, but has symptoms of "asthenia" (apathy, fatigue, blunted affect, etc.) and for whom adding a stimulant, bupropion, atomoxetine, or modafinil may be helpful. Finally, checking for psychotic symptoms that can often be subtle in many patients and the addition of an antipsychotic may bring the patient who fails to optimally respond to treatment to a complete response. All of these are examples of the art and science of managing patients who are failing to remit on the current antidepressant. Data concerning these strategies is limited but will be covered later in this chapter.

If the clinician chooses to switch an antidepressant, it should be considered whether to overlap the two antidepressants or to wash out the first antidepressant before starting the second. The disadvantages of washing out may be the possibility of worsening of underlying symptoms, prolonging the depressive symptoms, and the patient experiencing a possible antidepressant discontinuation syndrome. On the other hand, the advantages of washing out medications may be the prevention of potential drug interactions or additive side effects in some patients. Clearly, there are some antidepressants that are absolutely prohibited owing to tolerability issues and, more importantly, safety concerns. Examples of these include the use of MAOIs with most other antidepressants without an adequate washout to avoid the potential for hypertensive reactions, a serotonin syndrome, or cardiovascular effect (8–10). Overlapping treatments may help avoid the possibility of an antidepressant discontinuation syndrome when moving to the use of an anti-depressant with a similar pharmacodynamical profile. Titrating down the first antidepressant, while titrating up the second antidepressant is another alternative. Combining antidepressants during a switch may give the patient an opportunity to show an enhanced efficacy, particularly when using anti-depressants with different pharmacological profiles. An example may be when moving from an SSRI to bupropion. In summary, the clinician should not only take into consideration the issue of efficacy, but it is imperative that they be aware of drug interactions, safety, tolerability, cost, and issues around adherence.

DOCUMENTATION DURING THE MANAGEMENT OF COMBINATION STRATEGIES

It is important for clinicians to keep written records of past and current treatments (including the doses, duration of each dose, and descriptions of tolerability as well as efficacy) available at all times. Our group finds it helpful for patients to use some form of life charting techniques to ascertain the level of subjective and objective improvement that the patient experiences, as well as to serve as an additional tool to show patterns of response, adherence, and other potential factors that may impact the outcome (e.g., menstrual cycle, substance use, and other factors). It is important to obtain informed consent before all interventions, especially when using combination strategies that are not Food and Drug Administration (FDA) approved. This informed consent should describe the risk and benefit to the patient, explaining in detail the nonapproved status of these combinations and their side effects, even though they may be well documented in the literature. It is important to let the patient ask questions, and to involve significant others whenever possible. The patient should be kept updated with information and it should be documented that the information was provided to the patient. When there is an absence of literature, clinicians may rely on theoretical ideas of clinical utility which suggests that certain deficiencies in specific neurotransmitter systems may be the underlying cause of specific depressive symptoms. For example, a MDD patient who remains fatigued and unable to concentrate may preferentially benefit from the use of a drug that enhances noradrenergic activity. The modern psycho-pharmacologist must become adept in this art and science of treating depression, stay informed about innovative treatment strategies including combination strategies, and finally be able to explain these options coherently to the patient.

Clinicians should feel comfortable when seeking second opinions or consultations either to confirm diagnoses or to confer with experts on the use of particular combination treatment strategies, including expertise in particular somatic, psychosocial treatments, or investigational treatments.

Tailoring the treatment to the needs of the individual over time is part of the art and science of treating any patient with major depression to achieve optimal recovery.

AUGMENTATION

Lithium

Since the serendipitous discovery of the use of lithium as a mood-stabilizing compound in 1948, few individual psychotropics have been able to match lithium's contribution to biological psychiatry.

The antidepressant mechanism of lithium is thought to result from the potentiation of sensitization on the postsynaptic serotonergic receptors and from the presynaptic enhancement of serotonin transmission by lithium (11). Other hypotheses include effects on monoamine receptor sensitivity, simple additive effects of two antidepressants, and lithium's effect on noradrenergic and dopaminergic systems (12).

The literature is full of studies documenting the effect of lithium on TCA-resistant depression. The first report of the use of adjunct lithium in the treatment of TCA-resistant depression comes from deMontigny et al. (13) who conducted an open, uncontrolled study of unipolar depressives. The response to lithium potentiation was reported to be dramatic and occurred within 48 hours of its initiation. Since that report, there have been numerous uncontrolled studies or anecdotal reports on the effectiveness of lithium in TCA-resistant patients. Results from double-blind, controlled studies subsequently supported the data from the previous studies (11,12). One study evaluated the effects of lithium potentiation on TCA compared to placebo to rule out direct antidepressant effects of lithium; the results support the hypothetical synergism of lithium and TCA, rather than the antidepressant effects of lithium alone (11). However, in both of these studies, the small number of subjects is a methodological shortcoming (14).

Lithium augmentation for psychotic depression is reported in the literature. Several case reports suggest the efficacy of lithium potentiation in either TCA or TCA/neuroleptic treatment failures (15–17). As suggested in antidepressant monotherapy with lithium, a more favorable efficacy for lithium augmentation is suggested in bipolar rather than unipolar depression (15). The utilization of lithium potentiation on depressed geriatric patients who are either unresponsive to conventional treatment or who cannot tolerate the side effects of increased doses of TCA is reported to be beneficial (18,19). A review of the literature reports no significant adverse events from the combination of TCA and lithium.

With the beginning of a new era in the treatment of depressive disorders in the early 1980s, lithium quickly became one of the most accepted choices of augmentation to SSRIs and, subsequently, SNRIs. As a result, the literature is full of case reports, open-label studies, retrospective analyses, and some randomized controlled trials on the subject matter. To be fair, the majority of patients included in studies where lithium was added to a conventional antidepressant medication are classified as "treatment failures" on the primary antidepressant medication, or "treatment resistant"/ "treatment refractory." As a result, methodological drawbacks make it difficult to compare patient populations to those studies that are simply evaluating the efficacy of a primary antidepressant medication.

A review of 23 controlled and uncontrolled studies evaluating the efficacy of monotherapy with lithium for the treatment of depression suggests that lithium has reasonable antidepressant properties (20). Unfortunately, many of the studies have methodological flaws that fail to uniformly select for previous failures to other treatment.

Bauer et al. reviewed 27 studies including double-blind, placebo-controlled, randomized comparator, and open-label trials, and a total of 803 patients with refractory depression who were augmented with either lithium or placebo (21). In the acute-treatment trials, the average response rate in the lithium-augmented group was 45% versus 18% in the placebo-controlled (21). The trials noted that lithium augmentation should be continued for a minimum of 12 months (21). Unfortunately, only a few placebo-controlled trials examined lithium's efficacy with SSRIs or other antidepressants (21).

With particular interest on remission, Bauer et al. conducted a four-month randomized, parallel-group, double-blind, placebo-controlled trial of lithium augmentation during the continuation treatment of 30 patients with a refractory major depressive episode who had responded to acute lithium augmentation during a six-week open study (22). Relapses (including one suicide) occurred in 47% of patients who had received placebo in addition to antidepressants (22). None of the patients who received lithium suffered a relapse (22).

Nierenberg et al. conducted a systematic follow up of depressed patients with documented refractoriness to antidepressants, treated with lithium augmentation (23). Sixty-six patients were followed in a retrospective, naturalistic design for approximately 29 months to assess their longitudinal course (23). At followup, 29% had poor outcomes (e.g., hospitalization, suicide/death, or attempt), 23% fair outcomes (return of depressive symptoms only after two weeks), and 48% had good outcomes (did not meet criteria for poor or fair) (23). An important finding in this report suggested that an acute positive response to lithium augmentation predicted a good maintenance course (23).

Choosing lithium as an augmentation strategy to an antidepressant medication can be challenging. Despite lithium's well-documented augmentation data regarding efficacy, it is also associated with potential tolerability issues. In addition, truths and misconceptions regarding lithium have developed throughout the years of its use. With the availability of a large and growing number of treatment strategies, it is not uncommon for patients to associate lithium with negative misperceptions as an older, less commonly used medication; therefore, it is crucial that the clinician address these issues to increase patient comfort.

Although dosing strategies need to be clarified, augmentation can be carried out initially with 300 mg at bedtime, increasing to a range between 600 and 1200 mg/day in twice daily dosing within two to three weeks. While clinical correlation is best in determining efficacy, checking a predose morning lithium level approximately four to five days after the last adjustment is warranted. A typical "therapeutic window" for lithium is between 0.8 and 1.2 in the treatment of bipolar disorder, although significantly lower levels can be effective in unipolar depression when lithium is added to an antidepressant. Lithium's negative effects on organ systems include its ability to impede the release of thyroid hormones, to impair cardiac sinus mode function, and the urine-concentrating mechanism of the kidneys (24). As a result, the clinician should perform routine laboratory testing, including serum creatinine concentrations, electrolytes, thyroid function, a complete blood count, electocardiogram, and a pregnancy test in women of childbearing age (24). It should be noted that lithium may be quite useful in the treatment of the depressed patient with a history of "soft" bipolar symptoms or a family history of bipolarity.

There is an extensive literature on the use of lithium, suggesting positive acute and long-term efficacy. The use of lithium remains among the most well-documented augmentation strategies in the treatment resistant/refractory patient. However, more randomized controlled trials are needed to assess the efficacy of lithium potentiation, especially with newer antidepressants. In addition, more data are needed on dosing acutely and chronically, duration of treatment, and the addition of lithium to unique present-day, first-line strategies.

Thyroid Hormone

For over a century, it has been reported that depression is associated with thyroid abnormalities. Both hypo- and hyperthyroid states are correlated with affective disturbances, and the correction of the underlying thyroid dysfunction often alleviates affective symptoms. This association has led to the utilization of thyroid hormones in the treatment of depression. The first studies examining the effects of thyroid hormones in depression were conducted in the 1950s and showed an improvement in the symptoms following the use of triiodothyronine (T_3) (25,26). In 1969, Prange et al. (27) reported on the effects of thyroid hormones in depression using controlled, double-blind designs. Results suggest shortening the latency of TCA action (at least in women), and effective antidepressant activity in TCA-resistant patients (men and women). Replication of these findings shows that the addition of thyroid hormone to TCA in euthyroid patients can increase the efficacy of TCA and accelerate the onset of action (28–30). Many reports on uncontrolled studies in the 1970s are suggestive of TCA/T_3 combination being effective in a substantial number of patients who were unresponsive to monotherapy with a TCA. The usual dose of T_3 was 25 µg/day, and imipramine and amitriptyline were the TCAs most often used (31–35). Goodwin et al. (36) in a double-blind, but not placebo-controlled study reported that depressed patients unresponsive to TCA benefit from the addition of T_3. Thase et al. (37) reported on a sample of 20 depressed outpatients who were unresponsive to 12 weeks or more of imipramine administration, as well as to potentiation of imipramine with T_3 at 25 µg/day. This study did not validate the previous findings.

Sokolov et al. reported on a nonrandomized study of 24 patients without placebo control (38). Thyroid function was measured before antidepressant treatment following failure of acute desipramine treatment, but before T_3 augmentation (38). T_3 augmentation responders were found to have lower levels of thyroid stimulating hormone (TSH) (2.36 ± 0.75 vs. 3.29 ± 0.88) and higher levels of T_4 and free thyroxine index than nonresponders (35.25 ± 4.63 vs. 29.92 ± 6.60) (38). After antidepressant failure, prior to augmentation, TSH was lower in patients who went on to respond to T_3 (38). The findings suggest that T_3 augmentation response is associated with lower levels of TSH and elevations in the levels of T_4 and free thyroxine index present before antidepressant treatment (38).

Aronson et al. completed a meta-analysis of eight studies and 292 patients, addressing the efficacy of liothyronine sodium therapy in euthyroid, nonpsychotic depressed patients refractory to TCA therapy (39). Patients treated with liothyronine sodium augmentation were twice as likely to respond as controls. This corresponded to a 23.3% improvement in response rates, and a moderately large improvement in depression (39).

Joffe et al. completed a two-week randomized, double-blind, placebo-controlled study of 50 patients with unipolar refractory depression to desipramine or imipramine, by comparing the efficacy of lithium and liothyronine as augmenting agents (40). Both augmenting agents were more effective than placebo in reducing HAM-D scores, although there were no statistically significant differences between lithium (9/17 responded) and liothyronine (10/17 responded) (40).

In another study, Joffe and Singer completed a three-week, 40-patient, randomized, double-blind study in which subjects who had failed a trial of imipramine or desipramine were given either T_3 or T_4 in addition to their antidepressant (41). Fifty-three percent of subjects responded to T_3, whereas 19% responded to T_4 (41). This study would suggest that the T_3 hormone may be a better choice as an augmenting agent.

There are three reported cases in the literature of MAOI/T_3 combination efficacy in MAOI-resistant depression. The first report involves a rapid alleviation of depressive symptoms when T_3 was added to a combination of phenelzine and thiothixene in a woman who had blunted TSH response to thyroid releasing hormone (TRH) stimulation (42). The other report involved amelioration of depressive symptoms in two patients after T_3 was added to phenelzine, or phenelzine and lithium (43). Further controlled studies are needed to clearly define the safety and efficacy of thyroid hormone enhancement in MAOI-refractory depression.

Nearly all of the reports of using T_3 in doses ranging between 25 and 50 µg/day added to TCAs have found this combination to be safe. There are no reports of increased serious side effects caused by the individual agents or any unusual side effects (27,35,36). T_3 does not have any apparent effect on the TCA blood levels (44). T_3 has the potential to be associated with cardiotoxic effects, and the use of catecholamine-enhancing antidepressants have increased cardiovascular effects in hyperthyroid states with that stated, the combination of TCA and T_3 in therapeutic doses does not appear to have any adverse effects on cardiac function (35,36). Additionally, long-term use may be associated with an increased risk of osteoporosis (10).

The mechanism of T_3 in potentiating antidepressant response is speculative. Other proposed mechanisms of the TCA/T_3 antidepressant combination include synergism between T_3 and catecholamines. Another mechanism suggests that thyroid hormones increase the sensitivity of beta-receptors and, thus, improve the existing pool of catecholamines thought to be involved in the onset of depression (45). It is suggested that depression may be characterized by changes in the hypothalamic–pituitary–thyroid axis. While overt hypothyroidism is not commonly found in depressed persons, occult thyroid abnormalities may be present in approximately 25% of depressed persons, based on a blunted TSH response to TRH stimulation (46).

Buspirone

Buspirone is a novel anxiolytic with agonist properties at the 5HT-1A receptor, and possible activity at the $5HT_2$ receptor, as well as the D2 receptor (9). Although it is used primarily in the treatment of generalized anxiety, buspirone has been considered a safe alternative in the treatment of depressive disorders (9,47). The efficacy of buspirone as a monotherapy for depression with comorbid generalized anxiety disorder (GAD) in doses up to 90 mg/day has been demonstrated (48,49). Buspirone has also been used to reduce SSRI-induced sexual dysfunction, with this ameliorating activity probably secondary to its unique receptor profile.

Landen et al. conducted a four-week 119-patient double-blind, placebo-controlled trial of buspirone in combination with an SSRI in the treatment of patients with treatment-refractory depression (50). A total of 50.9% of patients in the buspirone group and 46.7% in the placebo group responded after four weeks of treatment (50). While the study was limited by some methodological drawbacks, there was no statistically significant difference between treatment groups. However, 69.4% of the patients responded in the poststudy treatment phase with an SSRI plus buspirone (50), and there were no reported statistically significant differences in the frequency of adverse effects (50).

Appelberg et al. completed a placebo-controlled, randomized, double-blind, placebo wash-in study of 102 outpatients who had failed to respond to an SSRI for a minimum of six weeks (51). These patients were assigned to either placebo or buspirone (10–30 mg twice daily) augmentation for six weeks. At the end point of the study, it was found that there was no significant difference between buspirone and placebo (51). Patients with initially high Montgomery-Åsberg Depression Rating Scale (MADRS) scores (greater than 30) showed a greater reduction ($p = 0.26$) in the buspirone group compared to those in the placebo group (51). No significant side effects were noted in either the placebo or the buspirone groups (51).

It should be noted that there are at least three open-label trials that do show efficacy with this combination regimen. Inherent problems with these studies are the lack of a placebo group as well as blinding. While it is necessary to further study buspirone for potential antidepressant effect, it may be of great value for its safety and low incidence of adverse effects. In addition, this medication may be considered for use in patients who have residual or comorbid anxiety symptoms or iatrogenic sexual dysfunction associated with the use of the primary antidepressant.

Lamotrigine

Lamotrigine is currently FDA approved for use in the prevention of relapse/recurrence of both mania and depression in bipolar disorder patients (52). Additionally, lamotrigine may be efficacious either as a monotherapy or as an augmentation agent for depression—either bipolar or unipolar subtypes—and has shown efficacy in lengthening relapse into a depressive episode in individuals diagnosed with bipolar disorder at a dose of 200 mg/day (53). Its favorable adverse effect profile has catapulted this treatment into the realm of antidepressant augmentation and, in some cases, has been used successfully as a monotherapy in the treatment of depressive disorders. With that stated, lamotrigine has very little published data in the area of treatment of unipolar depression. Theoretically, lamotrigine makes sense in that it modulates glutamate and other transmitters and increases plasma serotonin levels, and is a weak inhibitor of $5HT_3$ receptors (54).

Barbee and Jamhour conducted a retrospective chart review of lamotrigine augmentation (for an average of 41.8 weeks; average dose 112.90 mg/day) in 37 individuals with chronic or recurrent unipolar major depression, who had failed to respond adequately to at least two previous trials of antidepressants (55). Based on intent-to-treat analysis, response rates were: 40.5% much or very much improved, 21.6% mildly improved, and 37.8% unchanged (55). The results suggest that lamotrigine is efficacious as an augmentation agent, especially in patients with shorter duration depression and with fewer antidepressant trials (55).

Further studies are warranted to ascertain lamotrigine's efficacy as a monotherapy as well as an augmenting agent to antidepressant in both unipolar and bipolar depression (56). In considering lamotrigine for the treatment of either bipolar or unipolar depression, doses as low as 50 mg may provide efficacy with additional benefit, with a target dose of 200 mg/day. The usual treatment regimen guidelines for bipolar disorders is 25 mg/day with increases of 25 to 50 mg increments every two weeks toward a target dose of 200 mg/day (52). While lamotrigine is generally well tolerated, patients need to be educated about the risk of potential rash and Stevens–Johnson syndrome (52). This drug must be dosed carefully and precisely in that drug interactions with carbamazepine, valproate, oxcarbazepine as well as atypical antipsychotics such as aripiprazole and risperidone, may occur. Lamotrigine's role in the treatment of the depressed patient who has "soft" symptoms of bipolarity such as persistent recurrent depression or a family history of bipolar disorder should be considered.

Stimulants

It has long been known that stimulants such as amphetamine, methylphenidate, and pemoline have mood-elevating effects. Amphetamine is an indirect-acting sympathomimetic agent with some direct agonist properties, which exerts its stimulant properties via direct neuronal release of dopamine and norepinephrine, blockade of catecholamine reuptake, and weak monoamine oxidase inhibition (57). Methylphenidate is structurally and mechanistically related to amphetamine (58), and pemoline is a stimulant hypothesized to augment catecholamine transmission (58).

A review of the use of stimulants in the treatment of depression demonstrates several uncontrolled reports and little controlled data supporting the antidepressant effects of this treatment, either as monotherapy or as an augmentation strategy. The data appear to support stimulants more as an augmentation rather than monotherapy for depression (10,59).

Augmentation of TCAs with methylphenidate is suggested to be effective in rectifying TCA monotherapy failures (60). This suggestion is based on the report of five out of seven tricyclic-resistant patients failing an adequate trial of either imipramine or nortriptyline when methylphenidate was added at a dose of 20 mg/day (60). However, one patient experienced a manic episode, and another died from a cerebral vascular accident after two years on the combination (60). While several patients in this report showed an increase in the TCA level, which may account for the antidepressant mechanism of the combination, the antidepressant mechanism may also be accounted for by an additive or synergistic effect.

Additionally, uncontrolled reports suggest efficacy of augmenting TCA partial responders with dextroamphetamine (5–20 mg/day) (61).

The combination of MAOIs with stimulants in treatment-resistant depression is frequently avoided following reported cases of hyperthermic and hypertensive crises (some fatal) cited in the literature (62–65). However, there is more recent evidence that the combination of MAOIs and stimulants may prove to be both safe and effective in treatment-resistant patients when used properly. Feighner et al. (66) treated 13 patients with intractable depression who responded to the addition of amphetamine or methylphenidate to an MAOI with or without a TCA. Clinically significant side effects included orthostatic hypotension and, in three patients, anxiety, restlessness, agitation, or irritability (66). Two patients complained of dizziness, nausea, impairment of short-term memory, and insomnia (66), while one patient developed hypomania (66).

Fawcett et al. reported a retrospective, naturalistic study of 32 treatment-resistant patients who were augmented with either pemoline or dextroamphetamine after a partial or complete nonresponse to an adequate trial of an MAOI for a mean time of 22.3 months (67). Based on clinical global impression (CGI) scores, 78% of the 32 patients had a good response to at least one stimulant plus MAOI, with 53.8% reporting being "very much" or "much improved" (67). It should be noted that 3 out of 32 patients developed manic episodes (67). There was no evidence of serious adverse events. It should be noted that these papers should be referenced carefully to use this combination, because there is risk of hypertensive crisis if inaccurate application is used.

In the attempt to avoid the typical two-to-four week latency associated with tricyclic antidepressants, Gwirtsman et al. conducted a three-to-four week open-label trial of 20 depressed patients, in which both tricyclic therapy and methylphenidate were started concurrently (68). By the end of week 1, 30% of the patients responded to the TCA + methylphenidate hydrochloride, and 63% responded by the end of week 2 (68). Ultimately, 85% demonstrated improvement, based on CGI scores at the time of discharge (68).

These studies were uncontrolled and used concomitant psychotropics, including TCAs, thyroid enhancement, lithium, and other mood stabilizers. It is possible that the safety of adding a stimulant to an MAOI may be enhanced with concomitant use of a TCA, because there is evidence that the use of amitriptyline may protect against potential tyramine reactions (69); however, not all of the patients were on TCAs in these trials.

There is a report in the literature of one case using amphetamine to potentiate the antidepressant effects of fluoxetine (70). The patient failed to respond to a combination of imipramine potentiated with amphetamine (45 mg three times a day). He subsequently responded to a combination of fluoxetine (60 mg/day) and amphetamine (45 mg three times a day). Relapse of depressive symptoms was reported with attempts to discontinue the use of the amphetamine. We reported eight patients who had been given methylphenidate (10–40 mg/day) in addition to fluoxetine (20–80 mg/day), with a sustained antidepressant response for at least six months in two patients (10). In addition, we reported on a case where pemoline (37.5 mg twice a day) was added to fluoxetine (80 mg/day) with a sustained antidepressant response in one patient who had failed a number of other adequate antidepressant trials, some of which included pemoline potentiation. None of the cases combining either methylphenidate or pemoline had significant adverse events. The use of stimulants for medically ill, depressed patients in uncontrolled reports indicates a potential therapeutic role for this population (57). Finally, evidence indicates that the use of stimulants may combat the hypotensive effects of conventional antidepressants (71).

On the whole, the use of stimulants in the treatment of depression demonstrate little evidence of tolerance (57). Our own experience with the use of stimulants also suggests little evidence for abuse potential when used judiciously. The use of stimulants plays a very important potential role in the treatment of depressive disorders, particularly in patients with treatment-resistant depressions and depression associated with low energy, anhedonia, and comorbid attention-deficit hyperactivity disorder (ADHD). Obviously, well-controlled studies are needed to elaborate on their potential safety and efficacy.

Atypical Antipsychotics

There is a growing literature on the use of atypical antipsychotics as augmentation to anti-depressant medications. Atypical anti-psychotics act primarily by blocking the D2 and $5HT_{2A}$ receptors. They may also modulate in varying degrees several additional serotonin sub-receptors (such as $5HT_3$, $5HT_{1B}$, $5HT_{2B}$) and inhibit the reuptake of norepinephrine and serotonin. Each drug in this class possesses a unique receptor profile which can help the physician pick the appropriate therapy for the individual patient. Some of the above mechanisms at serotonin sub-receptors also apply to certain FDA approved anti-depressants (e.g., mirtazapine, nefazodone, trazodone), increasing the possibility that the atypical antipsychotics may be effective treatments for anxiety and depression.

The net result of $5HT_{2A}$ antagonism is the reversal of D2 blockade in the nigrostiatal pathway (responsible for extrapyramidal symptoms), the tuberoinfundibular pathway responsible for hyperprolactinemia), and the mesocortical pathway (responsible for negative symptoms). This differentiates the atypicals from conventional antipsychotics, and greatly improves the side effect profile. This blockade may facilitate serotonergic activity comparable to conventional antidepressants and may allow for mesocortical dopaminergic activity to actually increase. Unfortunately, we have come to learn that the newer atypical antipsychotics that seemingly have less serious problems may actually have an entirely new set of issues to deal with. Possible type II diabetes mellitus (glucose intolerance, insulin resistance), increased lipids, and weight gain are some examples of the potential risk of developing "the metabolic syndrome" associated with some agents in this new class of drugs. While increasing data suggest that the use of some atypical antipsychotics appears to cause a higher incidence of these problems, it is uniformly recommended to monitor metabolic parameters at baseline and regular intervals with all atypical antipsychotics set forth according to the guidelines provided by the American Psychiatric Association and the American Diabetes Association (72). With regard to the above-stated suggestion, the clinician must use careful judgment in the administration of these drugs in combination with antidepressant medications, coupled with patient education and regular monitoring. Moreover, because these are dopamine-blocking drugs, the typical warnings exist for the monitoring of all extrapyramidal syndromes.

Olanzapine

Shelton et al. conducted an eight-week, randomized, double-blind trial of 28 patients with treatment-resistant unipolar depression, to assess the efficacy and safety of olanzapine with fluoxetine or either agent alone (73). Olanzapine plus fluoxetine produced significantly greater improvement than either monotherapy from baseline—Montgomery-Asberg Depression Rating: combination, –13.6; olanzapine, –2.8; fluoxetine, –1.2 and CGI: combination, –2.0; olanzapine, 0.0; fluoxetine, –0.4 (73). Increased appetite and weight gain occurred significantly among patients treated with olanzapine (73). There were no significant differences between treatment groups with regard to extrapyramidal symptoms or adverse drug interactions.

Risperidone

Hirose and Ashby completed a six-week, 36-patient open-pilot study of fluvoxamine plus risperidone as an initial antidepressant therapy (74). Among the study completers, 76% achieved remission (vs. 20–30% remission rate of six-week SSRI treatment), 17% achieved response, and two were not responsive (74). Adverse effects were mild, without cases of extra pyramidal symptoms (EPS), nausea, or vomiting (74).

Ziprasidone

In an open-label trial conducted by Papakostas et al., 20 patients with MDD who had failed to respond to an adequate trial of an SSRI were treated with ziprasidone for six weeks (75). At the end of the trial, 61.5% were classified as responders with 38.5% remittance (75). Intent-to-treat analysis showed a 50% response and 25% remittance (75). The use of ziprasidone appeared safe with no severe adverse events and no clinically significant QTc prolongation (75).

Other Studies with Atypical Antipsychotics

Barbee et al. conducted a retrospective chart review of 76 medication trials in 49 patients to determine the effectiveness of olanzapine, risperidone, quetiapine, and ziprasidone as augmentation agents in patients with treatment-resistant depression (76). The overall response rate was 65%. The difference between baseline and final global assessment of functioning scores was statistically significant only in the olanzapine (57%) and risperidone (33%) groups (76). With regard to side effects it was found that weight gain was associated with olanzapine; nausea, anxiety, and depression were associated with risperidone; and sedation was associated with quetiapine and ziprasidone (76).

Our group has completed open-label studies of escitalopram plus quetiapine as well as SSRI or SNRI plus aripiprazole with significant improvement in rating scales such as the HAM-D17, HAM-A, CGI, and MADRS.

Although not specific to the treatment of unipolar depression, quetiapine and olanzapine have strong data in support of their use in the treatment of bipolar depression. Quetiapine has been shown to provide good efficacy at doses of 300 mg/day as well as 600 mg/day as a monotherapy with good tolerability in bipolar depression (77). Tohen et al., have completed a randomized, controlled study assessing olanzapine and placebo versus olanzapine combined with fluoxetine (78). Both groups showed statistically significant improvement in depressive symptoms.

Our group routinely uses all of the atypical antipsychotics in combination with antidepressants from all classes in varying dosages, with good success. As with other augmenting strategies, the inherent nature or treatment profile of the drug may be helpful in the treatment of a depressive disorder. An example would be the use of an atypical antipsychotic with sedation property to improve a case of sleep disturbance associated with depression. Another example would be the case of a depressed patient who presents clinically in a nonpsychotic fashion, but may have an underlying degree of psychosis, as in delusional guilt or rumination. In addition, the inherent receptor profile of the atypical antipsychotic drugs may be reason enough to use them as an antidepressant strategy. The pharmacodynamic profile of each second generation antipsychotic should allow reasonable serotonergic modulation. The two most recently approved atypicals, ziprasidone and aripiprazole, have the greatest propensity to manipulate multiple serotonin targets.

Benzodiazepines

Over 60% of patients with depression suffer from anxiety symptoms. Residual anxiety symptoms are common, yet can potentially aggravate the depression, and anxiety remains one of the greatest predictors of imminent suicide in depression. Benzodiazepines are effective anxiolytic medications offering rapid reduction in anxiety symptoms. Many negative perceptions secondary to potential abuse can be a barrier in the use of these highly effective medications. The role of acute reduction in anxious symptoms in the treatment of depression is important. There is little data on long-term use or in the treatment of residual and/or comorbid anxiety.

Benzodiazepine augmentation may be one of the more popular strategies employed by physicians, although there are little data to support it as well as little data to refute this strategy. If one were to consider the HAM-D, about one third of the items on this scale would count as "anxiety symptoms." The use of benzodiazepines will often lower the score on this scale to 30% within a few days if adequate doses of sedative are used. The ability to increase gamma-aminobutyric acid (GABA) activity with these medications may allow for an abrupt cessation of some key depressive symptoms.

Furukawa et al. completed a meta-analysis of nine randomized, controlled studies with 679 adult patients who were followed for up to eight weeks to determine whether antidepressant–benzodiazepine treatment was more efficacious than treatment with antidepressant alone in treating major depression (79). Based on intent-to-treat analysis, the treatment with the combination group was more likely, 63% versus 38%, to show response in four weeks (79).

Smith et al. completed an eight-week, double-blind, randomized study of 80 patients rated as markedly or moderately ill given fluoxetine (20–40 mg/day) plus placebo, or fluoxetine plus clonazepam (0.5–1.0 mg/day) (80). Patients in both treatment groups improved over the course of the study with regard to HAM-D scores, although the change in scores was more significant in the augmentation group within the first week ($p = 0.002$), at day 10, and at day 21 ($p < 0.001$) (80). No serious adverse events were found in either treatment group. Taper effects were modest and transitory (80).

Our group favors alprazolam (immediate- and long-acting preparations), lorazepam, and clonazepam for the above-stated purpose with the emphasis on rapid relief of depression-associated anxiety symptoms, and commonly for long-term maintenance to sustain recovery. Treatment with these medications can be short-term (approximately four to six weeks), or sustained as above, and is scheduled once daily to three times daily at relatively low doses. We have found that those patients who suggest continuation of the benzodiazepine medication beyond the initial acute treatment may be suffering from a comorbid anxiety disorder. We have also found that collaborating with patients on dosing and frequency is an effective strategy in determining an appropriate schedule with additional doses as needed for "breakthrough anxiety." This needs to be balanced with abuse potential, sedation, alcohol intake, and coadministration with other central nervous system–sedating agents.

Pindolol

Pindolol is a beta-adrenergic blocker that is also an antagonist and partial agonist at 5HT1A receptors (54). It has been theorized that pindolol can immediately disinhibit serotonin neurons, leading to the proposal that it may be a rapid onset antidepressant, or facilitating or augmenting agent (54). There are clinical studies that do suggest that pindolol augmentation may speed the onset of action of SSRIs, but there is little additionally supportive data (54).

Isaac conducted a 42-day randomized, double-blind, placebo-controlled study of 80 patients who were given milnacipran plus pindolol or milnacipran plus placebo (81). Improvement in MADRS total score was greater in the pindolol group from day 7 (mean change from baseline: –9.6 vs. –5.3) (81). CGI improvement was significant with 97.2% in the pindolol group and 60.6% in the placebo group (81).

Perez et al. conducted a single-blind placebo lead-in phase followed by a six-week randomized 111-patient, double-blind, parallel study with two treatment arms—fluoxetine plus pindolol and fluoxetine plus placebo (82). At endpoint, the response rate in the fluoxetine plus pindolol group and percentage of remitted patients was 15.6% and 15.4% greater than the placebo arm, respectively (82). The median time to sustained response with pindolol was significantly reduced when compared to that of placebo (19 days vs. 29 days) (82). There was no difference in side effects between groups in this study (82).

Perez et al. conducted a six-week double-blind, randomized, placebo-controlled trial of pindolol augmentation in 80 depressive patients resistant to SSRIs (83). At the endpoint, HAM-D and Montgomery-Asberg change from baseline were not significantly different between the placebo and pindolol arms of the study (12.5% change in both) (83).

Berman et al. completed a nine-week, 43-patient, double-blind, placebo-controlled trial in which patients were concurrently treated with fluoxetine and either placebo or pindolol for six weeks (84). From week 6 to week 9, all patients received fluoxetine and placebo (84). After two weeks, the rate of partial remission was 3% greater in the placebo group (84). At the time of completion of study, 65% of the patients demonstrated at least partial remission without any significant difference between the groups (84).

Limitations of the use of pindolol are the lack of replicated data, as well as adverse effects such as hypotension and exacerbation of asthma symptoms. This strategy may be useful for reducing time to antidepressant response, but more supportive data is warranted because the current evidence base is controversial.

Modafinil

Modafinil is a novel stimulant medication that is FDA approved for the treatment of narcolepsy, obstructive sleep apnea syndrome, and shift work sleep disorder, and is often used in the treatment of fatigue associated with multiple sclerosis. A putative minor mechanism of action is thought to occur by increasing the level of dopamine by inhibiting its reuptake, because this drug needs an intact dopamine system to function. It has no other pharmacodynamic of clinical similarities to typical stimulants (54). It may also enhance histamine release from the tuberomammilary nucleus into the frontal cortex in a system that parallels the reticular activating system where true stimulants work. The net effect may be the enhancement of cognitive arousal, alertness, and concentration (54). It has, therefore, been called a "histamine alerter." In addition, modafinil may decrease GABA transmission (85). Modafinil is well tolerated with minimal abuse potential. It is metabolized by the P450 system, and may cause a modest induction of the CYP3A4 system. Our group has found modafinil to be quite helpful in the treatment of fatigue associated with depression, or fatigue associated with the use of other psychotropic medications, or other comorbid illness. Schwartz et al. have completed small, uncontrolled studies in this area (86–88). It is generally administered after initiation of antidepressant therapy in a dose range of approximately 50 to 400 mg/day, administered once daily in the morning.

DeBattista et al. completed a study in which 136 patients with a partial response to six-week antidepressant therapy were enrolled in a six-week randomized, double-blind, placebo-controlled, parallel-group study (89). Patients received once-daily modafinil (100–400 mg/day) or matching placebo, as an adjunct to antidepressant therapy. Modafinil rapidly improved fatigue and daytime wakefulness from weeks 2 through 6 when compared with placebo; however, there were no statistically significant differences after the sixth week (89). Augmentation effects of modafinil versus placebo were not significant (89). Modafinil was well tolerated when administered in combination with a variety of antidepressants (89). This data suggest that modafinil is a response-facilitating agent, which has been replicated by Ninan et al. (90).

Menza et al. described a retrospective case series of seven patients with depression treated with modafinil to augment a partial or nonresponse to antidepressants (91). At doses of 100 to 200 mg/day, all seven patients achieved full or partial remission within one to two weeks, with five to seven patients achieving a 50% decrease in HAM-D scores (91). All patients had residual tiredness or fatigue that was particularly responsive to augmentation (91).

DeBattista et al. completed a four-week, prospective, open-label study of 33 patients with major depression and partial responses to antidepressant therapy. These patients received an antidepressant plus modafinil titrated from 100 to 400 mg/day, by week 4 (92). Changes from baseline to two weeks were significant [$p < 0.001$ for Beck Depression Inventory (BDI) and HAM-D] while changes from two to four weeks were not ($p = 0.69$ and 0.441) (92). The study suggested that modafinil is effective in facilitating anti-depressant response and could also address fatigue, effort, and overall depression level (92). Mean CGI changes were similar with improvements attributed to the changes in the first two weeks (92). On the neurocognitive battery, the Stroop interference test showed significant differences between weeks 1 and 4. No significant adverse events were noted (92). The Eppworth Sleepiness Scale and Fatigue Severity Scale showed consistent statistical improvement when sleep and fatigue were specifically studied.

Modafinil appears to have beneficial effects, especially regarding fatigue-like symptoms. It is generally well tolerated, with doses in the range of 100 to 400 mg/day. Further studies are needed to ascertain effects on other core depressive symptoms, and long-term efficacy, safety, and tolerability.

Steroid Hormones

Dysfunction of the hypothalamic–pituitary–adrenal (HPA) axis has been implicated in the pathophysiology of depression. Depression associated with thyroid abnormalities, and the depressogenic effects of progesterone (i.e., oral contraceptives) (93) and other steroids, support a link between the endocrine system and affective disorders. The use of estrogens in females for the treatment of postmenopausal depression has also been reported to be effective (94,95). The use of estrogens for the treatment of depressed women is also of theoretical interest in that there is evidence for increased monoamine oxidase activity in premenopausal depressed women, and estrogen (Premarin 0.125 mg/day) normalizes this activity as well as the depressed mood (96,97). These results suggest that a decrease in estrogen level may increase the metabolism of monoamines (a lowering of serotonin, norepinephrine, or dopamine, which may ultimately cause receptor upregulation). It is further suggested that the combination of antidepressants to increase available monoamine, when combined with estrogen which decreases monoamine oxidase activity, may be an effective treatment for depressed female patients of premenopausal or menopausal age (98).

Estrogen

There are mixed reports in the literature on the use of estrogen for depressed women, in varying phases of their reproductive life cycle. The idea of using estrogen for depression was first introduced based on the observations that estrogen levels diminish during menopause, and show fluctuations at other periods of the reproductive cycle. Some models suggest that estrogen may modulate serotonin, catecholamines, and even cortisol activity, all implicated to play a role in depression (9,96,97,99–101).

While it is possible from examination of current data that the onset of major depression is increased after menopause, there is little evidence that estrogen alone is effective in the treatment of depression in postmenopausal women (9). Four significant studies have found no improvement of depression in response to treatment with estrogen as a monotherapy (102–106).

There is evidence that estrogen might be effective as an augmentation to the treatment of depression in postmenopausal women and in postmenopausal women resistant to TCAs or SSRIs (101,102).

Schneider et al. pooled 127 women over 60 years old who were treated with sertraline with and without estrogen-replacement therapy, and reported on two 12-week, randomized, double-blind, multicenter trials for treatment of major depression (107). At endpoint, sertraline-treated women taking estrogen had significantly greater global improvement (79% vs. 58%) and better quality of life than those not receiving estrogen (mean ± SD: 73.5 ± 13 vs. 68.2 ± 14) (107). There was no reported difference in side effects between the estrogen and nonestrogen groups (107).

Clinicians should consider the potential risks and benefits of using estrogen replacement in peri- and postmenopausal females (e.g., personal/family history of breast cancer), especially in women who have residual symptoms or exacerbation of symptoms.

Testosterone

There is very little data on the use of testosterone as an augmenting agent in the treatment of depression. Testosterone is used to enhance libido in both men and women. In hypogonadal men, testosterone may improve mood and energy. In general, the use of testosterone alone as an antidepressant has shown inconclusive results.

Nineteen subjects completed an eight-week, randomized, placebo-controlled study in which Pope et al. administered either transdermal testosterone gel or placebo to men with refractory depression and low or normal testosterone levels (108). Each subject continued his existing antidepressant regimen. Efficacy analysis revealed that the testosterone-treated patients had a significantly greater rate of decrease in scores on both the HAM-D and CGI than the placebo-treated patients (108). One report demonstrated onset of paranoia and aggression when methyltestosterone was added to augment imipramine (109).

Cortisol Blockers

A developing antidepressant strategy directly targets the HPA axis. Abnormalities of the HPA axis were among the first and most consistently identified findings in depressed subjects. Such findings include elevated CSF corticotrophin-releasing hormone levels, elevated cortisol levels, and diminished sensitivity to dexamethasone suppression. In preclinical and clinical studies, chronic antidepressant treatment normalized these conditions. Therefore, agents that directly reduce the hypercortisolemia in depressed subjects were tested for antidepressant activity (9,110).

Two open trial studies (Murphy et al. 1991 and Wolkowitz et al. 1993) have evaluated steroid suppressant therapy (including metyrapone, ketoconazole, and aminoglutethimide) in treatment-refractory patients. Results are promising but preliminary, with the need for more data.

There is one randomized, controlled study in the literature, evaluating the effect of metyrapone or placebo plus SSRI in 63 patients. Primary outcome criteria were the number of responders and the time to onset of action. Patients were evaluated at baseline, three weeks, and five weeks with the HAM-D (17). Results showed that a statistically significant higher proportion of patients receiving metyrapone had a positive treatment response at days 21 and 35 compared to placebo patients. While this study supports the use of metyrapone as an accelerant to the onset of antidepressant action when added to an SSRI, further study on long-term efficacy is warranted (111).

Other Pharmacological Augmenting Agents

Yohimbine

Sanacora et al. conducted a six-week, 50-patient, randomized, double-blind controlled trial to determine if the combination of α2-antagonist yohimbine (doses 5.4–10.8 mg TID) with fluoxetine results in quicker antidepressant action than an SSRI agent alone (112). At the final visit, 69% of the subjects treated with fluoxetine plus yohimbine (F/Y), met the response criteria for CGI compared to 42% of those treated with fluoxetine plus placebo (F/P) (112). Using HDRS criteria, 65% and 42% were responders in the F/Y and F/P groups, respectively (112). Yohimbine dose increases were limited in four subjects owing to increases in blood pressure, tremulousness, and light-headedness (112).

Cappiello et al. completed a single-blind, randomized, three-week study of nine subjects to determine the efficacy of adding yohimbine (doses 5.4–10.8 mg TID) versus placebo to current fluvoxamine treatment in refractory depression patients (113). Yohimbine was associated with a reduction in HDRS of 24% ± 14% from baseline, thus meeting criteria for clinically significant categorical improvement (113). Yohimbine was generally well tolerated (113).

Inositol

Levine et al. completed a 27-patient, double-blind, controlled, four-week trial comparing SSRI plus placebo, and SSRI (inositol) in the treatment of depression (114). No significant differences were found between the two treatment groups, because 6/13 patients in the inositol and 7/14 in the placebo group showed more than 50% improvement in HDRS (114). No significant adverse events were noted.

SAMe

S-adenosyl-l-methionine (SAMe) is an endogenous substance in mammalian tissue that shows potential mood-elevating effects in man (115). Available for use in Europe, SAMe has medicinal usefulness in the treatment of several disorders, particularly, osteoarthritis (116). The first mood-elevating effects of SAM were discovered serendipitously in the 1970s, when the substance was being investigated for use in the treatment of schizophrenia, and was found to have mood-elevating properties (117,118). Several open-label and single-blind trials suggest antidepressant effects of SAMe on using intravenous or intramuscular routes of administration (118,119). Several double-blind trials report that SAMe has equal or more effective antidepressant effects when compared with amitriptyline, imipramine, and clomipramine (120–122). In general, these studies show a trend toward a more rapid onset of action and less, if any, side effects with the use of SAMe. Precipitation of mania/ hypomania has been reported with the use of SAMe as well (123). Its mechanism of antidepressant action remains unknown; however, the substance is an endogenous methyl donor for several CNS neurotransmitters, including serotonin, norepinephrine, and dopamine, all of which are implicated in the pathophysiology of depression (118). SAMe also affects the lipid composition of cell membranes, which may also be involved in the pathophysiology of affective disorders (124). SAMe increases folate activity that may also be involved in the pathogenesis of depressive disorders (125). All of the above-mentioned studies are based on the use of intramuscular or intravenous routes of administration. The reason for the preference of this route of administration over the oral route is based on limited investigation of the pharmacokinetics of SAMe suggesting that it has an unstable oral bioavailability. However, a recent open-label study using oral SAMe, suggests antidepressant efficacy (117). Further investigation into its oral bioavailability, as well as further controlled studies regarding its use in oral form are now proceeding. The evidence thus far suggests that SAM is a novel antidepressant agent.

Berlanga et al. completed a 63-patient, eight-week, double-blind clinical trial in 1992 to evaluate the efficacy of SAMe in accelerating the onset of action of imipramine. Forty placebo nonresponders were given either dissolved SAMe intramuscular (IM) or dissolved placebo IM with peroral imipramine 150 mg/day (126). Depressive symptoms decreased earlier with SAMe-imipramine than with placebo, but this difference was only significant through the second week (126). No adverse effects were noted in either the SAMe or placebo group (126).

ANTIDEPRESSANT COMBINATIONS

Mirtazapine

Mirtazapine is a novel anti-depressant with a proposed mechanism that involves blockade of alpha 2 heteroreceptors. The result is norepinephrine and possibly dopamine release increases, combined with unique actions on several serotonin sub-receptor and histamine blockade (127). Mirtazapine ultimately seems to have mixed agonism and antagonism at the $5HT_{1A}$ receptor, as well as blockade at the $5HT_{2c}$ and $5HT_3$ receptors (54).

Carpenter et al. completed a 26-subject, four-week, double-blind, placebo-controlled augmentation study where mirtazapine (15–30 mg at bed time) was added to current antidepressant medication (secondary to treatment failure) for the treatment of major depression (128). Forty-four percent of the subjects had clinical response to mirtazapine, demonstrating statistical significance (128). There was no difference in side effects between groups in this short four-week study.

Carpenter et al. completed an open-label study of 20 patients who had failed four weeks of standard antidepressant treatment, and were then subjected to four weeks of mirtazapine (15–30 mg) augmentation (129). At the four-week follow up, 55% were responders, 30% were nonresponders, and 15% had discontinued, owing to weight gain and sedation (129).

Because it is novel in its pharmacological action, and can reduce depressive and anxiety symptoms, as well as adverse effects from the use of other antidepressants, our group has found mirtazapine to be of particular benefit. Mirtazapine can help decrease insomnia symptoms, sexual dysfunctions, and GI upset associated with SSRIs and SNRIs. The potent $5HT_3$ blockade can reduce nausea associated with acute SSRI treatment. Potential appetite increase secondary to antihistamine properties as well as potential sedation can be limitations, whereas they may be beneficial for the treatment of residual poor appetite or insomnia or when nausea may accompany depression. Given the $5HT_3$ antagonism of this compound, however, higher doses may be associated with less sedation in some patients.

Bupropion

Bupropion, a norepinephrine–dopamine reuptake inhibitor (NDRI) may be the most widely used augmentation strategy in the treatment of depression. It is speculated to have little to no activity on 5HT. However, there is little controlled data to support its use. With that stated, many clinicians believe that the combination of bupropion plus a serotonergic agent can be quite successful not only in terms of efficacy, but also in reducing prominent adverse effects such as sexual dysfunction, weight gain, and fatigue. Bupropion theoretically "fits together" nicely when combined with a serotonergic agent. Our group generally initiates bupropion at a low dose and gradually builds up the dosage to 300 to 450 mg/day (once daily preparation) over a period of approximately two weeks. This two-week period acts to reduce the likelihood of anxiety and activation as a prominent adverse event.

While no randomized, controlled trials were found in the literature, four open-label design studies are described below.

DeBattista et al. conducted a six-week prospective, open-label trial of 28 patients to establish the efficacy of bupropion augmentation of SSRI and venlafaxine partial and nonresponders (52). At week 6, HAM-D and BDI scores were significantly reduced when compared with that at baseline (39% and 44%, respectively) (52). Sixty-four percent of the patients had ratings corresponding to that of the "much improved" or "very much improved" state by week 6 on the clinician-rated CGI (52). Headache and insomnia were the most commonly reported adverse effects with the incidence of 56% and 44%, respectively. One patient discontinued the study owing to the side effect of increased anxiety (52).

Lam et al. conducted a six-week naturalistic, open-label cohort study of 61 patients, comparing the effects of combining citalopram and bupropion sustained release versus switching to the other monotherapy in treatment-resistant depression (130). The combination option showed superiority to the monotherapy switch in the Structured Interview guide for the HAMD-17, the Seasonal Affective Disorders version change score (–14.8 vs. –10.1), and the proportion of patients in clinical remission (28% vs. 7%) (130). There were no differences in the proportion of patients who had side effects or in the severity of the side effects experienced.

Bodkin et al. conducted a chart review of 27 patients treated with the combination of an SSRI and bupropion (131). These patients were first observed in treatment with either SSRI or bupropion alone and were found to be partial responders. The second agent was added to the first for a mean time of 11.1 months (131). Ultimately, greater symptomatic improvement was found in 70% of the 27 subjects within the first 11 ± 14 months of combined daily use of bupropion (243 ± 99 mg) with SSRI (31 ± 16 mg fluoxetine-equivalents) than with either agent alone (131). Adverse effect risks were similar to those of monotherapy (131).

Spier treated 25 consecutive patients with bupropion in combination with an SSRI or venlafaxine after monotherapy failure or venlafaxine-induced side effect development (132). Fifty-six percent of the patients responded to combination therapy based on CGI score changes at an average follow up time of 21.3 months (132). Eighty percent of subjects receiving combination therapy responded, while only 20% responded when the combination was given to treat monotherapy-induced side effects (132). Combination therapy was generally well tolerated, with headache, nausea, diaphoresis, and decreased concentration being limited to only three cases (132).

HCAs/Tricyclics (TCAs)/MAOIs

The combined use of TCAs and MAOIs has been suggested for years as an alternative treatment for persons with resistant depression. Theoretically, the rationale for using both antidepressant agents would be to combine the effect of the TCA-mediated neurotransmitter reuptake inhibition with enzyme inhibition of the MAOI and thus bring about an increased amount of neurotransmission at the postsynaptic receptor for all three major amines involved in the pathogenesis of depression. However, the combined use of a TCA and an MAOI is warned against in the Physician's Desk Reference (133) on the basis of the possibility of the occurrence of hypertensive and hyperthermic episodes reported with such combinations. It is recommended to wait for 10 days before starting a TCA after discontinuation of an MAOI or before starting an MAOI after discontinuation of a TCA (133). However, there are several reports of safely switching from a TCA to an MAOI within a four-day period, and of this drug combination being used safely (134–137). In fact, there is evidence to suggest that certain TCAs, particularly amitriptyline, may help protect against tyramine-induced hypertensive reactions seen with MAOIs (67); however, such a drug combination should not keep the patient from adhering to a low-tyramine diet.

Early evidence of TCA/MAOI efficacy in treatment-resistant depression is derived from anecdotal reports and uncontrolled studies. Although not performed under controlled conditions, there are reports of depressed persons who failed to respond to monotherapy with TCAs or MAOIs, or failed sustained improvement with ECT responding to TCA/MAOI combinations (135,138,139).

Several controlled trials report that the TCA/MAOI treatment combination is not superior to either treatment alone (140,141). However, even these trials do not adequately study treatment-resistant depression specifically.

While the actual efficacy of the TCA/MAOI combination for treatment-resistant patients remains to be demonstrated in controlled studies, this treatment should be utilized only when the patients fail other conventional treatments. The TCAs recommended for use are the more serotonergic agents amitriptyline, trimipramine, and doxepin (142). Although tranylcypromine is noted for increased risk of hypertensive reactions, it is reported to be safe when used in combination with TCAs, as are phenelzine and isocarboxazid (137,140). It is generally not recommended to use imipramine, desipramine, or clomipramine, all of which possess at least some noradrenergic properties. Based on reports on the safety of TCA/MAOI combination, it can be started simultaneously, or the TCA started first and then treatment with the MAOI initiated. The use of lower doses—lower than when either drug was used alone—is recommended when initiating such a combination.

SSRIs

SSRIs have claimed the status of first-line treatment for depression since the 1980s. However, some patients do not fully remit and require further pharmacological action beyond serotonin. In the early years of the use of SSRIs, clinicians remained familiar with the use of TCAs/heterocyclics (HCAs) and commonly "overlapped" or combined treatments to achieve a "broader" pharmacological effect. Animal models and controlled/open-label reports suggested possible rapidity of response and, perhaps, a more robust response with combination relative to that achieved with monotherapy. HCAs are metabolized via the CYP2D6 pathway and, therefore, necessitate caution when being combined with other "2D6" drugs such as SSRIs/ SNRIs (fluoxetine, paroxetine, duloxetine, etc.). As with other TCAs, drug levels can be obtained five to seven days after the dosage is initiated and 8 to 12 hours after the last dose.

In an open, four-week, not controlled trial completed in 1991 by Nelson et al., 14 inpatients with major depression were administered both desipramine and fluoxetine, and their responses were retrospectively compared with those of 52 inpatients who were previously treated with desipramine alone (143). At weeks 1, 2, and 4 of the study, the response to the desipramine plus fluoxetine combination was better than that obtained when desipramine was given alone (week 1, 42% vs. 20%; week 2, 62% vs. 30%, week 4, 71% vs. 0%, complete remission defined as a change in HAM-D score $> 75\%$) (153). Hypotension, tachycardia, and allergic rash were noted as consequences of inappropriate tricyclic dose and imprecise monitoring of plasma drug levels (143).

Weilburg et al. (144) report the effects of fluoxetine added to the treatment of 30 depressed outpatients who showed a poor response to an adequate trial of an HCA. Improvement was seen in 86.7% of the patients. In all of the cases reported, the dose of the HCA was lowered after fluoxetine was added, with an average HCA maintenance dose (in imipramine equivalences) of 70.6 mg/day. Fluoxetine dose ranged from 20 to 60 mg/day. The HCA was discontinued for 12 of the 26 responders, of whom 8 relapsed but recovered when the use of HCA was restarted. The HCA antidepressants used included amitriptyline, desipramine, doxepin, imipramine, maprotiline, nortriptyline, trazodone, and trimipramine. No adverse events were reported.

Levitt et al. completed an eight-week, noncontrolled study in which 13 patients with major depression, who had failed treatment with desipramine or imipramine and were currently unsuccessfully being treated with fluoxetine, were given desipramine or imipramine along with their dose of fluoxetine (145). Of the 13 subjects, 54% had a greater than 40% decrease in HAM-D scores, and 31% of this group had a greater than 50% decrease in HAM-D (145). At week 3, responders had a higher mean tricyclic level when compared with nonresponders (145). No adverse events were reported.

Seth et al. examined eight cases of treatment-resistant depression treated with a combination of nortriptyline and a new SSRI, with or without concurrent lithium therapy (146). Notable improvement was seen in all patients in whom other drug regimes, such as MAOIs, TCAs, neuroleptics, and ECT had been ineffective (146). There were no reported significant side effects among the eight cases, seven of whom were elderly patients

(156). In each case, combination treatment was more effective than single treatment modalities.

Zajecka et al. reported 25 nonresponders to at least four weeks of open-label fluoxetine treatment. An HCA was added to fluoxetine, with dosages then titrated up (147). A retrospective analysis demonstrated that 35% of subjects who demonstrated a partial response to fluoxetine responded fully when an HCA was added to fluoxetine (147). Five of the responders (71%) who previously failed monotherapy with HCA had responded when HCA was used with fluoxetine. Five subjects who demonstrated significant improvement with the use of fluoxetine, but had mild residual depression symptoms experienced a partial improvement with the addition of HCA (42.7% HAM-D change) (147). One nonresponder subject experienced a generalized seizure with fluoxetine and maprotiline, which was then discontinued without significant sequelae (147).

Maes et al. completed a five-week, double-blind, placebo-controlled study of 26 patients with treatment-resistant depression (148). After one week of trazodone treatment, patients were randomized to receive placebo, pindolol, or fluoxetine in addition to the trazodone for four weeks (148). With the outcome measure being a 50% reduction in HDRS, 72.5% of patients treated with trazodone plus pindolol, 75% of patients treated with trazodone plus fluoxetine, and 20% treated with trazodone plus placebo showed a clinically significant response (148). No unique adverse events were noted (148).

Dual Serotonin-2 Antagonists and Reuptake Inhibitors (Trazodone and Nefazodone)

Nefazodone and trazodone are novel agents with dual serotonin-2 antagonism and reuptake inhibition. Both act by potent blockade at the $5HT_{2A}$, and weak serotonin reuptake inhibition. Nefazodone also has weak norepinephrine reuptake inhibition as well as weak alpha1-adrenergic–blocking properties. Trazodone also contains alpha1-antagonist properties, but lacks the norepinephrine reuptake inhibition capability of nefazodone (54). In many patients, trazodone produces sedation that can be poorly tolerated at therapeutic doses. It is for this reason that many clinicians choose to combine this drug in low doses (25–150 mg at bedtime) with other antidepressants, as an off-label hypnotic. Trazodone can improve overall sleep, and thus theoretically reduce depressive symptoms associated with insomnia. In addition, the 5HT2 antagonism may produce anxiolytic effects as well as potential sexual dysfunction reversal associated with SSRIs. Apart from marked sedation, priapism is also a side effect that the patient should be made aware of, and informed consent must be obtained from the patient before initiating treatment with trazodone.

Nefazodone is a unique antidepressant, but recent reports regarding its use are rare. Potential liver damage has resulted in a decline in its use in the

United States. As seen in the case of trazodone, nefazodone's receptor profile with $5HT_2$ blockade can be quite helpful in reducing adverse effects such as sleep and sexual dysfunction associated with the use of SSRIs. If $5HT_2$ blockade is desired, safer alternatives may include the use of mirtazapine or second-generation antipsychotics in low to moderate doses. In addition, the lack of antihistamine activity reduces the likelihood of sedation and increases the tolerability profile.

Taylor and Prather completed a non–placebo-controlled, nonrandomized cohort study of 11 patients with treatment-resistant depression and/or comorbid anxiety disorders, who were given increasing dosages of nefazodone, in addition to their previous regimen, until an optimum response was achieved (149). After augmentation, 63% achieved complete remission of depressive symptoms (149). In each of the 11 cases, nefazodone was efficacious and well tolerated in the treatment of depression and anxiety (149).

Our group tends to dose this drug once daily at bedtime, as opposed to twice daily, mainly for compliance and to reduce the relatively small likelihood of sedation during the day. This drug may also improve sleep and normalize sleep architecture in this augmentive strategy.

Atomoxetine

As a drug marketed for ADHD, this norepinephrine reuptake inhibitor may also increase dopamine secondarily in the frontal cortex (both transmitters share reuptake via the norepinephrine transporter here) (150). Given its lack of FDA approval, it should be classified as an augmentation drug, though it acts similarly to certain TCAs. There is no published data available for this drug in the treatment of depression. However, our group has anecdotally begun to combine this medication with serotonergic agents. Initial starting dose is approximately 40 mg/day, slowly increasing to 80 to 120 mg/day. If results are not seen at these doses, we will consider increasing up to 160 mg/day. Adverse effects include anxiety, activation and somnolence. Patients may experience a stimulant-like reaction with increased energy and motivation. Blood pressure should be monitored, especially if multiple noradrenergic agents are being combined.

CONCLUSION

This chapter started with a basic clinical introduction regarding the pros and cons of polypharmacy in MDD. We have now completed a thorough review of the evidence base that is used to support this common practice. Polypharmacy may be the rule rather than the exception when a clinician attempts to help a patient reach full remission of MDD symptoms and is gaining popularity when side effects need to be alleviated for the patient to remain adherent to long-term medication management. This form of polypharmacy will be covered in the following chapter. Finally, as you have noticed, the evidence base is somewhat lacking when compared to monotherapy data. Clinicians should always take each individual case into account and weigh the risks/benefits accordingly. The key to successful rational polypharmacy is to understand how each medication facilitates certain transmitter pathways and to attempt to match up residual symptoms with those malfunctioning pathways.

REFERENCES

1. Nierenberg AA, Keefe BR, Leslie VC, et al. Residual symptoms in depressed patients who respond acutely to fluoxetine. J Clin Psychiat 1999; 60:221–225.
2. Paykel ES. Residual symptoms after partial remission. Psychol Med 1995; 25:1171–1180.
3. Thase ME. Introduction: defining remission in patients treated with antidepressants. J Clin Psychiat 1999; 60(suppl 22):3–6.
4. Hirschfeld RM, Keller MB, Panico S, et al. The National Depressive and Manic Depressive Association consensus statement on the undertreatment of depression. JAMA 1997; 277:333–340.
5. Thase ME, Ninan PT. New goals in the treatment of depression: moving toward recovery. Psychopharm Bull 2002; 36(suppl 2):24–35.
6. Depression Guideline Panel No. 5. AHCPR Guidelines. American Psychiatric Association, 2000.
7. Dunner DL. Treatment-resistant depression: an overview of the problem. Primary Psychiat 2005; 12(2):27–29.
8. Janicak PG, Davis JM, Preskorn SH, Ayd FJ. Principles and Practice of Psychopharmacology. 3rd ed. Lippincott Williams & Wilkins, 2001.
9. Schatzberg AF, Nemeroff CB. Textbook of Psychopharmacology. 2d ed. American Psychiatric. In press.
10. Zajecka JM, Fawcett J. Antidepressant Combination and Potentiation. Psychiatric Medicine. Vol. 9. No. 1. Ryandic Publishing Inc., 1991.
11. deMontigny C, Cournoyer G, Morrissette R, et al. Lithium carbonate addition in tricyclic antidepressant-resistant depression. Arch Gen Psychiat 1983; 40:1327–1334.
12. Heninger G, Chorney DS, Sternberg DE. Lithium carbonate augmentation of antidepressant treatment. Arch Gen Psychiat 1983; 40:1335–1342.
13. deMontigny C, Grunberg F, Morrissette R, et al. Lithium carbonate induces rapid relief of depression in tricyclic antidepressant drug responders. Br J Psychiat 1981; 138:252–256.
14. Kantor D, McNevin S, Leichner P, et al. The benefit of lithium carbonate adjunct in refractory depression—fact or fiction? Can J Psychiat 1986; 31:416–418.
15. Nelson JC, Magure CM. Lithium augmentation in psychotic depression refractory to combined drug treatment. Am J Psychiat 1986; 13:363–366.
16. Pai M, White AC, Deane AG. Lithium augmentation in the treatment of delusional depression. Br J Psychiat 1986; 148:736–738.
17. Price LH, Yeates C, Nelson JC. Lithium augmentation of combined neuroleptic-tricyclic treatment in delusional depression. Am J Psychiat 1983; 140:318–322.

18. Kushnir SL. Lithium antidepressant combinations in the treatment of depressed, physically ill geriatric patients. Am J Psychiat 1986; 143:378–379.
19. Lafferman J, Solomon K, Ruskin P. Lithium augmentation for treatment-resistant depression in the elderly. Geriatr Psychiat Neurol 1988; 1:49–52.
20. Katona CLE. Lithium augmentation in refractory depression. Psychiatr Dev 1988; 2:153–171.
21. Bauer M, Adli M, Baethge C, et al. Lithium augmentation therapy in refractory depression: clinical evidence and neurobiological mechanisms. Can J Psychiat 2003; 48(7):440–446.
22. Bauer M, Bschor T, Kunz D, Berghofer A, Strohle A, Muller-Oerlinghausen B. Double-blind, placebo-controlled trial of the use of lithium to augment antidepressant medication in continuation treatment of unipolar major depression. Am J Psychiat 2000; 157:1429–1435.
23. Nierenberg AA, Price LH, Charney DS, Heninger GR. After lithium augmentation: a retrospective follow-up of patients with antidepressant-refractory depression. J Affect Disord 1990; 18:167–175.
24. Sadock BJ, Sadock VA. Kaplan & Sadock's Synopsis of Psychiat. 9th ed. New York, NY: Lippincott Williams & Wilkins, 2003.
25. Flach FF, Celian CI, Rawson RW. Treatment of psychiatric disorders with triiodothyronine. Am J Psychiat 1958; 114:841–842.
26. Feldmesser-Reiss EE. The application of triiodothyronine in the treatment of mental disorders. J Nerv Ment Dis 1958; 127:540–545.
27. Prange AJ Jr, Wilson IC, Rabon AM, et al. Enhancement of imipramine antidepressant activity by thyroid hormone. Am J Psychiat 1969; 126: 457–469.
28. Wilson IC, Prange AJ Jr, McClane TK, et al. Thyroid hormone enhancement of imipramine in non-retarded depression. N Engl J Med 1970; 282:1063–1067.
29. Wheatley D. Potentiation of amitriptyline by thyroid hormone. Arch Gen Psychiat 1972; 26:229–233.
30. Coppen A, Whybrow PC, Noguera R, et al. The comparative antidepressant value of L-tryptophan and imipramine with and without potentiation by liothyronine. Arch Gen Psychiat 1972; 26:234–241.
31. Banki CM. Triiodothyronine in the treatment of depression. Orv Hetil 1975; 116:2543–2546.
32. Banki CM. Cerebrospinal fluid amine metabolites after combined amitriptyline-triiodothyronine treatment of depressed women. Eur J Pharmacol 1977; 11: 311–315.
33. Earle BV. Thyroid hormone and tricyclic atidepressants in resistant depressions. Am J Psychiatr 1970; 126:1667–1669.
34. Ogura C, Okuma T, Uchida Y, et al. Combined thyroid (triiodothyronine) antidepressant treatment in depressive states. Folia Psychiatr Neurol Jpn 1974; 28:179–186.
35. Tsutsui S, Yamazaki Y, Namba T, et al. Combined therapy of T_3 and antidepressants in depression. J Int Med Res 1979; 7:138–146.
36. Goodwin FK, Prange AJ Jr, Post RM, et al. Potentiation of antidepressant effects by L-triiodothyronine in tricyclic nonresponders. Am J Psychiatr 1982; 139:34–38.

37. Thaes ME, Kupfer DJ, Jarrett DB. Treatment of imipramine-resistant recurrent depression. An open clinical trial of adjunctive L triiodothyronine. J Clin Psychiatr 1989; 50:385–388.
38. Sokolov ST, Levitt AJ, Joffe RT. Thyroid hormone levels before unsuccessful antidepressant therapy are associated with later response to T3 augmentation. Psychiat Res 1997; 69(2–3):203–206.
39. Aronson R, Offman HJ, Joffe RT, Naylor CD. Triiodothyronine augmentation in the treatment of refractory depression. Arch Gen Psychiat 1996; 53:842–848.
40. Joffe R, Singer W, Levitt AJ, MacDonald C. A placebo-controlled comparison of lithium and triiodothyronine augmentation of tricyclic antidepressants in unipolar refractory depression. Arch Gen Psychiat 1993; 50:387–393.
41. Joffe R, Singer W. A comparison of triiodothyronine and thyroxine in the potentiation of tricyclic antidepressants. Psychiat Res 1990; 32:241–251.
42. Hullett FJ, Bidder TG. Phenelzine plus triiodothyronine combination in a case of refractory depression. J Nerv Ment Dis 1983; 171:318–321.
43. Jaffe RT. Triiodothyronine potentiation of the antidepressant effect of phenelzine. J Clin Psychiatr 1988; 49:409–410.
44. Glassman AH, Perel JM. The clinical pharmacology of imipramine. Arch Gen Psychiat 1973; 28:649–653.
45. Whybrow PC, Prange AJ Jr. A hypothesis of thyroid-catecholamine-receptor interaction. Arch Gen Psychiatr 1981; 38:106–113.
46. Loosen PT, Prange AJ Jr. Serum thyrotropin-response to thyrotropin releasing hormone in psychiatric patients: a review. Am J Psychiat 1982; 139:405–416.
47. Sramek JJ, Tansman M, Suri A, et al. Efficacy of buspirone in generalized anxiety disorder with coexisting mild depressive symptoms. J Clin Psychiat 1996; 57(7):28–91.
48. Rickles K, Amsterdam J, Clary C, et al. Buspirone in depressed outpatients: a controlled study. Psychopharm Bull 1990; 26:163–167.
49. Robinson DS, Rickles R, Feighner J, et al. Clinical effects of 5HT$_{1a}$ partial agonists in depression: a composite analysis of buspirone in the treatment of depression. J Clin Psychopharm 1990; 10(suppl 3):67S–76S.
50. Landen M, Bjorling G, Agren H, Fahlen T. A randomized, double-blind, placebo-controlled trial of buspirone in combination with an SSRI in patients with treatment-refractory depression. J Clin Psychiat 1998; 59(12):664–668.
51. Appelberg B, Syvalahti EK, Koskinen TE, Mehtonen OP, Muhonen TT, Naukkarinen HH. Patients with severe depression may benefit from buspirone augmentation of selective serotonin reuptake inhibitors: results from a placebo-controlled, randomized, double-blind, placebo wash-in study. J Clin Psychiat 2001; 62(6):448–452.
52. DeBattista C, Solvason HB, Poirier J, Kendrick E, Schatzberg AF. A prospective trial of bupropion sr augmentation of partial and non-responders to serotonergic antidepressants. J Clin Psychopharmacol 2003; 23(1):27–30.

53. Calabrese JR, Bowden CL, Sachs G, et al. A placebo-controlled 18-month trial of lamotrigine and lithium maintenance treatment in recently depressed patients with bipolar I disorder. J Clin Psychiat 2003; 64(9):1013–1024.

54. Stahl SM. Essential Psychopharmacology. 2d ed. Cambridge, UK: Cambridge University Press, 2000.

55. Barbee JG, Jamhour NJ. Lamotrigine as an augmentation agent in treatment-resistant depression. J Clin Psychiat 2002; 63(8):737–741.

56. Calabrese JR, Bowden CL, Sachs GS, et al. A double-blind placebo-controlled study of lamotrigine monotherapy in outpatients with bipolar I depression. J Clin Psychiat 1999; 60(2):79–88.

57. Biel JH, Boop BA. Amphetamines: structure–activity relationships. In: Iverson L, Iverson S, Snyder S, eds. Handbook of Psychopharmacology. Vol. II. New York: Plenum Press, 1978:137.

58. Chiarello RJ, Cole JO. The use of psychostimulants in general psychiatry. Arch Gen Psychiatr 1987; 44:286–295.

59. Satel SL, Nelson CJ. Stimulants in the treatment of depression: a critical overview. J Clin Psychiatr 1989; 50:24–249.

60. Wharton RN, Perel JM, Dayton PG, Malitz S. A potential use for methylphenidate with tricyclic antidepressants. Am J Psychiatr 1971; 127(12): 1619–1625.

61. Wagner SG, Klein DF. Treatment refractory patients: affective disorders. Psychopharm Bull 1988; 24:69–73.

62. Krisko I, Lewis E, Johnson JE III. Severe hyperpyrexia due to tranylcyopromine-amphetamine toxicity. Ann Intern Med 1968; 70:559–564.

63. Mason A. Fatal reaction associated with tranylcypromine and methylamphetamine. Lancet 1962; 1:1073.

64. Dally PJ. Fatal reaction associated with tranylcypromine and methylamphetamine. Lancet 1962; 1:1235–1236.

65. Zeck P. Dangers of some antidepressant drugs. Med J Aust 1961; 2:602–608.

66. Feighner JP, Herbstein J, Damlouji N. Combined MAOI, TCA and direct stimulant therapy of treatment-resistant depression. J Clin Psychiatr 1985; 46(6):206–209.

67. Fawcett J, Kravitz HM, Zajecka JM, Schaff MR. CNS stimulant potentiation of monoamine oxidase inhibitors in treatment refractory depression. J Clin Psychopharmacol 1991; 11(2):127–132.

68. Gwirtsman H, Szuba MP, Toren L, Feist M. The antidepressant response to tricyclics in major depressives is accelerated with adjunctive use of methylphenidate. Psychopharmacol Bull 1994; 30(2):157–164.

69. Pare CMB, Kline N, Hallstrom C, et al. Will amitriptyline prevent the "cheese" reaction of monoamine-oxidase inhibitors? Lancet 1982; 2:183–186.

70. Linet LS. Treatment of refractory depression with a combination of fluoxetine and d-amphetamine. Am J Psychiatr 1989; 146:803–804.

71. Wharton RN, Perel JM, Dayton PG, et al. A potential clinical use for methylphenidate with tricyclic antidepressants. Am J Psychiatr 1971; 127: 1619–1625.

72. American Diabetes Association, American Psychiatric Association. Consensus development conference on antipsychotic drugs and obesity and diabetes. J Clin Psychiat 2004; 65(2):267–272.
73. Shelton R, Tollefson GD, Tohen M, et al. A novel augmentation strategy for treating resistant major depression. Am J Psychiat 2001; 158(1):131–134.
74. Hirose S, Ashby CR Jr. An open pilot study combining risperidone and a selective serotonin reuptake inhibitor as initial antidepressant therapy. J Clin Psychiat 2002; 63(8):733–736.
75. Papakostas G, Petersen TJ, Nierenberg AA, et al. Ziprasidone augmentation of selective serotonin reuptake inhibitors (SSRIs) for SSRI-resistant major depressive disorder. J Clin Psychiat 2004; 65(2):217–221.
76. Barbee J, Conrad EJ, Jamhour NJ. The effectiveness of olanzapine, risperidone, quetiapine and ziprasidone as augmentation agents in treatment-resistant major depressive disorder. J Clin Psychiat 2004; 65(7):975–981.
77. Calabrese J, Macfadden W, McCoy R, et al. Double-blind, placebo-controlled study of quetiapine in bipolar depression. 157th Annual Meeting of the American Psychiatric Association, New York, New York, May 1–6, 2004 (NR756).
78. Tohen M, Vieta E, Calabrese J, et al. Efficacy of olanzapine and olanzapine-fluoxetine combination in the treatment of bipolar I depression. Arch Gen Psychiat 2003; 60(11):1079–1088.
79. Furukawa T, Streiner DL, Young LT. Is antidepressant-benzodiazepine combination therapy clinically more useful? A meta-analytic study. J Affect Disord 2001; 65:173–177.
80. Smith W, Londborg PD, Glaudin V, Painter JR. Short-term augmentation of fluoxetine with clonazepam in the treatment of depression: a double-blind study. Am J Psychiat 1998; 155(10):1339–1345.
81. Isaac M. Milnacipran and pindolol: a randomized trial of reduction of antidepressant latency. Hum Psychopharmacol Clin Exp 2003; 18:595–601.
82. Perez V, Puiigdemont D, Gilaberte I, Alvarez E, Artigas F, Grup de Recerca en Trastorns Afectius. Augmentation of fluoxetine's antidepressant action by pindolol: analysis of clinical, pharmacokinetic and methodological factors. J Clin Psychopharmacol 2001; 21(1):36–45.
83. Perez V, Soler J, Puigdemont D, Alvarez E, Artigas F. A double-blind, randomized, placebo-controlled trial of pindolol augmentation in depressive patients resistant to serotonin reuptake inhibitors. Arch Gen Psychiat 1999; 56: 375–379.
84. Berman R, Darnell AM, Miller HL, Anand A, Charney DS. Effect of pindolol in hastening response to fluoxetine in the treatment of major depression: a double-blind, placebo-controlled trial. Am J Psychiat 1997; 154:37–43.
85. Ferraro L, Tanganelli S, O'Connor WT, et al. The vigilance promoting drug modafinil decrease GABA release in the medial preoptic area and in the posterior hypothalamus of the awake rat: possible involvement of the serotonergic 5-HT3 receptor. Neuroscience Lett 1996; 220(1):5–8.
86. Schwartz TL. An open-label study of adjunctive modafinil in patients with sedation related to serotonergic antidepressant therapy. J Clin Psychiat 2004; 65(9):1223–1227.

87. Schwartz TL. Adjunctive modafinil reduces sedation caused by SSRI treatment in depressed patients. Primary Psychiat Noteworthy Briefs from the Field 2004; 11(8):13.

88. Schwartz TL, Leso L, Beale M, Ahmed R, Naprawa S. Modafinil in the treatment of depression with severe comorbid medical illness. Psychosomatics 2002; 43:336–337.

89. DeBattista C, Doghramji K, Menza MA, Rosenthal MH, Fieve RR. Modafinil in Depression Study Group. Adjunct modafinil for the short-term treatment of fatigue and sleepiness in patients with major depressive disorder: a preliminary double-blind, placebo-controlled study. J Clin Psychiat 2003; 64(9):1057–1064.

90. Ninan PT, Hassman HA, Glass SJ, McManus FC. Adjunctive modafinil at initiation of treatment with a selective serotonin reuptake inhibitor enhances the degree and onset of therapeutic effects in patients with major depressive disorder and fatigue [Clinical Trial]. J Clin Psychiat 2004; 65(3):414–420.

91. Menza M, Kaufman KR, Castellanos A. Modafinil augmentation of antidepressant treatment in depression. J Clin Psychiat 2000; 61(5):378–381.

92. DeBattista C, Lembke A, Solvason HB, Ghebremichael R, Poirier J. A prospective trial of modafinil as an adjunctive treatment of major depression. J Clin Psychopharmacol 2004; 24(1):87–90.

93. Malek-Ahmadi P, Behrmann PJ. Depressive syndrome induced by oral contraceptives. Dis Nerv Syst 1976; 37:406–408.

94. Frank RT, Goldberger MA, Salmon VJ. The menopause symptoms, hormonal status and treatment. NY J Med 1936; 36:1363–1375.

95. Vogel W, Klaiber EL, Bouerman DM. Roles of the gonadal steroid hormones in psychiatric depression in men and women. Prog Neuropsychopharmacol Bio Psychiatr 1978; 2:487–503.

96. Klaiber EL, Boverman DM, Vogel W. The effects of estrogen therapy on plasma MAO activity and EEG: driving responses of depressed women. Am J Psychiatr 1972; 128:1492–1498.

97. Wiesbader J, Koszrok R. The menopause: a consideration of symptoms, etiology, and treatment by means of estrogens. Endocrinology 1938; 23:32.

98. Ananth J, Ruskin R. Treatment of intractable depression. Int Pharmacopsychiat 1984; 9:218–229.

99. Fischette CT, Biegon A, McEwen B. Sex stressed modulation of the serotonin behavioral syndrome. Life Sci 1984; 35:1197–1206.

100. Klaiber EL, Boverman DM, Vogel W, et al. Estrogen therapy for sekere persistant depression in women. Arch Gen Psychiat 1979; 36:550–554.

101. Stahl S. Role of hormone therapies for refractory depression. American Psychiatric Association Annual Meeting, New York, NY, May 4, 1996.

102. Schneider MA, Brotherton PL, Hailes J. The effect of exogenous oestrogens on depression in menopausal women. Med J Aust 1977; 2:162–163.

103. Shapira B, Oppenheim G, Zohar J, et al. Lack of efficacy of estrogen supplementation to imipramine in resistant female depressives. Biol Psychiat 1985; 20:576–579.

104. Coope J. Is oestrogen therapy effective in the treatment of menopausal depression? J R Coll Gen Pract 1981; 31:134–140.

105. Coope J, Thomson J, Poller L. Effects of "natural estrogen" replacement therapy on menopausal symptoms and blood clotting. Br Med J 1975; 4:139–143.
106. Prange AJ. Estrogen may well affect response to antidepressant. JAMA 1972; 219:143–144.
107. Schneider L, Small GW, Clary CM. Estorgen replacement therapy and antidepressant response to sertraline in older depressed women. Am J Geriatr Psychiat 2001; 9(4):393–399.
108. Pope H Jr, Cohane GH, Kanayama G, Siegel AJ, Hudson JI. Testosterone gel supplementation for men with refractory depression. A randomized, placebo-controlled trial. Am J Psychiat 2003; 160:105–111.
109. Wilson IC, Prang AJ, Lard PP. Methyltestosterone in men: conversion of depression to paranoid reaction. Am J Psychiat 1974; 131:21–24.
110. Murphy BEP, Wolkowitz OM. The pathophysiologic significance of hyperadrenocorticism: antiglucocorticoid strategies. Psychiat Ann 1993; 23:682–690.
111. Jahn H, Schick M, Kiefer F, et al. Metyrapone as additive treatment in major depression: a double-blind and placebo-controlled trial. Arch Gen Psychiat 2004; 61:1235–1244.
112. Sanacora G, Berman RM, Cappiello A, et al. Addition of the α2-antagonist yohimbine to fluoxetine: effects on rate of antidepressant response. Neuropsychopharmacology 2004; 29:1166–1171.
113. Cappiello A, McDougle CJ, Malison RT, Heninger GR, Price LH. Yohimbine augmentation of fluvoxamine in refractory depression: a single-blind study. Biol Psychiat 1995; 38:765–767.
114. Levine J, Mishori A, Susnosky M, Martin M, Belmaker RH. Combination of inositol and serotonin reuptake inhibitors in the treatment of depression. Biol Psychiat 1999; 45:270–273.
115. Baldessarini RJ. The neuropharmacology of S-adenosyl-L-methionine. Am J Med 1987; 83:95–103.
116. Marcolongo R, Giordano N, Colombo B, et al. Double-blind multicentre study of the activity of S-adenosyl-methionine in hip and knee osteoarthritis. Curr Ther Res 1985; 37:82–94.
117. Rosenbaum JF, Fava M, Falk W, et al. An open-label pilot study of oral-S-adenosyl-L-methionine in major depression: interim results. Psychopharm Bull 1988; 24(1):189–194.
118. Lipinski JF, Cohen BM, Frankenberg F, et al. An open trial of S-adenosylmethionine for treatment of depression. Am J Psychiat 1984; 141:448–450.
119. Agnoli A, Andreoli V, Casacchia M, et al. Effect of S-adenosyl-L-methionine (SAM) upon depressive symptoms. J Psychiat Res 1976; 13:43–54.
120. Bell K, Plon L, Nobal M, et al. Antidepressant activity of S-adenosyl-L-methionine (SAMe) in depressed inpatients treated for 14 days, a double blind study. 14th Congress of the Collegium Internationale Neuro–Psychopharmacologicum, San Juan, Puerto Rico, December, 1986.
121. Miccoli L, Porro V, Bertolino A. Comparison between the antidepressant activity of S-adenosyl-L-methionine (SAMe) and that of some tricyclic drugs. Acta Neurol 1978; 33:243–255.

122. Scarzella R, Appiotti A. A double clinical comparison of SAMe versus chlorimipramine in depressive syndromes. VIth World Congress of Biological Psychiatry, Honolulu, 1977.
123. Carney MWP, Chary TKN, Bottiglieri EH, et al. The switch mechanism and the bipolar/unipolar dichotomy. Br J Psychiat 1989; 154:48–51.
124. Cimino M, Vantini G, Algeri S, et al. Age-related modification of dopaminergic and beta-adrenergic receptor system: restoration to normal activity by modifying membrane fluidity with S-adenosylmethionine. Life Sci 1984; 34:2029–3039.
125. Reynolds EH, Stramentinoli G. Folic acid, S-adenosyl-L-methionine and affective disorder. Psychol Med 1983; 13:705–710.
126. Berlanga C, Ortega-Soto HA, Ontiveros M, Senties H. Efficacy of S-adenosyl-L-methionine in speeding the onset of action of imipramine. Psychiat Res 1992; 44:257–262.
127. Millan MJ, et al. Mirtazapine enhances frontocortical dopaminergic and corticolimbic adrenergic, but not serotonergic, transmission by blockade of alpha-2 adrenergic and serotonin 2c receptors. European J Neuroscience 2000; 12(3):1079–1095.
128. Carpenter L, Yasmin S, Price LH. A double blind, placebo controlled study of antidepressant augmentation with mirtazapine. Soc Biol Psychiat 2002; 51: 183–188.
129. Carpenter L, Jocic Z, Hall JM, Rasmussen SA, Price LH. Mirtazapine augmentation in the treatment of refractory depression. J Clin Psychiat 1999; 60(1):45–49.
130. Lam R, Hossie H, Solomons K, Yatham LN. Citalopram and bupropion-sr: combining versus switching in patients with treatment-resistant depression. J Clin Psychiat 2004; 65(3):337–340.
131. Bodkin JA, Lasser RA, Wines JD Jr, Gardner DM, Baldessarini RJ Combining serotonin reuptake inhibitors and bupropion in partial responders to antidepressant monotherapy. J Clin Psychiat 1997; 58(4):137–145.
132. Spier S. Use of bupropion with SRIs and venlafaxine. Depress Anxiety 1998; 7:73–75.
133. Physician's Desk Reference 95th ed., Montvale, NJ:Thompson PDR; 2005.
134. Kahn D, Silver JM, Opler LA. The safety of switching rapidly from tricyclic antidepressants to monoamine oxidase inhibitors. J Clin Psychopharm 1989; 9:198–202.
135. Sethna ER. A study of refractory cases of depressive illnesses and their response to combined antidepressant treatment. Br J Psychiat 1974; 124:265–272.
136. Spiker DG, Pugh DD. Combining tricyclic and monoamine oxidase inhibitor antidepressants. Arch Gen Psychiat 1976; 33:828–830.
137. Schmauss M, Kapphammer HP, Meyr P, et al. Combined MAO inhibitor and tri-(tetra)cyclic antidepressant treatment in therapy resistant depression. Prog Neuro-Psychopharmacol Biol Psychiat 1988; 12:523–532.
138. Hynes B. Combining the antidepressant drugs. Br Med J 1965; 1:589–590.
139. Gander DR. Treatment of depressive illnesses with combined antidepressants. Lancet 1965; 2:107–109.

140. Razani J, White KL, White J, et al. The safety and efficacy of combined amitriptyline and tranylcypromine antidepressant treatment. Arch Gen Psychiat 1983; 40:652–661.
141. Young JPR, Lader MH, Hughes WC. Controlled trial of trimipramine, monoamine oxidase inhibitors and combined treatment in depressed outpatients. Br Med J 1979; 4:1315–1317.
142. White K, Simpson G. Combined monoamine oxidase inhibitor-tricyclic antidepressant treatment: a reevaluation. J Clin Psychopharmacol 1981; 1: 264–281.
143. Nelson JC, Mazure CM, Bowers MB Jr, Jatlow PI. A preliminary, open study of the combination of fluoxetine and desipramine for rapid treatment of major depression. Arch Gen Psychiat 1991; 48:303–307.
144. Weilburg JB, Rosenbaum JF, Biederman J, et al. Fluoxetine added to non-MAOI antidepressants converts nonresponders to responders: a preliminary report. J Clin Psychiat 1989; 50:447–449.
145. Levitt A, Joffe RT, Kamil R, McIntyre R. Do depressed subjects who have failed both fluoxetine and a tricyclic antidepressant respond to the combination? J Clin Psychiat 1999; 60(9):613–616.
146. Seth R, Jennings AL, Bindman J, Phillips J, Bergmann K. Combination treatment with noradrenalin and serotonin reuptake inhibitors in resistant depression. Br J Psychiat 1992; 161:562–565.
147. Zajecka J, Jeffries H, Fawcett J. The efficacy of fluoxetine combined with a heterocyclic antidepressant in treatment-resistant depression: a retrospective analysis. J Clin Psychiat 1995; 56(8):338–343.
148. Maes M, Vandoolaeghe E, Desnyder R. Efficacy of treatment with trazodone in combination with pindolol or fluoxetine in major depression. J Affect Disord 1996; 41:201–210.
149. Taylor FB, Prather MR. The efficacy of nefazodone augmentation for treatment-resistant depression with anxiety symptoms or anxiety disorder. Depression Anxiety 2003; 18(2):83–88.
150. Stahl SM. Neurotransmission of cognition, part 2. Selective NRIs are smart drugs: exploiting regionally selective actions on both dopamine and norepinephrine to enhance cognition. J Clin Psychiat 2003; 64(2):110–111.

7

Combining Drug Treatments to Achieve Better Tolerability and Adherence

George I. Papakostas

*Massachusetts General Hospital/Harvard Medical School,
Boston, Massachusetts, U.S.A.*

Thomas L. Schwartz

*Department of Psychiatry, SUNY Upstate Medical University,
Syracuse, New York, U.S.A.*

INTRODUCTION

Given the information provided in earlier chapters regarding acute outcomes and the potential prophylactic effects of long-term maintenance pharmacotherapy for major depressive disorder (MDD), it seems worthwhile to continue the development of safer and more tolerable antidepressant agents. Short of this and due to a narrow potential pipeline, we must often rely on polypharmacy techniques to achieve remission as noted in the last chapter. What about the use of polypharmacy to mitigate acute and chronic adverse events? The continuation of pharmacotherapy in patients who have experienced sufficient symptom improvement during the acute phase of treatment has been repeatedly shown to minimize the risk of recurrence of depression (1) as noted, and it appears that antidepressant remitters who continue to receive pharmacotherapy on a long-term basis and remain in remission experience an improvement in psychosocial functioning, while antidepressant remitters who were switched to placebo and sustained remission experience a worsening of psychosocial functioning (2). As a result, it is becoming increasingly apparent to clinicians and patients alike that long-term compliance with treatment is necessary to successfully recover from depression and restore the premorbid level of functioning or "wellness." Therefore, to increase the likelihood of adherence to treatment in addition to minimizing the degree of discomfort and impairment, it is important for physicians to identify and address side effects during the course of pharmacotherapy. In the following chapter, we will review the evidence reporting on the use of pharmacotherapeutic strategies for the treatment of antidepressant-associated side effects.

ADJUNCTIVE STRATEGIES

Sexual Dysfunction

Antidepressant-induced sexual dysfunction is among the most common adverse events reported during treatment with many of the antidepressants and, among the newer agents, most notably during treatment with the selective serotonin reuptake inhibitors (SSRIs) (3,4) but also with venlafaxine, mirtazapine,(4), and possibly duloxetine as well. A number of agents have been reported to alleviate antidepressant-associated sexual dysfunction in case reports or series or in small open-label trials. These agents include antidepressants such as bupropion (5–9), mianserin (10), trazodone and nefazodone (11–13), psychostimulants (14), dopaminergic agents such as ropinirole (15), amantadine (16–18), and other agents including yohimbine (19–23), granisetron (24), cyproheptadine (23,25–31), loratadine (32), bethanechol (33), pramipexole (34), and *Gingko biloba* (35–37). Finally, case reports (38–46), retrospective chart reviews (47), and open-label trials (3,46,48–50) report on the use of adjunct sildenafil for antidepressant-associated sexual dysfunction. These open-label trials cumulatively involve 40 men and 19 women, and report improvements in sexual function in 69% to 90% of patients following addition of sildenafil. However, only a fraction of these potential treatment strategies have been subject to stringent, controlled investigation that we will discuss below.

The promising, open-label trials involving sildenafil augmentation were soon followed by three double-blind, placebo-controlled trials reporting greater improvement in sexual function among adjunct [to SSRIs, tricyclic antidepressants (TCAs), venlafaxine] sildenafil-treated men than in placebo-treated men with antidepressant-associated sexual dysfunction (51–53). There is also a positive, double-blind, placebo-controlled trial for adjunctive vardenafil in SSRI-induced erectile dysfunction (54). Controlled studies of sildenafil or vardenafil for the treatment of antidepressant-associated sexual dysfunction in women are yet to be published.

An alternative adjunct strategy to sildenafil for antidepressant-induced sexual dysfunction is bupropion. In fact, adjunct bupropion was found to be the most popular strategy for antidepressant-associated sexual dysfunction in one survey of clinicians (55). Initial open-label trials of adjunctive bupropion for antidepressant-associated sexual dysfunction were soon followed by a negative, underdosed and underpowered, double-blind, placebo-controlled trial (56). However, a subsequent larger ($n = 42$) double-blind, randomized trial did report bupropion augmentation (300 mg/day) to be more effective than placebo in alleviating SSRI-associated sexual dysfunction (57). This study has yet to be replicated.

There have also been several negative double-blind studies with other agents. Michelson et al. (58) randomized 57 women successfully treated with SSRIs but who reported worsening of sexual function during treatment to receive adjunctive buspirone (15–30 mg), amantadine (50–100 mg), or placebo for eight weeks and found no difference between the three groups in terms of improvement in sexual functioning. Similarly, Michelson et al. (59) randomized 118 SSRI-treated women to receive adjunctive mirtazapine (15–30 mg), yohimbine (5.4–10.8 mg), olanzapine (2.5–5 mg), or placebo for six weeks. Again, there was no difference between the four groups in terms of improvement in sexual functioning. Finally, there are also negative placebo-controlled trials of granisetron (24,60–63) and ephedrine (63) for antidepressant-associated sexual dysfunction.

Fatigue and Hypersomnia

Case reports or series (64–70) and small, open-label trials (71–74) suggest the potential utility of modafinil augmentation for the treatment of depression and fatigue in MDD outpatients with antidepressant-associated or residual fatigue and hypersomnia. However, double-blind, placebo-controlled studies present equivocal results. DeBattista et al. (75) studied 136 MDD outpatients with incomplete response to a number of antidepressants and complaints of fatigue and/or hypersomnia who were randomized to receive modafinil augmentation (100–400 mg) versus placebo for a total of six weeks. Overall, there was no difference between the two groups at endpoint in terms of improvement in hypersomnia or fatigue. However, significantly greater improvement in hypersomnia and fatigue early on (weeks 1–2) in modafinil-treated patients than in placebo-treated patients was reported. Fava et al. (76) studied 311 MDD outpatients with an incomplete response to an SSRI also complaining of fatigue and hypersomnia who were randomized to receive modafinil augmentation (200 mg) versus placebo for eight weeks. Similarly, there were no significant differences in improvement in hypersomnia or fatigue between the two groups. However, there was a greater reduction in depressive symptoms and hypersomnia in modafinil- than placebo-treated patients who had a significant burden of depressive symptoms (17-item Hamilton Depression Rating scale (HAMD17) scores $\geq$14) at baseline, which would suggest that modafinil may be more effective in treating hypersomnia and fatigue that are secondary to depression rather than those that are antidepressant-induced. Finally, only anecdotal evidence supports the use of adjunct bupropion (77) or psychostimulants (78) for SSRI-associated fatigue.

Insomnia, Anxiety, Jitteriness and Agitation

Insomnia, anxiety, and jitteriness are among the most common adverse events reported during initial treatment with the SSRIs and are present in more than a third of patients treated with low-dose SSRIs (79). Amsterdam et al. (80) first reported a significant reduction in jitteriness and anxiety among 54 fluoxetine-treated MDD outpatients who received alprazolam augmentation (0.5–4 mg daily). Subsequently, a double-blind study of the use of clonazepam versus placebo co-initiation with fluoxetine revealed greater improvements in anxiety and insomnia in clonazepam-treated patients than in placebo-treated patients (81). Similarly, a double-blind study of the use of zolpidem versus placebo augmentation for MDD patients who were experiencing significant insomnia during treatment with SSRIs revealed improvement in the quality of sleep in zolpidem-treated patients than in placebo-treated patients (82).

That adjunctive treatment with benzodiazepines is effective in alleviating TCA-induced insomnia is also supported by several studies including a double-blind, placebo-controlled augmentation study of triazolam with various TCAs for MDD (83). A double-blind, placebo-controlled co-initiation study of alprazolam with desipramine for MDD (84), and a double-blind placebo-controlled co-initiation study of triazolam with imipramine for MDD (85). Adjunctive treatment with bentazepam was also reported to result in lower anxiety symptoms than placebo in clomipramine-treated MDD patients in one double-blind study (86). The amount of controlled studies for benzodiazepines in this area is second only to the amount of controlled data described previously for sexual dysfunction.

There are scant data regarding older neuroleptics, and two double-blind studies suggest greater decreases in symptoms of agitation and hostility among depressed outpatients randomized to receive treatment with a tricyclic antidepressant in addition to a typical neuroleptic than among patients treated with a tricyclic antidepressant alone (87,88).

Anecdotal reports supporting the use of melatonin for the treatment of sleep disturbance in depression (89,90) were soon followed by a positive double-blind, placebo-controlled trial of melatonin (5–10 mg, slow release formulation) as an adjunct to fluoxetine for the treatment of sleep disturbance of MDD and/or insomnia resulting from fluoxetine use (91). Case reports and open-label trials (91–96) suggesting the potential utility of trazodone for antidepressant-associated insomnia, the most popular adjunctive strategy for antidepressant-induced insomnia in one survey of clinicians (97), have been confirmed by a small positive, double-blind study of trazodone augmentation of SSRIs for SSRI-associated insomnia (98). Finally, *Gingko biloba* has been reported to increase sleep efficiency and decrease the number of nighttime awakenings in trimipramine-treated patients (99).

Akathisia and Bruxism

Akathisia and bruxism are commonly reported during treatment with a number of newer antidepressants (100). A series of reports of adjunctive buspirone for the treatment of bruxism associated with the use of SSRIs or the seratonin and norepinephrine reuptake inhibitor (SNRI) venlafaxine have been published (101–105). In addition, there is only anecdotal evidence for the usefulness of the anticholinergic benztropine (106), or the selective β-adrenergic receptor antagonists propranolol for SSRI-induced akathisia (107,108).

Gastrointestinal Distress

Nausea is commonly associated with premature discontinuation of treatment, while the incidence of antidepressant-induced nausea has been reported to range between 20% and 40% during the course of treatment with newer antidepressants such as the SSRIs, SNRIs, and bupropion (109). There have been reports of the use of adjunctive (5HT4)-selective agonists and cholinergic enhancers, cisapride or mosapride, in alleviating venlafaxine (110) or fluvoxamine-emergent nausea (111). Similarly, reports suggesting the use of the selective 5HT3-receptor antagonist ondansetron for bupropion-emergent nausea (112) exist. Finally, there is anecdotal evidence for the use of Gorei-san (TJ-17) (113,114) or mirtazapine (115) for the treatment of SSRI-associated nausea. The mechanism of action is purported to be 5HT3-receptor blockade.

Weight Gain

Weight gain is often associated with longer term use of serotonergic agents. This weight gain may be acutely amplified if antihistaminergic drug properties are also involved (e.g., mirtazapine). One could opt to use antidepressants that are relatively devoid of serotonergic activity (e.g., bupropion, desipramine, nortriptyline, protriptyline, etc.) to avoid this side effect. However, clinicians often like to utilize serotonin where comorbid anxiety exists in the depressed patient, which makes weight gain unavoidable.

Anorectic agents or appetite suppressants, do so by decreasing appetite or increasing satiety. They are classified as centrally acting sympathomimetic agents or serotonergic agents. Sympathomimetic agents include phendimetrazine, phentermine, mazindol, diethylpropion (all of which are schedule III and IV controlled substances), amphetamine and related compounds, and phenylpropanolamine. Of the serotonergic agents, fenfluramine and dexfenfluramine were withdrawn from the market in September 1997 over concerns about valvular heart disease (116). Because of their high potential for abuse, amphetamines are generally not recommended for treating obesity (117). Currently, sibutramine, a mixed serotonergic and noradrenergic reuptake inhibitor, is one of two appetite suppressants approved by the Food and Drug Administration (FDA) for treating obesity in general. There are no current studies involving these adjunctive agents with regard to depression and one must watch for serotonin syndrome when mixing this latter drug with other serotonergic antidepressants.

Orlistat, a fat or lipase blocker, was also recently approved by the FDA for general weight loss. Orlistat may be a better option than sibutramine for patients already taking other drugs because it does not act systemically, and so there is less risk of interaction with centrally acting medications.

Only a positive case series by Schwartz and Beale exists where the average weight loss within this relatively short time period was 5.6 kg, or 34.6% of the weight gained as a result of psychotropic drug use (118). Schwartz et al. have completed extensive reviews within this area as a follow up to their pilot work (119–121).

Amantadine, nizatadine, topiramate, and metformin (122–126) have been researched in small open-label studies and show weight loss induced by neuroleptics and mood stabilizers, but no such data exists for antidepressant augmentation.

Finally, in two small pilot studies, adjunctive naltrexone, an opioid antagonist, has decreased weight by reversing the observed hunger and craving for sweet, fatty foods caused by tricyclic antidepressants and lithium. Hunger and eating disinhibition subscales declined significantly (127).

SWITCHING ANTIDEPRESSANTS OWING TO INTOLERANCE

An alternative strategy to targeting side effects with adjunctive pharmacotherapeutic strategies is to switch to a different agent altogether. This practice, however, is grossly understudied. Specifically, open-label trials focusing on the acute phase of treatment support switching from one SSRI to another owing to intolerance (128–134), or switching to bupropion for fluoxetine-associated sexual dysfunction (135). Double-blind studies are yet to be conducted. In addition, there is an even greater need for studies focusing on switching from one agent to another during the continuation and maintenance phase in remitted patients. In a small chart review, Posternak and Zimmerman (136) reported a 0% relapse rate among nine (mostly SSRI) remitted patients switched to another SSRI or a non-SSRI antidepressant.

In conclusion, during the course of the past few years, there appears to be a dramatic increase in the number of controlled trials focusing on the use of adjunctive pharmacotherapeutic strategies to alleviate a number of side effects of antidepressants. Specifically, of the 25 double-blind, placebo-controlled trials reviewed, 16 have been published since 2000. The majority of these studies focus on the treatment of antidepressant-induced sexual dysfunction (43), with the remaining on insomnia, jitteriness and anxiety (37), or fatigue and hypersomnia (80). Of these, sildenafil and vardenafil augmentation for antidepressant-induced sexual dysfunction in men as well as adjunctive benzodiazepines for antidepressant-induced anxiety or jitteriness and insomnia appear to be best-supported strategies, with several positive, double-blind, placebo-controlled studies each. However, double-blind studies of sildenafil for sexual dysfunction in women treated with antidepressants are yet to be published. Melatonin and trazodone appear promising for SSRI-associated insomnia although evidence supporting their use has yet to be replicated. For bupropion augmentation in sexual dysfunction there is one positive and one negative study, while for modafinil augmentation for hypersomnia and fatigue, two equivocal studies have been reported. Finally, the use of adjunctive buspirone, amantadine, mirtazapine, yohimbine, olanzapine, granisetron, ephedrine, and *Gingko biloba* for antidepressant-induced sexual dysfunction is not supported by published double-blind studies. Weight loss studies are positive, but grossly underpowered and uncontrolled in nature.

Despite the dramatic increase in double-blind studies, numerous practices, many of which appear promising, are yet to be subject to controlled comparison including switching from one antidepressant to another because of poor tolerability. In parallel, there is a paucity of uncontrolled or controlled studies for a number of side effects including weight gain and cognitive slowing. In addition, it appears that the strategies best supported by the existing literature are not necessarily the ones most often chosen by clinicians (97). Therefore, a sustained effort in conducting controlled trials of adjunctive pharmacotherapeutic strategies for antidepressant-associated adverse events and educating clinicians regarding the timely identification, and evidence-based treatment of such adverse events is necessary to improve the standard of care for depression.

REFERENCES

1. Nierenberg AA, Petersen TJ, Alpert JE. Prevention of relapse and recurrence in depression: the role of long-term pharmacotherapy and psychotherapy. J Clin Psychiat 2003; 64(suppl 15):13–17.
2. Kocsis JH, Schatzberg A, Rush AJ, et al. Psychosocial outcomes following long-term, double-blind treatment of chronic depression with sertraline versus placebo. Arch Gen Psychiat 2002; 59(8):723–728.
3. Fava M, Rankin MA, Alpert JE, Nierenberg AA, Worthington JJ. An open trial of oral sildenafil in antidepressant-induced sexual dysfunction. Psychother Psychosom 1998; 67(6):328–331.
4. Clayton AH, Pradko JF, Croft HA, et al. Prevalence of sexual dysfunction among newer antidepressants. J Clin Psychiat 2002; 63(4):357–366.

5. Labbate LA, Pollack MH. Treatment of fluoxetine-induced sexual dysfunction with bupropion: a case report. Ann Clin Psychiat 1994; 6(1):13–15.

6. Labbate LA, Grimes JB, Hines A, Pollack MH. Bupropion treatment of serotonin reuptake antidepressant-associated sexual dysfunction. Ann Clin Psychiat 1997; 9(4):241–245.

7. Ashton AK, Rosen RC. Bupropion as an antidote for serotonin reuptake inhibitor-induced sexual dysfunction. J Clin Psychiat 1998; 59(3):112–115.

8. Chengappa KN, Kambhampati RK, Perkins K, et al. Bupropion sustained release as a smoking cessation treatment in remitted depressed patients maintained on treatment with selective serotonin reuptake inhibitor antidepressants. J Clin Psychiat 2001; 62(7):503–508.

9. Gitlin MJ, Suri R, Altshuler L, Zuckerbrow-Miller J, Fairbanks L. Bupropion-sustained release as a treatment for SSRI-induced sexual side effects. J Sex Marital Ther 2002; 28(2):131–138.

10. Dolberg OT, Klag E, Gross Y, Schreiber S. Relief of serotonin selective reuptake inhibitor induced sexual dysfunction with low-dose mianserin in patients with traumatic brain injury. Psychopharmacology (Berl) 2002; 161(4): 404–407.

11. Reynolds RD. Sertraline-induced anorgasmia treated with intermittent nefazodone. J Clin Psychiat 1997; 58(2):89.

12. Michael A, Tubbe PA, Praseedom A. Sertraline-induced anorgasmia reversed by nefazodone. Br J Psychiat 1999; 175:491.

13. Michael A, O'Donnell EA. Fluoxetine-induced sexual dysfunction reversed by trazodone. Can J Psychiat 2000; 45(9):847–848.

14. Bartlik BD, Kaplan P, Kaplan HS. Psychostimulants apparently reverse sexual dysfunction secondary to selective serotonin reuptake inhibitors. J Sex Marital Ther 1995; 21(4):264–271.

15. Worthington JJ III, Simon NM, Korbly NB, Perlis RH, Pollack MH. Anxiety disorders research program. Ropinirole for antidepressant-induced sexual dysfunction. Int Clin Psychopharmacol 2002; 17(6):307–310.

16. Balogh S, Hendricks SE, Kang J. Treatment of fluoxetine-induced anorgasmia with amantadine. J Clin Psychiat 1992; 53(6):212–213.

17. Shrivastava RK, Shrivastava S, Overweg N, Schmitt M. Amantadine in the treatment of sexual dysfunction associated with selective serotonin reuptake inhibitors. J Clin Psychopharmacol 1995; 15(1):83–84.

18. Balon R. Intermittent amantadine for fluoxetine-induced anorgasmia. J Sex Marital Ther 1996; 22(4):290–292.

19. Price J, Grunhaus LJ. Treatment of clomipramine-induced anorgasmia with yohimbine: a case report. J Clin Psychiat 1990; 51(1):32–33.

20. Balon R. Fluoxetine-induced sexual dysfunction and yohimbine. J Clin Psychiat 1993; 54(4):161–162.

21. Hollander E, McCarley A. Yohimbine treatment of sexual side effects induced by serotonin reuptake blockers. J Clin Psychiat 1992; 53(6):207–209.

22. Jacobsen FM. Fluoxetine-induced sexual dysfunction and an open trial of yohimbine. J Clin Psychiat 1992; 53(4):119–122.

23. Keller Ashton A, Hamer R, Rosen RC. Serotonin reuptake inhibitor-induced sexual dysfunction and its treatment: a large-scale retrospective study of 596 psychiatric outpatients. J Sex Marital Ther 1997; 23(3):165–175.

24. Nelson EB, Shah VN, Welge JA, Keck PE Jr. A placebo-controlled, crossover trial of granisetron in SRI-induced sexual dysfunction. J Clin Psychiat 2001; 62(6):469–473.
25. Lauerma H. Successful treatment of citalopram-induced anorgasmia by cyproheptadine. Acta Psychiatr Scand 1996; 93(1):69–70.
26. Aizenberg D, Zemishlany Z, Weizman A. Cyproheptadine treatment of sexual dysfunction induced by serotonin reuptake inhibitors. Clin Neuropharmacol 1995; 18(4):320–324.
27. Arnott S, Nutt D. Successful treatment of fluvoxamine-induced anorgasmia by cyproheptadine. Br J Psychiat 1994; 164(6):838–839.
28. Cohen AJ. Fluoxetine-induced yawning and anorgasmia reversed by cyproheptadine treatment. J Clin Psychiat 1992; 53(5):174.
29. McCormick S, Olin J, Brotman AW. Reversal of fluoxetine-induced anorgasmia by cyproheptadine in two patients. J Clin Psychiat 1990; 51(9): 383–384.
30. Steele TE, Howell EF. Cyproheptadine for imipramine-induced anorgasmia. J Clin Psychopharmacol 1986; 6(5):326–327.
31. Sovner R. Treatment of tricyclic antidepressant-induced orgasmic inhibition with cyproheptadine. J Clin Psychopharmacol 1984; 4(3):169.
32. Brubaker RV. Fluoxetine-induced sexual dysfunction reversed by loratadine. J Clin Psychiat 2002; 63(6):534.
33. Gross MD. Reversal by bethanechol of sexual dysfunction caused by anticholinergic antidepressants. Am J Psychiat 1982; 139(9):1193–1194.
34. Sporn J, Ghaemi SN, Sambur MR, et al. Pramipexole augmentation in the treatment of unipolar and bipolar depression: a retrospective chart review. Ann Clin Psychiat 2000; 12(3):137–140.
35. Cohen AJ, Bartlik B. *Ginkgo biloba* for antidepressant-induced sexual dysfunction. J Sex Marital Ther 1998; 24(2):139–143.
36. Ellison JM, DeLuca P. Fluoxetine-induced genital anesthesia relieved by *Ginkgo biloba* extract. J Clin Psychiat 1998; 59(4):199–200.
37. Ashton AK, Ahrens K, Gupta S, Masand PS. Antidepressant-induced sexual dysfunction and *Ginkgo biloba*. Am J Psychiat 2000; 157(5):836–837.
38. Gupta S, Droney T, Masand P, Ashton AK. SSRI-induced sexual dysfunction treated with sildenafil. Depress Anxiety 1999; 9(4):180–182.
39. Gupta S, Masand P, Ashton AK, Berry SL. Phenelzine-induced sexual dysfunction treated with sildenafil. J Sex Marital Ther 1999; 25(2):131–135.
40. Ashton AK. Sildenafil treatment of paroxetine-induced anorgasmia in a woman. Am J Psychiat 1999; 156(5):800.
41. Ashton AK, Bennett RG. Sildenafil treatment of serotonin reuptake inhibitor-induced sexual dysfunction. J Clin Psychiat 1999; 60(3):194–195.
42. Balon R. Fluvoxamine-induced erectile dysfunction responding to sildenafil. J Sex Marital Ther 1998; 24(4):313–317.
43. Balon R. Sildenafil and sexual dysfunction associated with antidepressants. J Sex Marital Ther 1999; 25(4):259–264.
44. Schaller JL, Behar D. Sildenafil citrate for SSRI-induced sexual side effects. Am J Psychiat 1999; 156(1):156–157.
45. Rosenberg KP. Sildenafil citrate for SSRI-induced sexual side effects. Am J Psychiat 1999; 156(1):157.

46. Nurnberg HG, Lauriello J, Hensley PL, Parker LM, Keith SJ. Sildenafil for sexual dysfunction in women taking antidepressants. Am J Psychiatr 1999; 156(10):1664.

47. Price D. Sildenafil (Viagra): efficacy in the treatment of erectile dysfunction in depressed patients treated with common concomitant conditions. J Impot Res 1998; 10:584.

48. Nurnberg HG, Hensley PL, Lauriello J, Parker LM, Keith SJ. Sildenafil for women patients with antidepressant-induced sexual dysfunction. Psychiatr Serv 1999; 50(8):1076–1078.

49. Damis M, Patel Y, Simpson GM. Sildenafil in the treatment of SSRI-induced sexual dysfunction: a pilot study. Prim Care Companion J Clin Psychiat 1999; 1(6):184–187.

50. Seidman SN, Pesce VC, Roose SP. High-dose sildenafil citrate for selective serotonin reuptake inhibitor-associated ejaculatory delay: open clinical trial. J Clin Psychiat 2003; 64(6):721–725.

51. Seidman SN, Roose SP, Menza MA, Shabsigh R, Rosen RC. Treatment of erectile dysfunction in men with depressive symptoms: results of a placebo-controlled trial with sildenafil citrate. Am J Psychiat 2001; 158(10):1623–1630.

52. Nurnberg HG, Hensley PL, Gelenberg AJ, Fava M, Lauriello J, Paine S. Treatment of antidepressant-associated sexual dysfunction with sildenafil: a randomized controlled trial. JAMA 2003; 289(1):56–64.

53. Tignol J, Furlan PM, Gomez-Beneyto M, et al. Efficacy of sildenafil citrate (Viagra) for the treatment of erectile dysfunction in men in remission from depression. Int Clin Psychopharmacol 2004; 19(4):191–199.

54. Shabsigh R, Bakish D, Goldstein I, et al. Vardenafil temporarily improves erectile dysfunction and depression intensity in men with mild major depressive disorder and erectile dysfunction. Eur Neuropsychopharmacol 2004; 14s1:S208–S209.

55. Dording CM, Mischoulon D, Petersen TJ, et al. The pharmacologic management of SSRI-induced side effects: a survey of psychiatrists. Ann Clin Psychiat 2002; 14(3):143–147.

56. Masand PS, Ashton AK, Gupta S, Frank B. Sustained-release bupropion for selective serotonin reuptake inhibitor-induced sexual dysfunction: a randomized, double-blind, placebo-controlled, parallel-group study. Am J Psychiat 2001; 158(5):805–807.

57. Clayton AH, Warnock JK, Kornstein SG, Pinkerton R, Sheldon-Keller A, McGarvey EL. A placebo-controlled trial of bupropion SR as an antidote for selective serotonin reuptake inhibitor-induced sexual dysfunction. J Clin Psychiat 2004; 65(1):62–67.

58. Michelson D, Bancroft J, Targum S, Kim Y, Tepner R. Female sexual dysfunction associated with antidepressant administration: a randomized, placebo-controlled study of pharmacologic intervention. Am J Psychiat 2000; 157(2):239–243.

59. Michelson D, Kociban K, Tamura R, Morrison MF. Mirtazapine, yohimbine or olanzapine augmentation therapy for serotonin reuptake-associated female sexual dysfunction: a randomized, placebo controlled trial. J Psychiatr Res 2002; 36(3):147–152.

60. Jespersen S, Berk M, Wyk CV, et al. A pilot randomized, double-blind, placebo-controlled study of granisetron in the treatment of sexual dysfunction in women associated with antidepressant use. Int Clin Psychopharmacol 2004; 19(3):161–164.

61. Kang BJ, Lee SJ, Kim MD, Cho MJ. A placebo-controlled, double-blind trial of *Ginkgo biloba* for antidepressant-induced sexual dysfunction. Hum Psychopharmacol 2002; 17(6):279–284.

62. Wheatley D. Triple-blind, placebo-controlled trial of *Ginkgo biloba* in sexual dysfunction due to antidepressant drugs. Hum Psychopharmacol 2004; 19(8): 545–548.

63. Meston CM. A randomized, placebo-controlled, crossover study of ephedrine for SSRI-induced female sexual dysfunction. J Sex Marital Ther 2004; 30(2): 57–68.

64. Menza MA, Kaufman KR, Castellanos A. Modafinil augmentation of antidepressant treatment in depression. J Clin Psychiat 2000; 61(5):378–381.

65. Berigan TR. Augmentation with modafinil to achieve remission in depression: a case report. Prim Care Companion J Clin Psychiat 2001; 3(1):32.

66. Schwarz TL, Leso L, Beale M, Ahmed R, Naprawa S. Modafinil in the treatment of depression with severe comorbid medical illness. Psychosomatics 2002; 43(4):336–337.

67. Even C, Friedman S, Dardennes R, Guelfi JD. Modafinil as an alternative to light therapy for winter depression. Eur Psychiat 2004; 19(1):66.

68. Holder G, Brand S, Hatzinger M, Holsboer-Trachsler E. Reduction of daytime sleepiness in a depressive patient during adjunct treatment with modafinil. J Psychiatr Res 2002; 36(1):49–52.

69. Nasr S. Modafinil as adjunctive therapy in depressed outpatients. Ann Clin Psychiat 2004; 16(3):133–138.

70. Ashton AK. Modafinil augmentation of phenelzine for residual fatigue in dysthymia. Am J Psychiat 2004; 161(9):1716–1717.

71. Markovitz PJ, Wagner S. An open-label trial of modafinil augmentation in patients with partial response to antidepressant therapy. J Clin Psychopharmacol 2003; 23(2):207–209.

72. DeBattista C, Lembke A, Solvason HB, Ghebremichael R, Poirier J. A prospective trial of modafinil as an adjunctive treatment of major depression. J Clin Psychopharmacol 2004; 24(1):87–90.

73. Lundt L. Modafinil treatment in patients with seasonal affective disorder/ winter depression: an open-label pilot study. J Affect Disord 2004; 81(2):173–178.

74. Schwartz TL, Azhar N, Cole K, et al. An open-label study of adjunctive modafinil in patients with sedation related to serotonergic antidepressant therapy. J Clin Psychiat 2004; 65(9):1223–1227.

75. DeBattista C, Dighramji K, Menza M, Rosenthal MH, Fieve RR. The modafinil in depression study group. Adjunct modafinil for the short-term treatment of fatigue and sleepiness in patients with major depressive disorder: a preliminary double-blind, placebo-controlled study. J Clin Psychiat 2003; 64(9):1057–1064.

76. Fava M, Thase ME, DeBattista C. A multicenter, placebo-controled study of modafinil augmentation in partial responders to selective serotonin reuptake inhibitors with persistent fatigue and hypersomnia. J Clin Psychiat 2005; 66(1): 85–93.

77. Green TR. Bupropion for SSRI-induced fatigue. J Clin Psychiat 1997; 58(4):174.

78. Masand PS, Anand VS, Tanquary JF. Psychostimulant augmentation of second generation antidepressants: a case series. Depress Anxiety 1998; 7(2): 89–91.

79. Papakostas GI, Petersen T, Denninger JW, et al. Treatment-related adverse events and outcome in a clinical trial of fluoxetine for major depressive disorder. Ann Clin Psychiat 2003; 15(3–4):187–192.

80. Amsterdam JD, Hornig-Rohan M, Maislin G. Efficacy of alprazolam in reducing fluoxetine-induced jitteriness in patients with major depression. J Clin Psychiat 1994; 55(9):394–400.

81. Londborg PD, Smith WT, Glaudin V, Painter JR. Short-term cotherapy with clonazepam and fluoxetine: anxiety, sleep disturbance and core symptoms of depression. J Affect Disord 2000; 61(1–2):73–79.

82. Asnis GM, Chakraburtty A, DuBoff EA, et al. Zolpidem for persistent insomnia in SSRI-treated depressed patients. J Clin Psychiat 1999; 60(10):668–676.

83. Cohn JB. Triazolam treatment of insomnia in depressed patients taking tricyclics. J Clin Psychiat 1983; 44(11):401–406.

84. Fawcett J, Edwards JH, Kravitz HM, Jeffriess H. Alprazolam: an antidepressant? Alprazolam, desipramine, and an alprazolam-desipramine combination in the treatment of adult depressed outpatients. J Clin Psychopharmacol 1987; 7(5):295–310.

85. Dominguez RA, Jacobson AF, Goldstein BJ, Steinbrook RM. Comparison of triazolam and placebo in the treatment of insomnia in depressed patients. Curr Ther Res 1984; 36(5):856–865.

86. Calcedo Ordonez A, Arosamene X, Otero Perez FJ, et al. Clomipramine/ bentazepam combination in the treatment of major depressive disorders. Hum Psychopharmacol 1992; 7:115–122.

87. Rickels K, Jenkins BW, Zamostien B, Raab E, Kanther M. Pharmacotherapy in neurotic depression. Differential population responses. J Nerv Ment Dis 1967; 145(6):475–485.

88. Rickels K, Hutchison JC, Weise CC, Csanalosi I, Chung HR, Case WG. Doxepin and amitriptyline-perphenazine in mixed anxious-depressed neurotic outpatients: a collaborative controlled study. Psychopharmacologia 1972; 23(4):305–318.

89. deVries MW, Peeters FP. Melatonin as a therapeutic agent in the treatment of sleep disturbance in depression. J Nerv Ment Dis 1997; 185(3):201–202.

90. Dalton EJ, Rotondi D, Levitan RD, Kennedy SH, Brown GM. Use of slow-release melatonin in treatment-resistant depression. J Psychiat Neurosci 2000; 25(1):48–52.

91. Dolberg OT, Hirschmann S, Grunhaus L. Melatonin for the treatment of sleep disturbances in major depressive disorder. Am J Psychiat 1998; 155(8): 1119–1121.

92. Metz A, Shader RI. Adverse interactions encountered when using trazodone to treat insomnia associated with fluoxetine. Int Clin Psychopharmacol 1990; 5(3):191–194.

93. Jacobsen FM. Low-dose trazodone as a hypnotic in patients treated with MAOIs and other psychotropics: a pilot study. J Clin Psychiat 1990; 51(7): 298–302.

94. Nierenberg AA, Keck PE Jr. Management of monoamine oxidase inhibitor-associated insomnia with trazodone. J Clin Psychopharmacol 1989; 9(1):42–45.

95. Nierenberg AA, Adler LA, Peselow E, Zornberg G, Rosenthal M. Trazodone for antidepressant-associated insomnia. Am J Psychiat 1994; 151(7): 1069–1072.

96. Bertschy G, Ragama-Pardos E, Muscionico M, et al. Trazodone addition for insomnia in venlafaxine-treated, depressed inpatients: a semi-naturalistic study. Pharmacol Res 2005; 51(1):79–84.

97. Dording CM, Mischoulon D, Petersen TJ, et al. The pharmacologic management of SSRI-induced side effects: a survey of psychiatrists. Ann Clin Psychiat 2002; 14(3): 143–147.

98. Kaynak H, Kaynak D, Gozukirmizi E, Guilleminault C. The effects of trazodone on sleep in patients treated with stimulant antidepressants. Sleep Med 2004; 5(1):15–20.

99. Hemmeter U, Annen B, Bischof R, et al. Polysomnographic effects of adjuvant *Ginkgo biloba* therapy in patients with major depression medicated with trimipramine. Pharmacopsychiatry 2001; 34(2):50–59.

100. Lane RM. SSRI-induced extrapyramidal side-effects and akathisia: implications for treatment. J Psychopharmacol 1998; 12(2):192–214.

101. Ellison JM, Stanziani P. SSRI-associated nocturnal bruxism in four patients. J Clin Psychiat 1993; 54(11):432–434.

102. Romanelli F, Adler DA, Bungay KM. Possible paroxetine-induced bruxism. Ann Pharmacother 1996; 30(11):1246–1248.

103. Bostwick JM, Jaffee MS. Buspirone as an antidote to SSRI-induced bruxism in 4 cases. J Clin Psychiat 1999; 60(12):857–860.

104. Jaffee MS, Bostwick JM. Buspirone as an antidote to venlafaxine-induced bruxism. Psychosomatics 2000; 41(6):535–536.

105. Pavlovic ZM. Buspirone to improve compliance in venlafaxine-induced movement disorder. Int J Neuropsychopharmacol 2004;7(4):523–524.

106. Diler RS, Yolga AY, Avci A. Fluoxetine-induced extrapyramidal symptoms in an adolescent: a case report. Swiss Med Wkly 2002; 132(9–10):125–126.

107. Lipinski JF, Hudson JI, Cunningham SL, et al. Polysomnographic characteristics of neuroleptic-induced akathisia. Clin Neuropharmacology 1991; 14(5):413–419.

108. Fleischhacker WW. Propanolol for fluoxetine-induced akathisia. Biol Psychiat 1991; 30(5):531–532.

109. DeVane CL. Immediate-release versus controlled-release formulations: pharmacokinetics of newer antidepressants in relation to nausea. J Clin Psychiat 2003; 64(suppl 18):14–19.

110. Johnna RL. Relatively low doses of cisapride in the treatment of nausea in patients treated with venlafaxine for treatment-refractory depression. J Clin Psychopharmacol 1996; 16(1):35–37.

111. Ueda N, Yoshimura R, Shinkai K, Terao T, Nakamura JL. Characteristics of fluvoxamine-induced nausea. Psychiat Res 104(3):259–264.

112. Lara DR, Busnello ED, Souza DO. Ondansetron rather than metoclopramide for bupropion-induced nausea. Can J Psychiat 2001; 46(4):371.

113. Yamada K, Kanba S, Yagi G, Asai M. Herbal medicine in the treatment of fluvoxamine-induced nausea and dyspepsia. Psychiat Clin Neurosci 1999; 53(6):681.

114. Yamada K, Yagi G, Kanba S. Effectiveness of Gorei-san (TJ-17) for treatment of SSRI-induced nausea and dyspepsia: preliminary observations. Clin Neuropharmacol 2003; 26(3):112–114.

115. Caldis EV, Gair RD. Mirtazapine for treatment of nausea induced by selective serotonin reuptake inhibitors. Can J Psychiat 2004; 49(10):707.

116. Connolly HM, Crary JL, McGoon MD, et al. Valvular heart disease associated with fenfluramine-phentermine. N Engl J Med 1997; 227:581–588.

117. Bray GA. Use and abuse of appetite supressant drugs in the treatment of obesity. Ann Int Med 1993; 119:707–713.

118. Schwartz TL, Beale M. Psychotropic induced weight gain alleviated with orlistat. Psychopharm Bull 2003; 37(1):5–8.

119. Schwartz TL, Nihalani N, Jindal S, Virk S, Jones N. Psychiatric medication induced obesity: an epidemiologic review. Obes Rev 2004; 5:115–121.

120. Schwartz TL, Virk S, Jindal S, Nihalani N, Jones N. Psychiatric medication induced obesity: an etiologic review. Obes Rev 2004; 5:167–170.

121. Schwartz TL, Nihalani N, Virk S, Jindal S, Chilton M. Psychiatric medication induced obesity: treatment options. Obes Rev 2004; 5:233–238.

122. Floris M, Lejeune J, Deberdt W. Effect of amantadine on weight gain during olanzapine treatment. Eur Neuropsychopharmacol 2001; 11:181–182.

123. Breier A, Tanaka Y, Roychowdhury S, et al. Nizatidine for the prevention of weight gain during olanzapine treatment in schizophrenia and related disorders: a randomised controlled double blind study. Presented at the Meeting of the Colleges of Psychiatric and Neurologic Pharmacists, San Antonio, Tex, Mar 23–26, 2001.

124. Ghaemi SN, Manwani SG, Katzow JJ, Ko JY, Goodwin FK. Topiramate treatment of bipolar spectrum disorders: a retrospective chart review. Ann Clin Psychiat 2001; 13(4):185–189.

125. Vieta E, Torrent C, Garcia-Ribas G, et al. Use of topiramate in treatment-resistant bipolar spectrum disorders. J Clin Psychopharmacol 2002; 22(4):431–435.

126. Morrison JA, Cottingham EM, Barton BA. Metformin for weight loss in pediatric patients taking psychotropic drugs. Am J Psych 2002; 159:655–657.

127. Zimmermann U. Soc of Biol Psych 1997; 41:747–749.

128. Brown WA, Harrison W. Are patients who are intolerant to one serotonin selective reuptake inhibitor intolerant to another? J Clin Psychiat 1995; 56(1):30–34.

129. Zarate CA, Kando JC, Tohen M, Weiss MK, Cole JO. Does intolerance or lack of response with fluoxetine predict the same will happen with sertraline? J Clin Psychiat 1996; 57(2):67–71.

130. Thase ME, Blomgren SL, Birkett MA, Apter JT, Tepner RG. Fluoxetine treatment of patients with major depressive disorder who failed initial treatment with sertraline. J Clin Psychiat 1997; 58(1):16–21.

131. Thase ME, Ferguson JM, Lydiard RB, Wilcox CS. Citalopram treatment of paroxetine-intolerant depressed patients. Depress Anxiety 2002; 16(3):128–133.

132. Calabrese JR, Londborg PD, Shelton MD, Thase ME. Citalopram treatment of fluoxetine-intolerant depressed patients. J Clin Psychiat 2003; 64(5):562–567.

133. Burke WJ, Bose A, Wang J, Stahl S. Switching depressed patients from citalopram to escitalopram is well tolerated and effective. 42nd Annual Meeting of the American College of Neuropsychopharmacology, San Juan, Puerto Rico, 2003.

134. Schaefer DM, Ruggiero LD, Iyengar MK, Lipschitz A. Tolerability of controlled release paroxetine in patients with previously intolerant SSRI/ SNRI therapy. New Clinical Drug Evaluation Unit (NCDEU) Annual Meeting, 2004.

135. Walker PW, Cole JO, Gardner EA, et al. Improvement in fluoxetine-associated sexual dysfunction in patients switched to bupropion. J Clin Psychiat 1993; 54(12):459–465.

136. Posternak MA, Zimmerman M. The effectiveness of switching antidepressants during remission: a case series of depressed patients who experienced intolerable side effects. J Affect Disord 2002; 69(1–3):237–240.

8

Depression and Genetics

Francisco Moreno

Department of Psychiatry, College of Medicine,
The University of Arizona Health Sciences Center,
Tucson, Arizona, U.S.A.

Holly Garriock

Interdisciplinary Program in Genetics and Psychiatry,
University of Arizona, Tucson, Arizona, U.S.A.

INTRODUCTION

The field of genetics represents one of the most promising approaches to understanding the mechanisms underlying disease and behavior. Over the last several decades, we have moved from thinking of genetic disorders as rare conditions that dramatically affect a small fraction of the population, to the understanding that genes influence most aspects of a person's life and death. Well-evidenced examples of this influence include genetic associations with personality traits, cognitive style, temperament, intellect, and of course serious mental illnesses. Our knowledge of the genetic bases for major depressive disorder (MDD) and most other mental illnesses has progressed significantly, but remains poorly understood due in part to a number of complicating factors relevant to the field of psychiatric genetics.

LIMITATIONS IN PSYCHIATRIC GENETICS

Although the adoption of standardized diagnostic schemes such as the Diagnostic and Statistical Manual for Mental Disorders (DSM) represented a major advance in clinical psychiatry facilitating uniform nomenclature for descriptive syndromes, DSM is by definition non-etiology driven. The limited availability of quantifiable biological markers such as those available in other areas of medicine (clinical laboratory parameters, histopathological findings, etc.) further compromises our ability to explore genetic determinants of mental illness.

MDD is a syndrome defined by the presence of subjective symptoms, and consequent suffering or dysfunction. Aside from its intrinsic challenge to diagnostic consistency, depression is a phenotype that does not follow a classic Mendelian pattern of inheritance. A Mendelian disease runs in families in a strict dominant–recessive or X-linked fashion, and although there are a thousand known disease genes, almost no psychiatric diseases are clearly established among them by way of one single gene equaling one single mental disorder.

A pattern of inheritance that does not follow a traditional Mendelian model is considered "complex." Complex models commonly possess the following features: (a) Incomplete penetrance (of those carrying the gene, some may never express the disorder, while others may do so very late in life), (b) Phenocopies (the same illness may have a nongenetic cause), (c) Heterogeneity (different gene mutations can give the same syndrome), (d) Pleogenic inheritance (the same gene can be involved with several disorders such as schizophrenia or autism), and (e) Multiple susceptibility genes (the higher the complexity of the disorder, the higher the number of genes that would account for only a fraction of the observed phenotype). As was noted in an earlier chapter about the etiology of MDD, this is a very heterogenous disorder with complex etiologic interplay between genetics and the environment.

TRADITIONAL GENETIC APPROACHES

Segregation studies explore patterns of disease expression in pedigrees that may provide information on the mode of inheritance of a given disorder. Earlier studies suggested against "single major locus" inheritance (1–3). Two subsequent reports were able to reject nongenetic models of inheritance but could not discriminate between single major locus and polygenic inheritance (4,5). In a more recent study focusing on subjects with early life onset (by age 25 years), recurrent, or nonpsychotic unipolar MDD, when a restrictive definition of affection status for relatives of probands was used (i.e., requiring recurrent MDD), there was evidence for a non-Mendelian recessive major gene effect, while under a more relaxed definition of affliction status (any major affective illness) the best fitting model implied a codominant major locus (6). Given the lack of consistent segregation study findings in MDD, it is presumed that fairly complex inheritance models involving multiple genes with different modes of transmission may contribute to disease vulnerability. It has also been hypothesized that other genes may exert a protective influence and foster resiliency in face of social stress.

GENETIC EPIDEMIOLOGY

Findings from modern genetic research involving family, twin, and adoption studies consistently support a familial and genetic influence in depression. There is however a fair amount of variability in the results between studies, perhaps due in part to the range of ascertainment methods utilized (e.g., family history vs. direct-interview assessments), the selection of proband groups (e.g., parents and children), and diagnostic criteria (e.g., DSM or other methods) among others.

In multiple family studies, the risk of depression in relatives of depressed probands has been substantially and significantly higher than the risk in relatives of normal controls, with relative risks ranging from approximately two- to six-fold (7–10). Family studies have also provided important evidence about clinical features of depression that are associated with greater familiality. Well-replicated reports indicate that the familial risk of depression is inversely related to the age of onset of depression in the proband (11–16). The familial risk of MDD in particular for early onset depression has been replicated in studies of depressed adults, children of depressed parents, and relatives of depressed children (17–22). Similarly, the number of prior depressive episodes in the proband has been associated with a higher familial risk than single episodes, Bland et al. (23). Interestingly, rates of MDD are elevated in family members of bipolar disorder (BD) probands, and rates of BD are elevated in relatives of MDD probands. Although family studies can indicate a familial component for MDD, the underlying genetic contribution cannot be clarified with this method.

Twin studies represent an important tool to assess the genetic versus environmental liability for a given disorder. Monozygotic (MZ) twins who possess an identical genetic load are compared to same sex dizygotic (DZ) twins who share 50% of their genes. Understanding that most twins share major aspects of their environment, twin studies take advantage of a naturally occurring laboratory to compare concordance rates between MZ and DZ twin pairs for a given diagnosis. Recurrent depression has been associated with a higher ratio of MZ than DZ concordance (49% vs. 20%) (24). The "heritability estimate" (h^2) is a well-accepted parameter for quantifying the proportional risk of a disorder that is attributable to genetics. Several clinical and population-based twin registries of large size have yielded h^2 ranging from 29% to 75%. The large variability in results is believed to be a consequence of methodological differences like corrections for reliability of diagnosis, assumed population risks, and other variables mentioned above (25–30). Several clinical features have been found to predict co-twin depression, including number of episodes, duration of longest episode, recurrent thoughts of death or suicide, and level of distress or impairment. These clinical features were similarly predictive regardless of sex, but had stronger prediction in MZ twins. Some twin studies have also suggested that severity of depressive symptoms and qualitative subtypes such as "atypicality" of neurovegetative symptoms, and seasonality of mood may be heritable (28,31–33).

Adoption studies can also help assess the effect of the environment in the liability to a given disorder by studying affected probands who were adopted at birth and comparing the rates of such disorders in both biological and adopted parents. Despite the limited number of studies reported to have utilized this approach, the findings inconsistently suggest an increase in occurrence of MDD among biological relatives of depressed adoptees (34–37).

Molecular biology techniques have allowed us to identify the base pair sequences for the entire human genome. Given that the function of a gene is to encode the structure of a specific protein, a mutation by omission, substitution, or insertion of one or more of the bases that form a gene may result in the alteration in function or the absence of a protein. These sequence variations abundantly observed in the general population are known as polymorphisms. Polymorphisms can be used as marker loci within a given genetic region. The "linkage" relationship between a disorder and a marker locus suggests genetic influence. Techniques geared to locate disease risk genes in MDD are compromised by the difficulty of assembling the large collections of samples (population-based) or families (pedigree-based) that would be required to identify susceptibility loci influencing this relatively common, heterogeneous phenotype. Although some large studies of BD have included unipolar MDD in the definition of affective illness, large-scale gene-mapping studies of unipolar MDD itself have not been reported. In an early linkage analysis, sib pairs were used in a linkage analysis of 30 markers in 13 families with MDD without significant results (38). Another linkage analysis of recurrent major depression was conducted in five large Swedish families. They tested linkage to chromosomes 4p, 16, 18, and 21, which have previously been claimed to harbor susceptibility loci for BD, but no evidence of significant linkage was detected either (39). In a study of 34 pedigrees ascertained through probands with early-onset recurrent unipolar depression, no evidence of linkage or association was found between MDD (or broader affective disorder phenotypes) and any of 38 polymorphisms in 12 genes related to neuroendocrine or serotonergic systems (40). The lack of definitive conclusions from classical linkage approaches in MDD may be improved by a dramatic expansion in size to several hundred nuclear families. However, because MDD may not segregate in families as in a true Mendelian disorder, it may be too heterogeneous and genetically complex, having many genes of small influence, further complicating the power to detect linkage.

The "candidate gene approach" has become a popular method in the last several years because of its greater likelihood of identifying disease genes in a more feasibly obtainable sample. A candidate gene for MDD is a gene that based either on its function (protein it encodes for) or on its location, might be related to MDD. Although our knowledge of genes that are important for normal behavior remains limited, there are now substantial data to support the utility of these methods for finding genes that affect illnesses. Thus, candidate gene association approaches are complementary to linkage approaches, and may offer advantages like efficiency and may sometimes increase knowledge gained about the illness even with negative studies; a positive study may identify a causative gene while enhancing our understanding of function, rather than just recognizing location. This approach should be utilized with caution given that many well-hypothesized candidate genes have yielded negative results due in part to limited sample sizes, phenotypic limitations, and environmental influences (41).

As a result, strategies utilized in other fields of science to deal with complex genetic disorders have also been incorporated to psychiatry. Examples include attempts to reduce genetic heterogeneity by avoiding largely admixed populations, narrow the phenotypic definition by the use of "endophenotypes," modify the phenotypic definition by selecting quantitative traits (clinical target symptoms) rather than the traditional categorical DSM diagnosis, and to assess the effect of environmental interactions like childhood trauma or recent life stressors. Examples of alternative phenotypes include the use of sensory motor gating, oculomotor function, measures of cognitive processing, and working memory in schizophrenia. To narrow the phenotypic scope of "depression," researchers have studied patients with stricter clinical specificity (subsyndromes or specifiers—psychotic depression, atypical depression, and melancholic depression), resulting in modest contributions to the genetic understanding of MDD. Newer alternative phenotypes selected based on valid etiological rationale may offer advantages over clinical subsyndromes. These include neurocognitive findings such as psychomotor dysfunction and impairments in attention, memory, and executive functioning. Biological markers may include electrophysiological abnormalities such as frontal electroencephalograph asymmetry, sleep architectural features in polysomnogram like decreased rapid eye movement latency or ultradian rhythms, structural and functional imaging findings like hippocampal volume, regional cerebral blood flow, and glucose utilization in the amygdala, and response to biological challenges (cognitive or depressive response to neurotransmitter depletions) (42).

The above-mentioned alternative phenotypes may provide better temporal stability supporting the presence of a "trait" quality as opposed to a transitional "state," and may facilitate relevant candidate gene association or linkage findings. Following these principles, several candidate gene association studies in MDD have reported interesting results. To exemplify some of the most commonly cited candidate genes, we will mention some key reports involving the 5-hydroxytryptamine (5-HT) transporter, the tryptophan hydroxylase (TPH), and the pro–brain-derived neurotrophic factor (BDNF) gene.

CANDIDATE GENES

Based on our current understanding of the mechanisms underlying vulnerability to stress and depression or antidepressant response, many candidate genes have been proposed for their role in the synthesis, transport, recognition, degradation, and regulation of monoamines neurotransmitters (most notably serotonin 5-HT) or a series of intracellular signaling molecules ultimately believed to influence the pathway of neurotrophic signaling (most notably BDNF).

The 5-HT transporter protein [serotonin transporter (SERT)] plays an important role in uptake of 5-HT into the presynaptic cell by a sodium-dependent mechanism. Blockade of this transporter is the basis for the mechanism of action of the selective serotonin reuptake inhibitors (SSRIs). The SERT gene (SLC6A4) is located on chromosome 17. A 44–base pair insertion or deletion polymorphism represents the long (l) and short (s) alleles in the promoter region of the gene (43). In vitro studies suggest that the "l" allele of the polymorphism is associated with higher transcriptional activity, greater levels of SERT mRNA, and higher uptake of labeled 5-HT (43,44). Polymorphic SLC6A4 variation has been extensively studied in a variety of behavioral phenotypes. Slightly higher scores in neurotic personality traits were initially reported in subjects with the "s" allele. Others failed to replicate these findings. Higher "l" allele frequencies have been reported in depressive suicide victims, and obsessive–compulsive disorder patients compared to control subjects. Greater depressive response during serotonin depletion has also been associated with the "ll" genotype in remitted depressive subjects (45). Association with "ls" also has been reported in a postmortem sample of MDD (46). Other studies have failed to find any association between alleles of SLC6A4 and mood disorders in European, Japanese, African, and other populations. Highly significant differences in SLC6A4 allele frequency exist between races. SLC6A4 polymorphisms have also been inconsistently associated with antidepressant response. Reports that European subjects with "ll" genotype respond better to SSRI antidepressants contrast with reports of "ss" genotype association with better response in Asian subjects. Although evidence of an association of SLC6A4 had been inconclusive, a prospective longitudinal study recently found intriguing results. In a sample of 847 Caucasian subjects, Caspi and colleagues (47) found a significant association of the "s" allele with depression, but this was only in the presence of stressful life events. This study is an illustrative example of the challenges observed in psychiatric genetics and in the field's increasing methodological sophistication and improved ability to address relevant variables such as the "nature and nurture" interaction.

Another polymorphism related to SERT is a variable nucleotide tandem repeat polymorphism in intron-2 (Stin-2). Multiple reports of association of this polymorphism with depression-related phenotypes, including evidence for linkage disequilibrium between the intron-2 and the promoter polymorphisms exist.

The TPH gene encodes the rate-limiting enzyme for the synthesis of 5-HT making it an ideal candidate gene to study in depression phenotypes. The allele "A" of the intron 7 (A218C) has been associated with BD, and higher incidence of suicide. The "C" homozygous genotype has lower frequency in MDD compared to healthy controls. Although transmission disequilibrium test (TDT) studies failed to replicate these findings, a series of reports continue to point attention to this gene and its role in the response to lithium prophylaxis in mood disorders, aggressive disposition, and influence in 5-HT turnover rate. Additional polymorphisms have been identified; two in the promoter region of the gene (A6526G and G5806T) are of particular interest. Suicide attempters and completers reportedly have increased frequencies of the haplotype–6526g–5806T–218C. Another marker in intron 3 has also been associated with a phenotype that combines mood, suicidality, and impulsive aggression.

An isoform of TPH (TPH-2) has recently received considerable attention as it selectively influences the rate of 5-HT synthesis in the brain (48). Although several variants have been reported for TPH-2, the "A" allele of the (G1463A) polymorphism leads to an amino acid alteration in the TPH-2 protein that results in an 80% loss of function (5-HT synthesis). The "A" allele was found to be over-represented in a sample of unipolar depressed subjects (6.9%) compared to bipolar patients and healthy controls (0.9%). The rare allele frequency of "A" in healthy and BD subjects suggested a role for this allele in MDD. Most striking was the fact that seven of the nine MDD patients with the "A" allele had treatment resistant depression and the other two had only responded to high doses of SSRIs. Although this report must be replicated, it also speaks to the importance of addressing endophenotypes such as the subpopulation of MDD patients with treatment resistance (49,50).

BDNF has been consistently implicated in the adaptation to stress exposure, cognitive function, and antidepressant response among other relevant central nervous system functions. It has been found to be decreased (both short- and long-term) in the hippocampus of animal models of depression. BDNF is reported to promote function, growth, and sprouting of brain 5-HT neurons and for all these reasons represents an ideal candidate gene for studies of depressive vulnerability. Interestingly, Val-66-Met has been associated with impacting intracellular trafficking and activity-dependent secretion of BDNF, with the "66-Met" form showing less depolarization-induced secretion of BDNF (51). The BDNF dinucleotide

G-Tn polymorphism, and Val-66-Met single nucleotide polymorphism were significantly associated with BD in a family-based association study of European descent probands (52). However, other studies involving Japanese and Chinese populations have failed to find a Val-66-Met association with mood disorders.

CONCLUSION

In this section, we offer a general overview of the rationale and common methodology for the study of genetic effects in MDD. We have discussed, among the most relevant findings, evidence that implicates genetic factors in the etiology of depression-related phenotypes. It has long been demonstrated that depression is a familial phenotype; also it is broadly accepted that MZ twins share higher concordance rates compared to DZ twins and that reports of heritability estimates for MDD range from 29% to 75% depending on methodological issues. The use of candidate genes and the incorporation of novel etiologically defined quantifiable phenotypes may prove to be an adequate complement to traditional psychiatric genetics approaches. Consistent findings with these methodologies may help clarify the underlying mechanisms required for normal brain function, disease states, or the continuum in specific quantitative traits. Recent findings further support the notion that identifying environmental risk or protective factors and assessing their interaction with genes must become a routine element in psychiatric genetic studies. Recent advances in biotechnology, bioinformatics, and biostatistics, coupled with improved phenotypes may facilitate progress despite the identified challenges in dealing with complex genetic traits in behavioral phenotypes.

REFERENCES

1. Crowe R, Namboodiri K, Ashby H, Elston R. Segregation analysis and linkage analysis of a large kindred of unipolar depression. Neuropsychopharmacology 1981; 7:20–25.
2. Goldin LR, Gershon ES, Targum SD, Sparkes RS, McGinnis M. Segregation and linkage analyses in families of patients with bipolar, unipolar, and schizoaffective mood disorders. Am J Hum Genet 1983; 35:274–287.
3. Tsuang M, Bucher K, Fleming J, Faraone S. Transmission of affective disorders: an application of segregation analysis to blind family study data. J Psychiat Res 1985; 19:23–29.
4. Price RA, Kidd KK, Weissman MM. Early onset (under age 30 years) and panic disorder as markers for etiologic homogeneity in major depression. Arch Gen Psychiat 1987; 44:434–440.
5. Cox N, Reich T, Rice J, Elston R, Schober J, Keats B. Segregation and linkage analysis of bipolar and major depressive illness in multigenerational pedigrees. J Psychiat Res 1989; 23:109–123.

6. Marazita ML, Neiswanger K, Cooper M, et al. Genetic segregation analysis of early-onset recurrent unipolar depression. Am J Hum Genet 1997; 61:1370–1378.

7. Andreasen NC, Rice J, Endicott J, Coryell W, Grove WM, Reich T. Familial rates of affective disorder: a report from the National Institute of Mental Health Collaborative Study. Arch Gen Psychiat 1987; 44:461–469.

8. McGuffin P, Katz R, Bebbington P. Hazard, heredity and depression: a family study. J Psychiat Res 1987; 21:365–375.

9. Merikangas KR, Prusoff BA, Weissman MM. Parental concordance for affective disorders: psychopathology in offspring. J Affect Disord 1988; 15: 279–290.

10. Gershon ES, Hamovit J, Guroff JJ, et al. A family study of schizoaffective, bipolar I, bipolar II, unipolar, and normal control probands. Arch Gen Psychiat 1982; 39:1157–1167.

11. Weissman MM, Gershon ES, Kidd KK, et al. Psychiatric disorders in the relatives of probands with affective disorders: the Yale University-National Institute of Mental Health Collaborative Study. Arch Gen Psychiat 1984; 41:13–21.

12. Weissman MM, Gammon GD, John K, et al. Children of depressed parents: increased psychopathology and early onset of major depression. Arch Gen Psychiat 1987; 44:847–853.

13. Weissman MM, Warner V, Wickramaratne P, Prusoff BA. Early-onset major depression in parents and their children. J Affect Disord 1988; 15:269–277.

14. Mitchell J, McCauley E, Burke P, Calderon R, Schloredt K. Psychopathology in parents of depressed children and adolescents. J Am Acad Child Adolesc Psychiat 1989; 28:352–357.

15. Rende R, Weissman M, Rutter M, Wickramaratne P, Harrington R, Pickles A. Psychiatric disorders in the relatives of depressed probands II. Familial loading for comorbid non-depressive disorders based upon age of onset. J Affect Disord 1997; 42:23–28.

16. Harrington R, Rutter M, Weissman M, et al. Psychiatric disorders in the relatives of depressed probands I. Comparison of prepubertal, adolescent and early adult onset cases. J Affect Disord 1997; 42:9–22.

17. Puig-Antich J, Goetz D, Davies M, et al. A controlled family history study of prepubertal major depressive disorder. Arch Gen Psychiat 1989; 46:406–418.

18. Kupfer DJ, Frank E, Carpenter LL, Neiswanger K. Family history of recurrent depression. J Affect Disord 1989; 17:113–119.

19. Kutcher S, Marton P. Affective disorders in first-degree relatives of adolescent onset bipolars, unipolars, and normal controls. J Am Acad Child Adolesc Psychiat 1991; 30:75–78.

20. Williamson DE, Ryan ND, Birmaher B, et al. A case-control family history study of depression in adolescents. J Am Acad Child Adolesc Psychiat 1995; 34:1596–1607.

21. Warner V, Mufson L, Weissman MM. Offspring at high and low risk for depression and anxiety: mechanisms of psychiatric disorder. J Am Acad Child Adolesc Psychiat 1995; 34:786–797.

22. Kovacs M, Devlin B, Pollock M, Richards C, Mukerji P. A controlled family history study of childhood-onset depressive disorder. Arch Gen Psychiat 1997; 54:613–623.

23. Bland RC, Newman SC, Orn H. Recurrent and non recurrent depression. A family study. Arch Gen Psychiat 1986; 43:1085–1089.

24. McGuffin P, Katz R, Rutherford J. Nature, nurture and depression: a twin study. Psychol Med 1991; 21:329–335.

25. Torgersen S. Genetic factors in moderately severe and mild affective disorders. Arch Gen Psychiat 1986; 43:222–226.

26. Englund SA, Klein DN. The genetics of neurotic-reactive depression: a reanalysis of Shapiro's (1970) twin study using diagnostic criteria. J Affect Disord 1990; 18:247–252.

27. Kendler KS, Neale MC, Kessler RC, Heath AC, Eaves LJ. A population-based twin study of major depression in women. Arch Gen Psychiat 1992; 49:257–266.

28. Kendler K, Eaves L, Walters E, Neale M, Heath A, Kessler R. The identification and validation of distinct depressive syndromes in a population-based sample of female twins. Arch Gen Psychiat 1996; 53:391–399.

29. Kendler KS, Prescott CA. A population-based twin study of lifetime major depression in men and women. Arch Gen Psychiat 1999; 56(1):39–44.

30. Lyons M, Eisen S, Goldberg J, et al. A registry-based twin study of depression in men. Arch Gen Psychiat 1998; 55:468–472.

31. Kendler KS, Gardner CO, Prescott CA. Clinic characteristics of major depression that predict risk of depression in relatives. Arch Gen Psychiat 1999; 56(4):322–327.

32. Madden P, Heath A, Rosenthal N, Martin N. Seasonal changes in mood and behavior: the role of genetic factors. Arch Gen Psychiat 1996; 53:47–55.

33. Thapar A, McGuffin P. A twin study of depressive symptoms in childhood. Br J Psychiat 1994; 165:259–265.

34. Wender PH, Kety SS, Rosenthal D, Schulsinger F, Ortmann J, Lunde I. Psychiatric disorders in the biological and adoptive families of adopted individuals with affective disorders. Arch Gen Psychiat 1986; 43:923–929.

35. Mendlewicz J, Rainer J. Adoption study supporting genetic transmission in manic-depressive illness. Nature 1977; 268:326–329.

36. Cadoret R. Evidence for genetic inheritance of primary affective disorder in adoptees. Am J Psychiat 1978; 133:463–466.

37. von Knorring AL, Cloninger C, Bohman M, Sigvardsson S. An adoption study of depressive disorders and substance abuse. Arch Gen Psychiat 1983; 40: 943–950.

38. Tanna VL, Wilson AF, Winokur G, Elston RC. Linkage analysis of pure depressive disease. J Psychiatr Res 1989; 23(2):99–107.

39. Balciuniene J, Yuan QP, Engstrom C, et al. Linkage analysis of candidate loci in families with recurrent major depression. Mol Psychiat 1998; 3:162–168.

40. Neiswanger K, Zubenko G, Giles D, Frank E, Kupfer D, Kaplan B. Linkage and association analysis of chromosomal regions containing genes related to neuroendocrine or serotonin function in families with early onset, recurrent major depression. Am J Med Genet 1998; 81:443–449.

41. Risch N, Merikangas K. The future of genetic studies of human complex diseases. Science 1996; 273:1516–1517.

42. Hasler G, Drevets WC, Manji HK, Charney DS. Discovering endophenotypes for major depression. Neuropsychopharmacology 2004; 29:1765–1791.

43. Lesch K, Bengel D, Heils A, et al. Association of anxiety-related traits with a polymorphism in the serotonin transporter gene regulatory region. Science 1996; 274:1527–1531.

44. Heils A, Teufel A, Petri S, et al. Allelic variation of human serotonin transporter gene expression. J Neurochem 1996; 66:2621–2624.

45. Moreno FA, Rowe DC, Kaiser B, et al. Association between a serotonin transporter promoter region polymorphism and mood response during tryptophan depletion. Mol Psychiat 2002; 7(2):213–216.

46. Mann JJ, Huang Y, Underwood MD, et al. A serotonin transporter gene promoter polymorphism (5-HTTLPR) and prefrontal cortical binding in major depression and suicide. Arch Gen Psychiat 2000; 57:729–738.

47. Caspi.

48. Zhang X, Beaulieu JM, Sotnikova TD, Gainetdinov RR, Caron MG. Tryptophan hydroxylase-2 controls brain serotonin synthesis. Science 2004; 305(5681):217.

49. Zhang X, Gainetdinov RR, Beaulieu JM, et al. Loss-of-function mutation in tryptophan hydroxylase-2 identified in unipolar major depression. Neuron 2005; 45:11–16.

50. Garriock HA, Allen JJB, Delgado P, et al. Lack of association of TPH2 exon XI polymorphisms with major depression and treatment resistance. Mol Psychiatry 2005; 10:976–977.

51. Egan MF, Kojima M, Callicott JH, et al. The BDNF val66met polymorphism affects activity-dependent secretion of BDNF and human memory and hippocampal function. Cell 2003; 112:257–269.

52. Neves-Pereira M, Mundo E, Muglia P, King N, Macciardo F, Kennedy J. The Brain-derived neurotrophic factor gene confers susceptibility to bipolar disorder: evidence from a family-based association study. Am J Hum Genet 2002; 71(3):651–655.

9

Depression, Neuroimaging and Neurophysiology

Dan V. Iosifescu

Depression Clinical and Research Program, Massachusetts General Hospital, Harvard Medical School, Boston, Massachusetts, U.S.A.

INTRODUCTION

Since the advent of the modern era of psychiatry, clinicians and investigators have sought biological tests as a means of diagnosing patients with psychiatric disorders, as well as discriminating between likely treatment-responders and nonresponders, or identifying those at greater risk for relapse. In the last decades, the widespread availability of neuroimaging and electrophysiology [electroencephalogram (EEG)] technology has led to new efforts to apply these techniques to improve diagnosis and to predict treatment response in psychiatric disorders.

The search for disease-specific neuroimaging and EEG abnormalities is driven by two related goals. The first is the identification of the underlying pathophysiology associated with a given disease. In the past, the utility of selective serotonin reuptake inhibitors (SSRIs) in major depression provided evidence for serotonergic dysregulation in some affective illnesses. Similarly, the discovery of disease-specific functional and/or metabolic changes in certain brain regions would implicate those structures in the process of disease development or recovery. These findings could then guide future diagnostic procedures or even drug development. The second goal is to find objective biological (e.g., neuroimaging and EEG) markers of treatment–response, which could potentially allow more targeted and focused clinical interventions. For example, while first-line antidepressant treatments have response rates of 50% or more, large numbers of patients still fail to respond to multiple interventions (1). Moreover, it takes 6 to 12 weeks to fully evaluate the efficacy of an antidepressant treatment. As each new pharmacotherapy is tried, patients are exposed to additional cost, side effects, and the potential for loss of function and risk of suicide. The ability to predict treatment–response before or shortly after a new treatment is initiated would translate into significant improvement of our initial treatment selection process, ultimately resulting in a significant increase in the efficacy of our treatments.

In the following sections, we will review studies in major depressive disorder (MDD) involving multiple imaging modalities [structural and functional neuroimaging, and magnetic resonance spectroscopy (MRS)] as well as electrophysiology studies. We will briefly interpret their results and address some of the problems and limitations associated with these approaches.

Original reports or reviews included in this chapter were identified by conducting a MEDLINE search using the terms "neuroimaging," "magnetic resonance imaging (MRI)," "functional MRI (fMRI)," "MRS," and "EEG" combined with either "depression," "MDD," "bipolar disorder," or "affective illness." References in the publications identified were then reviewed manually to locate additional relevant publications.

Imaging Studies

Morphologic and functional imaging studies have identified a number of abnormalities in MDD patients, but these findings are often inconsistent or difficult to replicate, possibly due to the small sample size of most imaging studies. However, taken together, the neuroimaging abnormalities in MDD point to an imbalance in the relative role and activity between regions that putatively mediate emotional and stress responses (such as the amygdala and hippocampus) and regions that appear to inhibit emotional expression (such as the posterior orbital cortex and cingulate gyrus) (2). This imbalance may be reflected in the morphologic and functional imaging studies, as well as in the MRS studies reviewed below.

STRUCTURAL IMAGING

In a typical protocol, imaging is performed comparing medication-free subjects having MDD with age- and gender-matched healthy volunteers. In some studies, MDD patients then enter pharmacotherapy trials, and the outcome measures are ultimately correlated with the size of brain structures, or presence and extent of lesions such as white matter abnormalities. The neuroanatomical abnormalities reported so far in MDD patients include morphological lesions and reductions in gray matter volume (3).

A number of researchers have identified decreased frontal lobe volumes in depression (4,5) or familial affective illness (6). Volume reductions in the anterior cingulate gyrus of MDD subjects were also reported (6,7) and were corroborated by postmortem studies showing glial reduction in the corresponding gray matter (8).

Reductions in hippocampal volumes associated with MDD have been reported consistently (9). Although some researchers did not replicate this finding (10), a meta-analysis of 17 MRI studies supports the finding of a reduced hippocampus size in MDD (11). Reduced hippocampal volumes have been associated with the effects of hypercortisolemia and chronic stress, as well as with longer duration of depression (9).

Changes in basal ganglia volumes have also been reported in depressed patients (12). There is much disagreement in the literature on amygdala volumes in MDD, which have been reported to be either decreased (13) or increased (14).

MRI also allows the identification of white matter abnormalities, which in some studies are associated with affective illness. Most MRI reports of an increased incidence of brain white matter lesions (WML) have involved elderly MDD subjects compared to age-matched controls (15,16). In younger MDD subjects, however, the results are still equivocal; some studies reported increased incidence of WML (17), while others did not (18). The presence of brain WML has been associated with cardiovascular risk factors such as age, prior cerebrovascular disease, smoking, arterial hypertension, and increased serum cholesterol (19,20). Neuropathological studies have reported a large proportion of WML in depressed subjects to be related to brain vascular disease (21).

Recognition of the increased prevalence of brain WML in major depression has led investigators to describe "vascular depression," a subtype of MDD characterized by the presence of cerebrovascular disease (demonstrated on neuroimaging by brain WML) (15,22). In some studies, the presence of brain WML in MDD subjects was associated with lower rates of response to antidepressant treatment, compared with MDD subjects with no WML (23,24) as well as with higher rates of relapse in long-term follow-up (25). However, other researchers did not find a difference in the outcome of antidepressant therapy in depressed subjects with or without WML (26).

These conflicting results may point toward specific brain regions where the presence of WML has an impact on MDD. Not all WML appear to have an equal role in the etiology of depression. Several studies appear to conclude that brain WML in the frontal lobes and/or basal ganglia structures are most likely associated with the presence of clinical depression and with poor response to antidepressant treatment (23,24,27).

Overall, structural imaging studies in MDD suggest the presence of volumetric abnormalities in brain areas that mediate emotional and stress responses (such as hippocampus and amygdala), as well as in brain regions that putatively inhibit and control emotional expression (such as the prefrontal cortex and the anterior cingulate gyrus). The presence of WML further disrupts white matter circuits linking the limbic structures with the anterior cingulate and the prefrontal cortex; this may explain the association between WML in specific brain areas, and higher prevalence of MDD and poor response to antidepressant treatment.

FUNCTIONAL IMAGING

Functional neuroimaging techniques assess changes in brain blood flow or metabolism and allow inferences to be drawn about brain areas that are hyper- or hypoactive in various disease states. Available technologies include single photon emission computed tomography (SPECT), positron–emission tomography (PET), and fMRI.

Early investigators have simply compared at rest (baseline), the blood flow and metabolic rates in MDD subjects and healthy volunteers. PET studies and SPECT studies have shown lower fluorodeoxyglucose (FDG) metabolic rates and decreased blood flow, respectively, in the frontal lobes of subjects with major depression imaged at rest (28). More recently, investigators have associated specific changes in blood flow or metabolic patterns with specific emotional and cognitive tasks. Compared with healthy volunteers, MDD subjects had a different pattern of amygdala activation when exposed to anger induction (29), emotional faces (30), or sad words (31).

In MDD, PET has revealed multiple abnormalities of regional cerebral blood flow (CBF) and glucose metabolism in limbic and prefrontal cortical structures. Relative to healthy controls, regional CBF and metabolism in depressed subjects have been increased in the amygdala, orbitofrontal cortex, and medial thalamus, and decreased in the dorsomedial or dorsal anterolateral prefrontal cortex and anterior cingulate gyrus. Moreover, metabolic abnormalities appear to improve after antidepressant treatment (32–35).

In the amygdala, during depressive episodes, the resting CBF and glucose metabolism are abnormally elevated, correlating with the depression severity consistent with this structure's role in organizing the autonomic, neuroendocrine, and behavioral manifestations of some types of emotional responses (36). These metabolic abnormalities are also associated, in depressed subjects, with abnormal amygdala CBF responses to emotional stimuli, such as anger induction (29), emotional faces (30), or sad words (31). CBF and glucose metabolism are also abnormally increased in the orbitofrontal and the ventrolateral prefrontal cortex in unmedicated subjects with MDD; the values tend to normalize after successful treatment (37). Dysfunction of this brain region has also been associated with impaired emotional processing and decreased hedonic response as well as increased stress (38).

In contrast, CBF and metabolism in the subgenual anterior cingulate gyrus are decreased at rest in depressive subjects compared to healthy volunteers (6,39). This abnormality is also associated with a volumetric reduction of the corresponding cortex, measured by MRI-based morphometry (7) and by postmortem neuropathological studies (8). Similarly, several PET studies of MDD reported abnormally decreased CBF and glucose metabolism in the dorsomedial and the dorsal anterolateral prefrontal cortex, which normalized after antidepressant treatment (3,40,41). This finding may be explained by the reported abnormal reductions in the density and size of neurons and glia seen in the same brain areas in postmortem studies of MDD (42).

Various lines of evidence from these functional studies implicate a specific brain network involved in the control and modulation of emotions. This network includes brain structures such as prefrontal and parietal cortex, anterior cingulate, hippocampus, amygdala, and other limbic and paralimbic structures in generating affective illness (43,44). Drevets (3) also postulated a series of interconnected neural circuits in the pathology of MDD. These circuits would include limbic–thalamic–cortical and limbic–cortical–striatal–pallidal–thalamic circuits, involving the amygdala, orbital and medial prefrontal cortex, and anatomically related parts of the striatum and thalamus. These circuits have also been implicated more generally in emotional behavior by the results of electrophysiological lesion analysis and brain-mapping studies of humans and experimental animals (3). Thus, the deficits characteristic of mood disorders would not be circumscribed necessarily to only one brain structure, but would represent a relative imbalance in the interaction of different structures participating in the brain network for emotional regulation.

Functional imaging studies (PET and SPECT) have also been used to study treatment response in MDD. The same brain areas involved in mood regulation have also been the locus of metabolic changes as a result of antidepressant treatment in MDD. Earlier studies of treatment response used measures such as global metabolism and left hemisphere to right hemisphere ratios to assess differences before and after treatment. Some authors demonstrated normalization of baseline cerebral hypometabolism after treatment (40,45), while others reported continuous hypometabolism despite clinical response (46,47). Other authors found that prefrontal and paralimbic hypometabolism predicted a positive response to antidepressant treatment (48,49). In contrast, Mayberg et al. (43) reported an increased glucose metabolism rate in the anterior cingulate gyrus predicted treatment response at six weeks, and decreased metabolism in the same region predicted treatment resistance. In this study of 18 MDD patients (43), treatment was not uniform (primarily SSRIs, but also tricyclic antidepressants or bupropion), and outcome was assessed by chart review, though a subset of patients also received a posttreatment Hamilton Depression Scale rating. Nonetheless, the finding of such a striking pattern in an area identified in prior studies and known to have important reciprocal connections with other limbic structures was intriguing. More recently, Brody et al. (50) and Saxena et al. (51) have reported that treatment response in MDD correlated with greater decreases in glucose metabolism in the ventrolateral prefrontal cortex from pre- to posttreatment. Mayberg et al. (52) confirmed metabolic changes during antidepressant treatment in MDD and found a specific pattern of activation (in the striatum, anterior insula, and hippocampus) differentiating true antidepressant response from placebo response in MDD. However, while these studies are very encouraging, the value of functional neuroimaging studies as predictors of treatment outcome in an individual subject is still to be determined.

SPECT or PET can also be used, with appropriate ligands, to examine the distribution or density of neurotransmitter receptors in vivo and to correlate changes with treatment response. In one such study, Larisch et al. (53) assessed dopamine-2 (D2) receptor binding before and after SSRI treatment in 13 MDD subjects. Responders demonstrated increased D2 receptor binding in striatum and anterior cingulate following treatment, compared with nonresponders.

Overall, the findings of functional neuroimaging studies suggest that MDD is associated with activation of regions that putatively mediate emotional and stress responses (such as the amygdala), while areas that appear to inhibit emotional expression (such as the prefrontal and orbital cortex) contain morphological and functional abnormalities that might interfere with the modulation of emotional or stress responses (2). This functional imbalance between limbic and cortical structures in MDD may be corrected by successful antidepressant treatment.

MAGNETIC RESONANCE SPECTROSCOPY

MRS, a noninvasive tool for in vivo chemical analysis, has also been used to correlate treatment response with brain levels of several neurochemicals. MRS has several important advantages in the study of mood disorders. PET and SPECT allow differentiating between hyper- and hypometabolic tissue, by measuring blood flow or FDG metabolic rate. But no information can be obtained about specific metabolic pathways involved. In contrast, MRS allows measuring concentrations for a large number of metabolites (54). Therefore, one can measure chemical abnormalities and the effect of medications on different metabolic pathways. Moreover, MRS permits the study of several brain chemicals without the introduction of exogenous tracers or exposure to ionizing radiation.

Most commonly, MRS studies in psychiatric disorders involve proton (^{1}H) and phosphorus (^{31}P) spectroscopy. Such protocols have been developed to enable the measurement of brain neurotransmitters [γ–aminobutyric acid (GABA) and glutamate] and structural components of cells (synaptic proteins and membrane phospholipids) (55). Less often, MRS is also used to measure brain levels of psychotropic drugs including lithium and fluorinated drugs such as SSRIs, and correlating such levels with observed clinical response. Lithium-7 MRS has been utilized to demonstrate the variability in brain lithium levels among bipolar patients during maintenance therapy, despite similar serum levels (56). Similarly, fluorine-19 MRS measurement of brain paroxetine levels showed a correlation between withdrawal–emergent side effects and paroxetine brain levels (57). Whether these levels would be useful in predicting clinical response, however, is unknown. One open trial of fluvoxamine in obsessive–compulsive disorder could not assess the predictive value of fluorine-19 MRS because seven of eight subjects responded (58).

^{1}H MRS Studies of Patients with MDD

^{1}H MRS may be useful in identifying MDD-specific differences in the chemical composition of brain structures, and correlations between such abnormalities and antidepressant treatment response. Studies utilizing ^{1}H MRS in MDD have generally focused on changes in cerebral concentrations of creatine, *N*-acetyl aspartate, cytosolic choline (Cho), myoinositol (MI), GABA, and glutamate.

Significant deficits in MDD subjects have been identified in the cellular membrane phospholipid metabolism, as measured by choline levels in the orbito-frontal cortex Steingard et al. (59). ^{1}H MRS studies have documented both increases (60,61) and decreases (62) in the intensity of the ^{1}H MRS Cho resonance in depressed populations. Variation in reported results may reflect differences in study methodology and in the brain region investigated. However, baseline estimates of choline signal intensity, as well as change with treatment, have been shown to correlate with clinical response (62). In a subsequent publication, the authors also reported that change in choline level correlated with "true" drug response, compared with "placebo-pattern" response or nonresponse, in MDD patients (63). Ende et al. (64) reported a significant increase in hippocampal choline after electroconvulsive therapy (ECT). As choline is a precursor in phospholipid metabolism as well as synthesis of acetylcholine, it may indicate metabolic differences associated with response to antidepressant treatment. Decreased MI levels in the right frontal lobe were also found in MDD subjects relative to healthy volunteers (65). Because the MI resonance reflects the concentration of cellular phosphatidylinositol, an important component of cellular second messenger system, this finding suggests that an abnormality of second messenger systems may be present in MDD.

^{1}H MRS was also used to identify abnormalities in neurotransmitter levels in patients with MDD. Sanacora et al. (66–69) reported dramatic reductions in occipital cortex GABA levels (greater than 50% reduction) in unmedicated MDD subjects compared with healthy volunteers. Moreover, two separate studies reported significant increases in GABA levels in the occipital cortex of MDD subjects, after treatment with SSRIs (67) and after ECT (68). Because most subjects had improved with antidepressant treatment, there was no statistically significant correlation in these small studies between brain GABA levels and antidepressant treatment response. These results are consistent with reports of decreased GABA function and decreased GABA-A receptor binding in animal models of depression (66) and with earlier reports of decreased GABA levels in the cerebrospinal fluid of MDD patients compared with normal controls (70). SSRIs are known to induce increases in brain allopregnenolone (71), a neurosteroid with high affinity for GABA-A receptors, which facilitates GABAergic activity. This is the mechanism by which Ketter and Wang (72) explain the role of SSRI in increasing brain GABA levels.

There is more disagreement in the literature on glutamate levels. In some studies glutamate levels were increased in the occipital lobe of MDD subjects compared with controls (69) but were reduced in the anterior cingulate of MDD subjects (73). While the differences in reported results may relate to the different brain regions studied, abnormal brain glutamate levels in MDD would be consistent with animal and postmortem studies on the role of glutamate and of N-methyl-D-aspartate receptors in MDD (74).

^{31}P MRS Studies of Energy Metabolism in MDD

^{31}P MRS is used to noninvasively determine cerebral levels of high-energy phosphates [such as phosphocreatine (PCr), gamma-, alpha-, and beta-nucleoside triphosphate], as well as phosphomonoesters (PME) and phosphodiesters (PDE), which are involved in brain phospholipid metabolism.

Abnormalities of brain energy metabolism have been reported in MDD subjects; decreased nucleotide triphosphate (NTP) levels in basal ganglia (75,76) and frontal lobes (77), as well as decreased PCr (78) have also been reported. Because NTP primarily reflects levels of intracellular adenosine triphosphate (ATP), decreased NTP signifies a reduction of cellular bioenergetic metabolism. Reduced levels of cellular ATP would also be consistent with previous observations of alterations in the brain phospholipid metabolism. PME and PDE levels were reported to be increased in MDD (77), and in bipolar disorder (79). As membrane anabolites, in normal cellular function, PME are incorporated into the phospholipid membrane at the expense of ATP (80). Consequently, increased PME in MDD patients may reflect increased breakdown and turnover of cellular membrane, which in turn might be related to a reduction in the availability of ATP. Additionally, these findings suggest that in MDD subjects, alterations in both phospholipid metabolism and mitochondrial function may be closely related to mood state.

The majority of these findings can fit into a more cohesive bioenergetic and neurochemical model that is focused on the central nervous system's energy metabolism (81). These findings suggest a model of mitochondrial dysfunction in MDD that involves a shift toward glycolytic energy production, a decrease in total energy production and/or substrate availability, and altered phospholipid metabolism. Specifically, a shift toward glycolytic production of ATP may be related to additional MRS findings of reduced concentrations of high-energy compounds in MDD subjects.

The decrease in bioenergetic metabolism appears to also be related to severity of depression and response to treatment. Kato et al. (78) found that PCr was significantly decreased in severely depressed patients compared with mildly depressed patients. Renshaw et al. (76) found there was a direct correlation between the severity of depressive symptoms Hamilton depression rating scale scores (HAM-D scores) and beta-NTP. In addition, beta-NTP was lower by 21% in MDD subjects who responded to antidepressant treatment, compared to nonresponders. Recent data suggests that after antidepressant treatment, total NTP and beta NTP increase in treatment responders but not in treatment nonresponders (82). This study raises the possibility that beta-NTP and other high-energy phosphates might be useful as predictors of treatment response in MDD.

Overall, MRS studies have suggested that multiple metabolic and neurotransmitter abnormalities are present in MDD. Understanding the relationship between these in vivo chemical abnormalities and MDD symptoms may help shed light on the pathophysiology of major depression. These chemical abnormalities may also represent useful targets for predicting treatment outcome in MDD.

EEG STUDIES

Most depressed subjects have visually normal EEG tracings (83). Most significant EEG abnormalities in MDD subjects have been associated with underlying comorbid pathology, such as cerebrovascular disease or early dementia (84).

Quantitative EEG (QEEG) has enabled computerized spectral analysis of EEG signals, providing information, which cannot be extracted through visual inspection of EEG. Cordance, a QEEG measure integrating absolute and relative power of the signal, was shown to be decreased in subjects with MDD, compared to normal subjects (85). However, cordance is lowered both by advanced age and by delirium or dementia, and is therefore not specific to MDD.

Multiple studies have supported QEEG as a predictor of the outcome of antidepressant treatment in individual MDD subjects. At baseline, the absolute and the relative power of the EEG signal have been statistically different between future responders and nonresponders to antidepressant treatment (86,87). Cordance, a QEEG measure which integrates the absolute and relative power of the EEG signal was found to predict clinical response to SSRI antidepressants (88). In a recent study, we have used a similar QEEG measure (relative frontal theta power) to successfully predict responders and nonresponders to SSRI antidepressants; this variable could correctly classify 83% of the patients (89). In our study with 76% accuracy, a QEEG model that includes relative theta power and the asymmetry between left and right hemispheres of combined theta + alpha power, was also predictive of emergent suicidal ideation during SSRI treatment (90).

Other researchers have used EEG to predict response to ECT. The emphasis in such studies has been on the analysis of the ictal EEG to discriminate "effective" from "ineffective" seizures (91). However, most studies also attempted to assess baseline EEG features that were predictive of subsequent response. For example, fractal analysis of EEG data from the initial induced seizure was significantly associated in one study with remission status at two weeks among 40 MDD patients receiving bilateral ECT (92). This result is consistent with earlier findings suggesting predictive value for postictal suppression (93). However, other studies have not supported the usefulness of QEEG analysis to predict response to ECT (94).

Low-resolution electromagnetic tomography in which QEEG data was used to create three-dimensional maps of cortical currents and to localize the sources of electrical impulses has also been used to investigate brain electrical activity in MDD. Pizzagalli et al. (95) reported that theta activity in the rostral anterior cingulated gyrus in MDD subjects was directly correlated with treatment improvement (measured with Beck Depression Inventory).

Event-related potentials (ERPs) measure voltage changes on the scalp surface that correspond to cortical or brainstem activity in response to sensory stimuli. One such technique is the loudness-dependence of the auditory evoked potential (LDAEP), which describes how one ERP component (N1/P2) changes with increasing loudness of the auditory stimulus. The LDAEP is believed to correspond to the magnitude of serotonergic neurotransmission in auditory cortex, particularly the primary auditory cortex (96). Several investigators have reported an association between LDAEP and antidepressant response with SSRIs (97,98) or buprorion (99).

Overall, EEG abnormalities are not specific for MDD, but computerized analysis of EEG signals appears to detect patterns of activity associated with response to antidepressant treatment.

In conclusion, neuroimaging and electrophysiology studies in MDD reveal multiple brain abnormalities at anatomical, metabolical, and functional levels. While the results summarized above represent a significant progress in understanding brain function in depression, no biological measure has yet shown clear clinical utility. Research findings have been suggestive but not yet conclusive. Results with functional neuroimaging techniques and MRS may be particularly promising in detecting MDD-specific abnormalities at the level of neurocircuits involved in emotional regulation, as well as brain metabolism. Different forms of QEEG show promise as predictors of treatment response, which might eventually provide objective and individualized criteria for antidepressant treatment selection. But future studies will be necessary to clarify the generalizability of the current findings and to validate (or not) their usefulness in clinical practice. Very likely, our understanding of the pathophysiology of MDD will depend on our ability to integrate, in a coherent model, the complex anatomical, metabolical, and functional brain abnormalities described in depression.

REFERENCES

1. Fava M, Davidson KG. Definition and epidemiology of treatment-resistant depression. Psychiatr Clin North Am 1996; 19:179–200.
2. Manji HK, Drevets WC, Charney DS. The cellular neurobiology of depression. Natl Med 2001; 7(5):541–547.
3. Drevets WC. Neuroimaging studies of mood disorders. Biol Psychiat 2000; 48(8):813–829.
4. Kumar A, Jin Z, Bilker W, Udupa J, Gottlieb G. Late-onset minor and major depression: early evidence for common neuroanatomical substrates detected by using MRI. Proc Natl Acad Sci USA 1998; 95(13):7654–7658.
5. Steingard RJ, Renshaw PF, Yurgelun-Todd D, et al. Structural abnormalities in brain magnetic resonance images of depressed children. J Am Acad Child Adolesc Psychiat 1996; 35(3):307–311.
6. Drevets WC, Price JL, Simpson JR, et al. Subgenual prefrontal cortex abnormalities in mood disorders. Nature 1997; 386:824–827.
7. Hirayasu Y, Shenton ME, Salisbury DF, et al. Subgenual cingulate cortex volume in first-episode psychosis. Am J Psychiat 1999; 156:1091–1093.
8. Öngür D, Drevets WC, Price JL. Glial reduction in the subgenual prefrontal cortex in mood disorders. Proc Natl Acad Sci USA 1998; 95:13290–13295.
9. Sheline YI, Sanghavi M, Mintun MA, Gado MH. Depression duration but not age predicts hippocampal volume loss in medically healthy women with recurrent major depression. J Neurosci 1999; 19(12):5034–5043.
10. Ashtari M, Greenwald BS, Kramer-Ginsberg E, et al. Hippocampal/amygdala volumes in geriatric depression. Psychol Med 1999; 29:629–638.
11. Campbell S, Marriott M, Nahmias C, MacQueen GM. Lower hippocampal volume in patients suffering from depression: a meta-analysis. Am J Psychiat 2004; 161(4):598–607.
12. Parashos IA, Tupler LA, Blitchington T, Krishnan KR. Magnetic-resonance morphometry in patients with major depression. Psychiat Res 1998; 84(1):7–15.
13. Sheline YI, Gado MH, Price JL. Amygdala core nuclei volumes are decreased in recurrent major depression. Neuroreport 1998; 9(9):2023–2028.
14. Van Elst LT, Ebert D, Trimble MR. Hippocampus and amygdala pathology in depression. Am J Psychiat 2001; 158(4):652–653.
15. Krishnan KR, Hays JC, Blazer DG. MRI-defined vascular depression. Am J Psychiat 1997; 154(4):497–501.
16. de Groot JC, de Leeuw FE, Oudkerk M, Hofman A, Jolles J, Breteler MM. Cerebral white matter lesions and depressive symptoms in elderly adults. Arch Gen Psychiat 2000; 57(11):1071–1076.
17. Lyoo IK, Lee HK, Jung JH, Noam GG, Renshaw PF. White matter hyperintensities on magnetic resonance imaging of the brain in children with psychiatric disorders. Compr Psychiat 2002; 43(5):361–368.
18. Lenze E, Cross D, McKeel D, Neuman RJ, Sheline YI. White matter hyperintensities and gray matter lesions in physically healthy depressed subjects. Am J Psychiat 1999; 156(10):1602–1607.

19. Breteler MM, van Swieten JC, Bots ML, et al. Cerebral white matter lesions, vascular risk factors, and cognitive function in a population-based study: the Rotterdam Study. Neurology 1994; 44:1246–1252.

20. Breeze JL, Hesdorffer DC, Hong X, Frazier JA, Renshaw PF. Clinical significance of brain white matter hyperintensities in young adults with psychiatric illness. Harv Rev Psychiat 2003; 11(5):269–283.

21. Thomas AJ, O'Brien JT, Davis S, et al. Ischemic basis for deep white matter hyperintensities in major depression: a neuropathological study. Arch Gen Psychiat 2002; 59(9):785–792.

22. Alexopoulos GS, Meyers BS, Young RC, Campbell S, Silbersweig D, Charlson M. "Vascular depression" hypothesis. Arch Gen Psychiat 1997; 54(10):915–922.

23. Simpson S, Baldwin RC, Jackson A, Burns AS. Is subcortical disease associated with a poor response to antidepressants? Neurological, neuropsychological and neuroradiological findings in late-life depression. Psychol Med 1998; 28(5):1015–1026.

24. Iosifescu DV, Renshaw PF, Lyoo IK, et al. Brain MRI white matter hyperintensities, cardiovascular risk factors, and treatment outcome in major depressive disorder. Brit J Psychiat. In press.

25. O'Brien J, Ames D, Chiu E, Schweitzer I, Desmond P, Tress B. Severe deep white matter lesions and outcome in elderly patients with major depressive disorder: follow up study. BMJ 1998; 317:982–984.

26. Krishnan KR, Hays JC, George LK, Blazer DG. Six-month outcomes for MRI-related vascular depression. Depress Anxiety 1998; 8(4):142–146.

27. Steffens DC, Krishnan KR, Crump C, Burke GL. Cerebrovascular disease and evolution of depressive symptoms in the cardiovascular health study. Stroke 2002; 33(6):1636–1644.

28. George MS, Ketter TA, Post RM. SPECT and PET imaging in mood disorders. J Clin Psychiat 1993; 54(suppl):6–13.

29. Dougherty DD, Rauch SL, Deckersbach T, et al. Ventromedial prefrontal cortex and amygdala dysfunction during an anger induction positron emission tomography study in patients with major depressive disorder with anger attacks. Arch Gen Psychiat 2004; 61(8):795–804.

30. Sheline YI, Barch DM, Donnelly JM, Ollinger JM, Snyder AZ, Mintun MA. Increased amygdala response to masked emotional faces in depressed subjects resolves with antidepressant treatment: an fMRI study. Biol Psychiat 2001; 50(9):651–658.

31. Siegle GJ, Steinhauer SR, Thase ME, Stenger VA, Carter CS. Can't shake that feeling: event-related fMRI assessment of sustained amygdala activity in response to emotional information in depressed individuals. Biol Psychiat 2002; 51(9):693–707.

32. Mayberg HS, Lewis PJ, Regenold W, Wagner HN Jr. Paralimbic hypoperfusion in unipolar depression. J Nucl Med 1994; 35(6):929–934.

33. Navarro V, Gasto C, Lomena F, Mateos JJ, Marcos T. Frontal cerebral perfusion dysfunction in elderly late-onset major depression assessed by 99MTC-HMPAO SPECT. Neuroimage 2001; 14(1 Pt 1):202–205.

34. Kennedy SH, Evans KR, Kruger S, et al. Changes in regional brain glucose metabolism measured with positron emission tomography after paroxetine treatment of major depression. Am J Psychiat 2001; 158(6):899–905.

35. Brody AL, Saxena S, Stoessel P, et al. Regional brain metabolic changes in patients with major depression treated with either paroxetine or interpersonal therapy: preliminary findings. Arch Gen Psychiat 2001; 58(7):631–640.

36. Drevets WC, Price JL, Bardgett ME, Reich T, Todd RD, Raichle ME. Glucose metabolism in the amygdala in depression: relationship to diagnostic subtype and plasma cortisol levels. Pharmacol Biochem Behav 2002; 71(3):431–447.

37. Mayberg HS, Liotti M, Brannan SK, et al. Reciprocal limbic-cortical function and negative mood: converging PET findings in depression and normal sadness. Am J Psychiat 1999; 156(5):675–682.

38. Pizzagalli DA, Oakes TR, Fox AS, et al. Functional but not structural subgenual prefrontal cortex abnormalities in melancholia. Mol Psychiat 2004; 9(4): 325, 393–405.

39. Kegeles LS, Malone KM, Slifstein M, et al. Response of cortical metabolic deficits to serotonergic challenges in mood disorders. Biol Psychiat 1999; 45:76S.

40. Baxter LR Jr, Schwartz JM, Phelps ME, et al. Reduction of prefrontal cortex glucose metabolism common to three types of depression. Arch Gen Psychiat 1989; 46(3):243–250.

41. Kegeles LS, Malone KM, Slifstein M, et al. Response of cortical metabolic deficits to serotonergic challenge in familial mood disorders. Am J Psychiatry 2003; 160(1):76–82.

42. Rajkowska G, Miguel-Hidalgo JJ, Wei J, et al. Morphometric evidence for neuronal and glial prefrontal cell pathology in major depression. Biol Psychiat 1999; 45(9):1085–1098.

43. Mayberg HS, Brannan SK, Mahurin RK, et al. Cingulate function in depression: a potential predictor of treatment response. Neuroreport 1997; 8(4):1057–1061.

44. Seminowicz DA, Mayberg HS, McIntosh AR, et al. Limbic-frontal circuitry in major depression: a path modeling metanalysis. Neuroimage 2004; 22(1):409–418.

45. Kanaya T, Yonekawa M. Regional cerebral blood flow in depression. Jpn J Psychiat Neurol 1990; 44(3):571–576.

46. Hurwitz TA, Clark C, Murphy E, Klonoff H, Martin WR, Pate BD. Regional cerebral glucose metabolism in major depressive disorder. Can J Psychiat 1990; 35(8):684–688.

47. Martinot JL, Hardy P, Feline A, et al. Left prefrontal glucose hypometabolism in the depressed state: a confirmation. Am J Psychiat 1990; 147(10):1313–1317.

48. Buchsbaum MS, Wu J, Siegel BV, et al. Effect of sertraline on regional metabolic rate in patients with affective disorder. Biol Psychiat 1997; 41(1):15–22.

49. Little JT, Ketter TA, Kimbrell TA, et al. Venlafaxine or bupropion responders but not nonresponders show baseline prefrontal and paralimbic hypometabolism compared with controls. Psychopharmacol Bull 1996; 32(4):629–635.

50. Brody AL, Saxena S, Silverman DH, et al. Brain metabolic changes in major depressive disorder from pre- to post-treatment with paroxetine. Psychiat Res 1999; 91(3):127–139.

51. Saxena S, Brody AL, Ho ML, et al. Differential cerebral metabolic changes with paroxetine treatment of obsessive-compulsive disorder versus major depression. Arch Gen Psychiat 2002; 59(3):250–261.

52. Mayberg HS, Silva JA, Brannan SK, et al. The functional neuroanatomy of the placebo effect. Am J Psychiat 2002; 159(5):728–737.

53. Larisch R, Klimke A, Vosberg H, Loffler S, Gaebel W, Muller-Gartner HW. In vivo evidence for the involvement of dopamine-D2 receptors in striatum and anterior cingulate gyrus in major depression. Neuroimage 1997; 5(4 Pt 1):251–260.

54. Kato T, Inubushi T, Kato N. Magnetic resonance spectroscopy in affective disorders. J Neuropsychiat Clin Neurosci 1998; 10(2):133–147.

55. Lyoo IK, Renshaw PF. Magnetic resonance spectroscopy: current and future applications in psychiatric research. Biol Psychiat 2002; 51(3):195–207.

56. Sachs GS, Renshaw PF, Lafer B, et al. Variability of brain lithium levels during maintenance treatment: a magnetic resonance spectroscopy study. Biol Psychiat 1995; 38(7):422–428.

57. Henry ME, Moore CM, Kaufman MJ, et al. Brain kinetics of paroxetine and fluoxetine on the third day of placebo substitution: a fluorine MRS study. Am J Psychiat 2000; 157(9):1506–1508.

58. Strauss WL, Layton ME, Hayes CE, Dager SR. 19F magnetic resonance spectroscopy investigation in vivo of acute and steady-state brain fluvoxamine levels in obsessive-compulsive disorder. Am J Psychiat 1997; 154(4):516–522.

59. Steingard RJ, Yurgelun-Todd DA, Hennen J, et al. increased orbitofrontal cortex levels of choline in depressed adolescents as detected by in vivo proton magnetic resonance spectroscopy. Biol Psychiatry 2000; 48(11):1053–1061.

60. Charles HC, Lazeyras F, Krishnan KR, Boyko OB, Payne M, Moore D. Brain choline in depression: in vivo detection of potential pharmacodynamic effects of antidepressant therapy using hydrogen localized spectroscopy. Prog Neuropsychopharmacol Biol Psychiat 1994; 18(7):1121–1127.

61. Hamakawa H, Kato T, Murashita J, Kato N. Quantitative proton magnetic resonance spectroscopy of the basal ganglia in patients with affective disorders. Eur Arch Psychiat Clin Neurosci 1998; 248(1):53–58.

62. Renshaw PF, Lafer B, Babb SM, et al. Basal ganglia choline levels in depression and response to fluoxetine treatment: an in vivo proton magnetic resonance spectroscopy study. Biol Psychiat 1997; 41(8):837–843.

63. Sonawalla SB, Renshaw PF, Moore CM, et al. Compounds containing cytosolic choline in the basal ganglia: a potential biological marker of true drug response to fluoxetine. Am J Psychiat 1999; 156(10):1638–1640.

64. Ende G, Braus DF, Walter S, Weber-Fahr W, Henn FA. The hippocampus in patients treated with electroconvulsive therapy: a proton magnetic resonance spectroscopic imaging study. Arch Gen Psychiat 2000; 57(10):937–943.

65. Frey R, Metzler D, Fischer P, et al. Myo-inositol in depressive and healthy subjects determined by frontal 1H-magnetic resonance spectroscopy at 1.5 tesla. J Psychiat Res 1998; 32(6):411–420.

66. Sanacora G, Mason GF, Krystal JH. Impairment of GABAergic transmission in depression: new insights from neuroimaging studies. Crit Rev Neurobiol 2000; 14(1):23–45.

67. Sanacora G, Mason GF, Rothman DL, Krystal JH. Increased occipital cortex GABA concentrations in depressed patients after therapy with selective serotonin reuptake inhibitors. Am J Psychiat 2002; 159(4):663–665.

68. Sanacora G, Mason GF, Rothman DL, et al. Increased cortical GABA concentrations in depressed patients receiving ECT. Am J Psychiat 2003; 160(3):577–579.

69. Sanacora G, Gueorguieva R, Epperson CN, et al. Subtype-specific alterations of gamma-aminobutyric acid and glutamate in patients with major depression. Arch Gen Psychiat 2004; 61(7):705–713.

70. Gerner RH, Fairbanks L, Anderson GM, et al. CSF neurochemistry in depressed, manic, and schizophrenic patients compared with that of normal controls. Am J Psychiat 1984; 141(12):1533–1540.

71. Uzunova V, Sheline Y, Davis JM, et al. Increase in the cerebrospinal fluid content of neurosteroids in patients with unipolar major depression who are receiving fluoxetine or fluvoxamine. Proc Natl Acad Sci USA 1998; 95(6): 3239–3244.

72. Ketter TA, Wang PW. The emerging differential roles of GABAergic and anti-glutamatergic agents in bipolar disorders. J Clin Psychiat 2003; 64(suppl 3): 15–20.

73. Auer DP, Putz B, Kraft E, Lipinski B, Schill J, Holsboer F. Reduced glutamate in the anterior cingulate cortex in depression: an in vivo proton magnetic resonance spectroscopy study. Biol Psychiat 2000; 47(4):305–313.

74. Petrie RX, Reid IC, Stewart CA. The N-methyl-D-aspartate receptor, synaptic plasticity, and depressive disorder. A critical review. Pharmacol Ther 2000; 87(1):11–25.

75. Moore CM, Christensen JD, Lafer B, Fava M, Renshaw PF. Lower levels of nucleoside triphosphate in the basal ganglia of depressed subjects: a phosphorous-31 magnetic resonance spectroscopy study. Am J Psychiat 1997; 154(1): 116–118.

76. Renshaw PF, Parow AM, Hirashima F, et al. Multinuclear magnetic resonance spectroscopy studies of brain purines in major depression. Am J Psychiat 2001; 158(12):2048–2055.

77. Volz HP, Rzanny R, Riehemann S, et al. ^{31}P magnetic resonance spectroscopy in the frontal lobe of major depressed patients. Eur Arch Psychiat Clin Neurosci 1998; 248(6):289–295.

78. Kato T, Takahashi S, Shioiri T, Inubushi T. Brain phosphorous metabolism in depressive disorders detected by phosphorus-31 magnetic resonance spectroscopy. J Affect Disord 1992; 26(4):223–230.

79. Kato T, Takahashi S, Shioiri T, Murashita J, Hamakawa H, Inubushi T. Reduction of brain phosphocreatine in bipolar II disorder detected by phosphorus-31 magnetic resonance spectroscopy. J Affect Disord 1994; 31(2):125–133.

80. Kennedy EP. The biological synthesis of phospholipids. Can J Biochem Physiol 1956; 34(2):334–348.

81. Iosifescu DV, Renshaw PF. ^{31}P-magnetic resonance spectroscopy thyroid hormones in major depressive disorder: towards a bioenergetic mechanism in depression? Harv Rev Psychiat 2003; 11(2):51–63.

82. Iosifescu DV, Bolo NR, Jensen JE, et al. Brain bioenergetics and thyroid hormone treatment in MDD. American Psychiatric Association 157th Annual Meeting, New York, NY, 2004.

83. Malaspina D, Devanand DP, Krueger RB, Prudic J, Sackeim HA. The significance of clinical EEG abnormalities in depressed patients treated with ECT. Convuls Ther 1994; 10(4):259–266.

84. Leuchter AF, Daly KA, Rosenberg-Thompson S, Abrams M. Prevalence and significance of electroencephalographic abnormalities in patients with suspected organic mental syndromes. J Am Geriatr Soc 1993; 41(6):605–611.

85. Cook IA, Leuchter AF, Uijtdehaage SH, et al. Altered cerebral energy utilization in late life depression. J Affect Disord 1998; 49(2):89–99.

86. Ulrich G, Haug HJ, Fahndrich E. Acute vs. chronic EEG effects in maprotiline- and in clomipramine-treated depressive inpatients and the prediction of therapeutic outcome. J Affect Disord 1994; 32(3):213–217.

87. Knott VJ, Telner JI, Lapierre YD, et al. Quantitative EEG in the prediction of antidepressant response to imipramine. J Affect Disord 1996; 39(3):175–184.

88. Cook IA, Leuchter AF, Witte EA, Stubbeman WF, Abrams M, Rosenberg S. Early changes in prefrontal activity characterize clinical responders to antidepressants. Neuropsychopharmacology 2002; 27:130–131.

89. Iosifescu DV, Greenwald S, Devlin P, Alpert JE, Hamill S, Fava M. Frontal EEG at 1 Week Predicts Clinical Response to SSRIs in MDD. American Psychiatric Association 158th Annual Meeting, Atlanta, GA, 2005.

90. Iosifescu DV, Greenwald S, Devlin P, et al. Pretreatment Frontal EEG Predicts Changes in Suicidal Ideation During SSRI Treatment in MDD. Annual New Clinical Drug Evaluation Unit (NCDEU) Meeting, Boca Raton, FL, 2005.

91. Krystal AD, Weiner RD, Coffey CE. The ictal EEG as a marker of adequate stimulus intensity with unilateral ECT. J Neuropsychiat Clin Neurosci 1995; 7(3):295–303.

92. Gangadhar BN, Subbakrishna DK, Janakiramaiah N, Motreja S, Narayana Dutt D, Paramehwara G. Post-seizure EEG fractal dimension of first ECT predicts antidepressant response at two weeks. J Affect Disord 1999; 52(1–3):235–238.

93. Suppes T, Webb A, Carmody T, et al. Is postictal electrical silence a predictor of response to electroconvulsive therapy? J Affect Disord 1996; 41(1):55–58.

94. Nobler MS, Luber B, Moeller JR, et al. Quantitative EEG during seizures induced by electroconvulsive therapy: relations to treatment modality and clinical features. I. Global analyses. J ECT 2000; 16(3):211–228.

95. Pizzagalli D, Pascual-Marqui RD, Nitschke JB, et al. Anterior cingulate activity as a predictor of degree of treatment response in major depression: evidence from brain electrical tomography analysis. Am J Psychiat 2001; 158(3):405–415.

96. Hegerl U, Gallinat J, Juckel G. Event-related potentials. Do they reflect central serotonergic neurotransmission and do they predict clinical response to serotonin agonists? J Affect Disord 2001; 62(1–2):93–100.

97. Gallinat J, Bottlender R, Juckel G, et al. The loudness dependency of the auditory evoked N1/P2-component as a predictor of the acute SSRI response in depression. Psychopharmacology (Berl) 2000; 148(4):404–411.

98. Paige SR, Fitzpatrick DF, Kline JP, Balogh SE, Hendricks SE. Event-related potential amplitude/intensity slopes predict response to antidepressants. Neuropsychobiology 1994; 30(4):197–201.

99. Paige SR, Hendricks SE, Fitzpatrick DF, et al. Amplitude/intensity functions of auditory event-related potentials predict responsiveness to bupropion in major depressive disorder. Psychopharmacol Bull 1995; 31(2):243–248.

10

Depression and Somatic Treatments

Antonio Mantovani

Department of Neuroscience, Division of Brain Stimulation and Neuromodulation, Columbia University, New York, New York, U.S.A. and Department of Neuroscience, Postgraduate School in Applied Neurological Sciences, Siena University, Siena, Italy

Mark Goldman

Brown University, Providence, Rhode Island, U.S.A.

INTRODUCTION

Advances in science and technology have made available several somatic treatments for depression that have rekindled clinical and research interest. Although electroconvulsive therapy (ECT) remains the only physical treatment with widespread acceptance and application, vagus nerve stimulation (VNS) has gathered approvals in western Europe, Canada, and now in the United States. Transcranial magnetic stimulation (TMS), deep brain stimulation (DBS), and magnetic seizure therapy (MST) could ultimately offer novel means of treating neuropsychiatric disorders and may provide a better understanding of the brain pathophysiology of these disorders. This chapter describes somatic treatments now available regulatory-wise and in experimental phases of investigation. We will review efficacy and future potential in the context of managing major depressive disorder (MDD) for these treatments.

ECT, TMS, AND MST IN THE TREATMENT OF
MAJOR DEPRESSION

Despite the unparalleled efficacy of ECT in major depression, its use is limited by its cognitive side effects that decrease its acceptance by patients and some clinicians (1–3). The antidepressant properties of ECT and its effects on cognition are uncorrelated (1,4–6) and considerable progress has been made in altering the ECT technique to maintain efficacy while reducing cognitive side effects. Nonetheless, the forms of ECT with the most well-established efficacy or side-effect profile still result in a substantial side-effect burden (7–11). A growing body of evidence suggests that ECT electrical dosage and the intracerebral pathway of the electrical current are critical for determining efficacy as well as side effects (7,8,11–17). Depending on the combination of stimulus intensity and electrode position, antidepressant response rates with ECT vary from 30% to 70% or higher (7,8,11,17,18). Right unilateral (RUL) ECT results in less intense and persistent adverse cognitive effects than bilateral (BL) ECT, but RUL ECT can either be highly ineffective or effective, depending upon the electrical dosage relative to the seizure threshold (7,8,19,20). Supporting these clinical findings, alterations in regional brain activity, as reflected in regional cerebral blood flow (rCBF) (13,21,22), cerebral metabolic rate for glucose (23,24), and electroencephalographic (EEG) measures (16,17,25), correlate with the efficacy and objective cognitive side effects of ECT. For example, antidepressant response has been linked to increased EEG δ power and decreased rCBF in prefrontal regions, while retrograde amnesia for autobiographical memories has been linked to increased left frontotemporal EEG τ power (16,17,25,26). These findings suggest a technique that can target the induced current to regions implicated in antidepressant response, while sparing regions implicated in adverse cognitive effects, would maintain efficacy and have a superior side-effect profile. This advantage would be accentuated if such a technique offered better control, not only over intracerebral current pathways (i.e., targeting of regions) but also over intracerebral current density.

The use of an electrical stimulus to induce seizures is a fundamental limitation in refining convulsive therapy. The high impedance of the skull (27–29) shunts the bulk of the electrical stimulus away from the brain. An unknown proportion of the electrical stimulus results in neuronal depolarization, with the shunting producing a nonfocal, widespread intracerebral current distribution regardless of electrode placement. Measurements in humans (30,31) and monkeys (32) of shunting across the scalp and skull range from 80% to 97%. The degree of shunting varies considerably among individuals, due to individual differences in skull thickness and anatomy (29). Skull inhomogeneities, for which there are also considerable individual differences, result in further regional variability in current density even when the anatomic positioning of electrodes is consistent across patients (31–34). For example, Law (31) measured resistance in bone plugs from 20 regions of the human skull and found a 16-fold range (1360–21400 Ωcm) in resistivity values (31). Thus, inherent in the application of an external electrical stimulus that must traverse the scalp, skull, and cerebrospinal fluid (CSF) to reach the brain, is the highly variable and widespread distribution of current and little control over the intracerebral current density. Stimulating the brain with repetitive transcranial magnetic stimulation (rTMS) could obviate some of the limitations of electrical stimulation by inducing intracerebral current noninvasively using rapidly alternating magnetic fields (35,36). The scalp and skull are transparent to magnetic fields, removing a major source of individual differences in the intensity and spatial distribution of intracerebral current density. In addition, depending principally on coil geometry, the magnetic field can be spatially targeted in cortical regions, offering further control over intracerebral current paths (37–40). However, the electrical field induced by nonconvulsive rTMS is capable of neural depolarization at a depth extending to approximately 2 cm below the scalp (i.e., gray–white matter junction), so direct effects are limited to the cortex (41). On the other hand, measurements in nonhuman primates with intracerebral multicontact electrodes support the hypothesis that rTMS-induced current and the resulting seizure are more focal than those obtained with ECT (42–45). Thus, magnetic stimulation holds the promise of more precise control over current paths and current density in neural tissue.

A growing number of studies have examined the effects of subconvulsive levels of rTMS in depression, mania, schizophrenia, obsessive–compulsive disorder (OCD), posttraumatic stress disorder, and panic disorder (46–50). While prior work had shown that subconvulsive levels of ECT are not effective (51–53), it was not known whether the same would hold true for rTMS, particularly because a single electrical train was applied for subconvulsive ECT while repeated trains within a session were given with subconvulsive rTMS. Indeed, recent clinical trials with subconvulsive rTMS challenge the view that a seizure is necessary for brain stimulation techniques to exert antidepressant effects (34,54), much as recent work with ECT challenged the dogma that a seizure was sufficient for efficacy (7,8,11,17).

ECT IN MDD

ECT is generally regarded as the most effective antidepressant treatment in both unipolar (UP) and bipolar (BP) depressive disorders (3,55). Despite scores of studies, few phenomenological or clinical features have shown significant relationships with the likelihood or speed of ECT response (56), and whether the polarity of a patient's illness (BP vs. UP) had prognostic significance for ECT outcome. The most consistent findings pertain to episode duration and medication resistance. Patients with longer duration of current depressive episodes tend to have inferior outcome (57,58), as do patients who have not responded to one or more adequate medication trials in the index episode (11,58). There is also some evidence that patients with delusional (psychotic) depression may have superior outcome compared with nondelusional patients (59,60).

In line with most observations, Daly et al. (61) found no difference between BP and UP patients in the likelihood of response or degree of symptomatic improvement following the ECT course. However, they found a powerful and consistent effect for BP patients to have a more rapid onset of response and to receive fewer treatments than UP patients to meet response criteria (four for BPs vs. six for UPs).

It is not known why BP patients respond more rapidly to ECT than UP patients. It is noteworthy that ECT is a powerful anticonvulsant, with greater anticonvulsant properties in some models than traditional anticonvulsant medications (62,63). In this study, there was a trend for the average increase in seizure threshold per treatment to be greater in BP than UP patients. This may indicate more rapid onset of anticonvulsant effects in BP than UP patients. If this were the case, it would suggest that BP patients show a more profound and cumulative inhibitory response to seizure induction than UP patients. The difference in the speed of response was independent of the form of ECT utilized (electrode placement and stimulus dosage condition), while both BP and UP patients had a higher final response rate to the BL relative to the RUL ECT.

For decades there has been a controversy concerning the use of RUL or BL ECT (64). It has been established that RUL ECT causes less severe cognitive adverse effects than BL ECT (4,6,7,15,65). However, despite 40 comparative trials, the relative efficacy of both RUL and BL ECT remains uncertain (66,67). When efficacy differences have been found, they consistently favored BL ECT (68–70). Most patients in the United States receive BL treatment. Farah and McCall (71) conducted a survey of U.S. ECT practitioners and found that 52% initiated ECT with the BL placement. Sackeim and coworkers (72) conducted a survey of ECT directors at 59 facilities in the tristate New York metropolitan area. The mean percentage of patients receiving BL ECT was 79%. Recently, it has been shown that the efficacy of RUL ECT is contingent on electrical dosage (7,12,19,73,74). In a four-group study randomizing patients to RUL and BL placement and to an electrical dosage just above 0% or 150% above the initial seizure threshold, Sackeim et al. (7) found that higher-dosage RUL ECT was considerably more effective than low-dosage RUL ECT and produced less severe cognitive effects than either form of BL ECT. In a subsequent double-blind study (8), they suggested that RUL ECT delivered with a high stimulus intensity relative to seizure threshold is equivalent in efficacy to a criterion standard form of BL ECT, yet retains important advantages with respect to cognitive adverse effects. At all time points and for all efficacy measures, high-dosage

RUL and BL ECT could not be distinguished with regard to their antidepressant effects. Both were considerably more effective than either low- or moderate-dosage RUL ECT. These findings confirm earlier reports that the efficacy of RUL ECT is influenced by electrical dosage, and that fixed high-dosage RUL ECT can be as effective as BL ECT. Specifically, this study indicates that at sufficiently high stimulus intensity (500%) above the seizure threshold, RUL matches BL ECT in efficacy.

Despite the use of high electrical intensity with high-dosage RUL ECT, this treatment produced less severe and persistent cognitive adverse effects than BL ECT. In the postictal period, recovery of orientation was prolonged with BL ECT, and BL treatment produced the greatest retrograde amnesia in selective measures. During the week after treatment, BL ECT resulted in more severe impairment than any of the RUL conditions in each of the primary cognitive measures. These effects were of clinical consequence. Capacity to recall words after a two-hour delay on the Buschke Selective Reminding Test improved by 20% relative to baseline in patients treated with high-dosage RUL ECT, but decreased by 22% in patients treated with BL ECT. At this point, those in the BL group were 71% more likely than those in the high-dosage RUL group not to remember facts about their lives that they had reported at baseline. During the week after treatment, BL ECT also resulted in more severe cognitive adverse effects than any of the RUL treatments in a variety of secondary measures assessing global cognitive status, anterograde learning and memory, and retrograde memory. At two-month follow-up, BL ECT, either as a single course or as a crossover treatment, resulted in greater retrograde amnesia than high-dosage RUL ECT. This long-term effect held for all primary measures. Thus, despite high stimulus intensity relative to seizure threshold, RUL ECT retained important cognitive advantages relative to BL ECT.

As in several recent studies the rate of relapse after response to ECT was high despite adequate continuation treatment. Naturalistic studies show that the relapse rate during the 6 to 12 months following ECT exceeds 50% (7,8,75–83). With the possible exception of the combination of a tricyclic antidepressant and lithium (35.3% relapsed vs. 67.9% with other pharmacological agents), strength or adequacy of either continuation or maintenance treatment had no relationship to relapse, a finding previously reported (78). Also in line with previous results, the type or dosage of ECT was independent of relapse. In contrast, medication-resistant patients were less likely to respond to ECT regardless of the type of ECT used, and if they did respond, were more than twice as likely to relapse. These findings confirm earlier reports that medication resistance predicts both ECT short-term outcome and relapse (58,78,84,85). Because resistance to antidepressant medications is the leading indication for the use of ECT (3), research is needed on methods to improve ECT response and prevent relapse in this subgroup.

The study conducted by Sackeim et al. (86) used a customized ECT device with an extended output range. Given the marked variability in seizure threshold (70,87), it will not be possible to treat some patients with RUL ECT at six times the threshold using standard devices in the United States (504–576 mC maximal output). The findings support consideration of higher electrical output for standard ECT devices to obtain a better clinical outcome.

In a prospective, naturalistic study involving 347 patients at seven hospitals, clinical outcomes immediately after ECT and over a 24-week follow-up period were examined in relation to patient characteristics and treatment variables. In contrast to the 70% to 90% remission rates expected with ECT, remission rates, depending on criteria, were 30.3% to 46.7%. Longer episode duration, comorbid personality disorder, and schizoaffective disorder were associated with poorer outcome. Among remitters, the relapse rate during follow-up was 64.3%. Relapse was more frequent in patients with psychotic depression or comorbid Axis I or Axis II disorders. Only 23.4% of ECT non-remitters had sustained remission during follow-up. The remission rate with ECT in community settings was substantially less than that in clinical trials, mostly because providers frequently end the ECT course with the view that patients have benefited fully, yet formal assessment shows significant residual symptoms. Patients who do not remit with ECT have a poor prognosis; this underscores the need to achieve maximal improvement with this modality (18).

Although the response and remission rates observed by Prudic and colleagues would be considered high for routine pharmacologic treatment of major depression, the remission rates were well below expectations for ECT. When coupled with the relapse rate, it was evident that only a small percentage of patients who received ECT achieved a sustained remission. This suggests that rather than intrinsically reflecting limitations of ECT, this pattern reflects limitations in the delivery of care, and in particular, the low remission rate might be due largely to premature termination of the acute ECT course in patients who show significant but incomplete benefit. The high relapse rate might be due to insufficient intensity of continuation treatment in ECT remitters.

In a recent multicenter study, of the 253 patients who entered, 86% completed the acute course of ECT. Sustained response occurred in 79% of the sample, and remission occurred in 75% of the sample; 34% of patients achieved remission at or before ECT No. 6 (week 2), and 65% achieved remission at or before ECT No. 10 (weeks 3–4). Over half (54%) had an initial first response by ECT No. 3 (end of week 1). BL ECT, delivered three times per week at 1.5 times the seizure threshold with a mean number of eight sessions for the total sample, was associated with rapid response and remission in a high percentage of severely depressed patients (88). These findings of rapid response and the high likelihood of remission stand in sharp contrast to the symptomatic outcomes reported in pharmacotherapy trials in typically less severely ill outpatients with MDD. Usually 50% to

60% of these patients achieve response, while only 35% to 45% achieve remission (89). Additionally, only about two-thirds of the medication responses occurred within four weeks of initiating treatment. In more chronically depressed patients, response to medication may not be seen for 8 to 10 weeks. Remission may not occur for weeks or months following response (90–92). Not only is the probability of symptomatic response and remission high, but the time to the onset of benefits is remarkably quick with ECT. Other reports also indicate that the response of patients with MDD to ECT is rapid (93,94). Patients with psychotic depression seemed to have a more robust response (88,95) that may warrant earlier intervention with ECT in treatment algorithms. The role of age in the outcome with ECT has been studied, and it has been found that elderly patients had better rates of remission than younger patients (96).

Several meta-analyses (97–99) have examined the antidepressant efficacy and safety of different forms of ECT, among themselves and in comparison to simulated ECT and pharmacotherapy. All concluded that real ECT was significantly more effective than simulated ECT and pharmacotherapy; BL ECT was more effective than unilateral ECT, and high dose ECT more effective than low dose.

In conclusion, there is a reasonable evidence base for the use of ECT as an important treatment option for the management of MDD, including severe and resistant forms. Future studies are needed to clarify whether and when such an intervention can be a first choice treatment for specific categories of depressed patients.

TMS IN MDD

MDD has been the focus of the bulk of the clinical trials with TMS to date. Initial work used nonfocal coils positioned over the vertex, and found some suggestions of clinical benefit. Based on evidence for prefrontal abnormalities in depression, it was thought that rTMS over prefrontal cortex could produce a more profound antidepressant effect than over other cortical areas. To test this hypothesis, using a within-subject crossover design, Pascual-Leone et al. (100) reported that fast (10 Hz) left dorsolateral prefrontal cortex (DLPFC) rTMS for five days had marked antidepressant effects even in psychotic depression. Stimulation at other sites (right DLPFC, and vertex) and sham had no effect. This remarkable result was superior to what could be expected with any medication regimen, or even ECT; but most of the following studies could not replicate the same magnitude or speed of response using similar parameters and length of stimulation.

Extending the treatment to 10 days and increasing the number of pulses per day, a 50% response rate was reported in medication-resistant UP depressed patients in an open trial (101). A double-blind, sham-controlled, single-crossover study of fast left DLPFC rTMS in medication-resistant outpatients found improvements with 10 days of active rTMS but the degree of improvement was modest (102). Herwig et al. (103) reported similar findings with a 30% response rate to real rTMS, and 0% with sham.

There are suggestions that a longer duration of treatment may result in a more significant improvement. Pridmore et al. (104) was the first to extend the period of treatment to three or four weeks. Patients with melancholic depression referred for ECT were treated with rTMS to the left DLPFC and resulted in remission in 88% of cases in an open study. An ongoing double-blind, sham-controlled multicenter study on the efficacy of rTMS applied to the left DLPFC for six weeks will test whether longer periods of stimulation are more effective in a controlled setting, according to data regarding the application of rTMS to treat MDD that a longer period of stimulation could be required to evoke a clinical response (105).

It is still an open question as to whether the antidepressant effects of rTMS are region or frequency dependent. Klein et al. (106) randomized depressed outpatients to two weeks of active or sham slow (1 Hz) rTMS over right prefrontal cortex using a round, nonfocal coil. In the active group 41% of patients responded compared to 17% with sham. This study suggested that right-sided stimulation might be effective. A much smaller double-blind study replicated these results with the active group showing a better clinical response compared to the sham (107).

If lower frequencies were indeed as effective as higher frequencies, this would have significant safety implications, as lower frequencies carry less risk of seizure. When low and high frequencies have been compared in the same study, there are suggestions that lower frequencies may actually fare better. Kimbrell et al. (108) found a trend toward better improvement following two weeks of 1 Hz rTMS compared to 20 Hz to the left DLPFC in a crossover design. There were suggestions that baseline metabolic activity in the DLPFC correlated with response. Similarly, Padberg et al. (109) tested nonpsychotic, depressed patients with sham treatment, slow rTMS, or fast rTMS, all over the left prefrontal cortex. After five days, 83% in the slow group and 50% in the fast group improved, with no change in the sham group. A parallel-design, blinded study from George et al. (110) suggests that slower (5 Hz) left prefrontal TMS may be as effective as faster (20 Hz) left stimulation. Fitzgerald et al. (111) demonstrated that both high-frequency left rTMS and low-frequency right rTMS have benefits in patients with medication-resistant MDD. They concluded that treatment for at least four weeks is necessary for clinically meaningful benefits to be achieved.

There has been great interest in determining whether rTMS could offer an alternative to ECT for severe or treatment-resistant depression (TRD), particularly because the adverse effect profile of rTMS is relatively benign. Using a parallel-group, nonblinded design, Grunhaus et al. (112) randomly assigned inpatients to treatment with fast left DLPFC rTMS or ECT. Among nonpsychotic patients, up to four weeks of daily rTMS was not different in efficacy to ECT, but ECT was superior among psychotically depressed patients. Dannon et al. (113) demonstrated that patients treated with rTMS or ECT showed the same percentage of clinical stabilization at three and six months follow-up. Janicak et al. (114) randomized severely depressed patients to be treated with rTMS or ECT. No significant difference in efficacy was found between the two treatments (rTMS, 55% and ECT, 64%). All of these studies have the limitation that the patients were not blinded to the form of treatment, and some have questioned whether the ECT comparison group represented optimal ECT practice. Nevertheless, it would be impossible to blind the patient to the treatment modality in this case (because sham ECT would not be considered ethically acceptable), and all studies have found the side-effect profile to favor rTMS.

Several meta-analyses have examined the antidepressant efficacy of rTMS (115–117), and concluded that there is evidence for statistical benefit of rTMS; however, the effect size could be described as moderate and in some cases of limited clinical significance. For example, Burt et al. (49) found that the average percent improvement with active TMS was 28.94% (SD = 23.19) and with sham was 6.63% (SD = 25.56). Relatively few patients met the standard criteria for response or remission. It is also true however that the meta-analyses are heavily weighted toward the earlier studies that used what may now be considered inadequate dosages and durations of rTMS.

Further work using controlled designs is needed to determine whether the antidepressant effects of rTMS are region-, frequency-, or intensity-dependent, and to test the efficacy of more robust parameters in a sample large-enough to provide adequate statistical power. Such work is presently underway, with multi-center trials sponsored both by industry and by the National Institute of Mental Health.

MST IN MDD

Seizures have been elicited with rTMS, both inadvertently in normal volunteers and in two patients with depression (36,118,119), and intentionally in epileptic patients in an attempt to identify seizure focus (120–124). These reports suggested that seizure induction is related to the extent that magnetic stimulus intensity exceeds the individual's motor threshold (i.e., minimum intensity required to elicit a movement of a specified amplitude in a distal hand muscle), and led to the development of guidelines to ensure that standard applications of rTMS remain subconvulsive (125). Thus, on both conceptual and empirical grounds, it should be possible to develop devices capable of seizure induction, despite the anticonvulsant effects of the anesthetic medications typically used during ECT.

The deliberate induction of tonic–clonic seizures in rhesus monkeys under general anesthesia using a custom-modified magnetic stimulator with heightened output capabilities has recently been reported (126). Clinical application of magnetic seizure induction as a form of convulsive therapy has so far been limited to a report of two single cases (127,128). The first trial to our knowledge of MST for the first four treatments followed by conventional ECT resulted in a decrease in the Hamilton Rating Scale for Depression (HRSD-21) score to 13 from a baseline of 20. The Mini-Mental State score remained unchanged at 30 throughout the treatment course. Following the MST sessions, the patient received eight conventional ECT treatments (RUL, 200% above initial seizure threshold), and had a final posttreatment HRSD-21 score of six. The second report on the treatment of a patient with refractory MDD, who underwent a series of 12 sessions of MST in an inpatient setting, resulted in baseline HRSD-21 of 33 and Beck Depression Inventory of 40 decreasing to 6 and 11, respectively, one week after completion of the MST trial. Measures of cognitive functions supported the hypothesis that MST is associated with a less severe profile of cognitive side effects. [^{99m}Tc]-HMPAO (hexamethyl propylene amine oxime) single photon emission computerized tomography (SPECT) studies (baseline and four days after the completion of the MST trial) pointed to a raise in blood flow at baseline in the left fronto-parietal region and the brainstem. Another study examined the feasibility of MST in depressed patients, and contrasted magnetically induced seizures with conventional ECT in acute cognitive side effects and electrophysiological characteristics. Based on the fact that the induced current is limited to a small volume of the cortex, it was hypothesized that MST would have a superior cognitive side-effect profile when compared to ECT. Given the more focal induction of seizure activity, it was also hypothesized that MST would result in weaker ictal EEG expression. Compared to ECT, MST seizures had shorter duration, lower ictal EEG amplitude, and less postictal suppression. Patients had fewer subjective side effects and recovered orientation more quickly with MST than with ECT. MST was also superior to ECT on measures of attention, retrograde amnesia, and category fluency. Magnetic seizure induction in patients with depression is feasible, and appears to have a superior acute side-effect profile than ECT (129). These preliminary data support the prospect of antidepressant efficacy of MST and point to a benign cognitive side-effect profile in patients suffering from severe treatment-resistant major depression.

MINIMALLY INVASIVE SOMATIC TECHNIQUES
IN MDD: DBS AND VNS

As commented above, MDD is often a difficult-to-treat chronic illness. It is the second most disabling condition in the United States (130); nearly 10 million patients are treated annually (131). Symptoms fully resolve in only about one-third of patients after the first treatment (131–133). Approximately 20% will not achieve remission even after undergoing three adequate antidepressant trials (131). Thus, about four million individuals have TRD (134). Polypharmacy and ECT are the standard of care for TRD. Suicide and comorbid general medical conditions are major complications (135). The most afflicted subset of TRD patients have chronic, treatment intractable illness—severe symptoms and disability—which sometimes do not resolve following aggressive treatment with medications, psychotherapy, and ECT.

For them, neurosurgical procedures may remain a therapeutic option. Psychiatric neurosurgery has a history plagued by controversy, largely because indiscriminate use of prefrontal lobotomy in the mid-20th century frequently produced tragic deficits in emotional responsiveness and motivation. While the historical experience remains an enduring caution, current stereotactic methods, using considerably smaller and more precisely located targets, are much better tolerated and have less morbidity.

An increasingly specific neurobiological rationale for psychiatric neurosurgery is being developed. Research with modern neuroimaging including functional magnetic resonance imaging (fMRI) and positron emission tomography (PET) has focused attention on the relationship between the activity in specific neuroanatomical networks and psychiatric symptoms and upon changes noted after effective treatment. Somatic treatments for refractory depression can be grouped into two broad categories: neurostimulation and ablative or lesioning neurosurgery. The two stimulatory techniques involve DBS and the recent U.S. Food and Drug Administration–approved VNS.

Neurosurgical treatment for intractable psychiatric illness has gradually become more visible to the general public, due to the recent attention paid by the media to the therapeutic potential of DBS in neurology for Parkinson's disease. Most psychiatrists, in contrast, have been aware that modern lesion procedures offered a last avenue of hope for patients with intractable OCD and possibly MDD for the last several decades (136). This awareness is based on past retrospective studies and, more recently, a small number of prospective investigations. For example, a survey published in 1984 found that 78% of adult psychiatrists in the United Kingdom had referred patients for subcaudate tractotomy, mainly for refractory MDD and OCD. Later data indicate that referrals for psychiatric neurosurgery in Britain continued at roughly the same rate from 1979 to 1993, although the proportion of patients accepted for surgery was reduced from 50% to 60% to approximately 20% during that period. This decline resulted from the institution of high-dose medication trials as a screening criterion, and more patients responded to such trials before surgery (137).

Treatments for depression have come a long way in the past decades. For those patients with TRD continuing work has been aimed at developing what might be termed "neuroanatomically based" treatments. Two of these treatments include DBS and VNS in addition to the three discussed above. The efficacy of these treatments can be attributed to the effects they produce on various cortico-limbic neuroanatomic pathways that have been implicated in depression.

Spiegel et al. (138) who began stereotactic neurosurgery in humans, were the first to report that dorsomedial thalamotomies improved OCD symptoms. Their stereotactic procedure was less radical than lobotomy, but still risky at times. Because the lesioning electrodes were placed in a highly vascular structure without modern imaging guidance, hemorrhages were frequent, and 10% of the patients died, mainly for this reason. Later, during the 1950s and 1960s, several groups of neurosurgeons and psychiatrists, mainly in Europe, explored the therapeutic effects of selective lesions made under stereotactic guidance. The development of these techniques was informed at first not by specific empirical evidence, but by the general idea that fronto-subcortical (and particularly fronto-thalamic) connections were important in higher brain function, and that limbic networks modulate emotion (139–143).

Historically, neurosurgical lesioning procedures have been employed in the treatment of refractory depression, mostly in Europe, and have targeted these same pathways (136). The aim was to sever connections between subcortical structures and the frontal lobes. This helps to disconnect higher cortical structures and lower limbic structures. This imbalance may be implicated in the pathogenesis of depressive and anxiety disorders. The procedures developed most successfully were subcaudate tractotomy, anterior capsulotomy, cingulotomy, and limbic leucotomy (a combination of subcaudate tractotomy and cingulotomy). Subcaudate tractotomy and anterior capsulotomy, in particular, interrupt connections of orbital and medial prefrontal cortex to the thalamus. The target of anterior cingulotomy, the most widely performed and recognized procedure in the United States, is within the cingulate cortex itself (136). In particular, three of the lesioning procedures, anterior capsulotomy, subcaudate tractotomy, and anterior cingulotomy are of key interest as they are targets for electrode placement in DBS for depression treatment.

Anterior Capsulotomy

This procedure targets the fiber bundles in the anterior limb of the internal capsule connecting the frontal lobes and thalamus (16,144). While therapeutic effects in schizophrenia were considered unsatisfactory, results in patients with severe anxiety were better. Capsulotomy was further developed and used in a large series of patients by Lars Leksell and colleagues at the Karolinska Institute in Sweden, starting in the 1950s (136). After craniotomy, thermocoagulation lesions were made bilaterally using BP electrodes placed in the anterior third of the capsule. This procedure is now called open capsulotomy or thermo-capsulotomy, in contrast to the newer technique of gamma knife capsulotomy. The particular intent of gamma knife capsulotomy in the United States has been to target connections between dorsomedial thalmus and orbital and medial prefrontal cortex. The efficacy of anterior capsulotomy was first reported by Leksell's group. They found that just under half (48%) of depressed patients (of a total sample of 116 which also included patients with schizophrenia and nonobsessional anxiety) had satisfactory outcomes. Although modern rating scales were not used, criteria for judging improvements were strict. Only patients who were free of symptoms or very much improved were judged as responders. Much of the remaining evidence with respect to the efficacy of anterior capsulotomy only deals with the response to the procedure of those patients treated for OCD. In the United States, gamma knife anterior capsulotomy has been used almost exclusively for intractable OCD. As discussed below, trials of DBS at the capsulotomy target site for intractable depression are underway.

Subcaudate Tractotomy

In this procedure, lesions intended to interrupt orbitofrontal–subcortical connections are made under the head of the caudate nucleus, in the substantia innominata (145). Depression has been the most common diagnosis for patients undergoing this procedure. In an early report, Strom-Olsen and Carlisle (146) described beneficial effects in depressed patients who underwent stereotactic subcaudate tractotomy. A subsequent report from this group, in which structured interviews were used, described a 55% response rate in a total of 96 depressed patients operated on through 1973 and followed for two-and-a-half years on average (145). More recently, in their review of the same group's experience from 1979 to 1991, Hodgkiss et al. (147) classified 34% of depressed patients as "recovered" or "well" and 32% as "improved," out of a total 183 such patients who had undergone the surgery. Malizia found similar rates of response (137). The most comprehensive review of responses to subcaudate tractotomy included 1300 cases. Published in 1994, it concluded that subcaudate tractotomy enables 40% to 60% of patients to lead normal or near-normal lives (148). As noted above, compared to a suicide rate of roughly 15% in patients with similar MDD, 1% of patients committed suicide after subcaudate tractotomy in a 1975 study of 208 patients who underwent subcaudate tractotomy, mainly for depression.

Anterior Cingulotomy

Originally conceived by Fulton (206) as a treatment for psychiatric disorders, cingulotomy's first use was actually for intractable pain. The procedure was later applied to psychiatric disorders when mood and anxiety symptoms were found to be responsive in pain patients. Whitty et al. (149) first reported effects of cingulotomy in OCD, followed by the work of Kullberg (150). However, it is the work of Ballantine and colleagues (207) at Massachusetts General Hospital that is responsible for cingulotomy being the best known and most widely used procedure for intractable psychiatric illness in

North America. Beginning in 1962, this group demonstrated that anterior cingulotomy had a favorable safety profile. The investigative team has performed approximately 1000 cingulotomies, studying its efficacy for a range of psychiatric indications. Current indications for anterior cingulotomy include intractable pain, MDD, and OCD. The targets for this procedure are the anterior cingulate cortex (Brodmann areas 24 and 32) adjacent to the underlying fibers of the cingulum bundle. Ballantine (151) reported that, of 118 depressed patients treated with stereotactic cingulotomy, 42% were "recovered" or "well" and 24% were "improved." A later review of 34 patients who underwent cingulotomy in the era of MRI guidance found that 60% of patients with UP depression had favorable responses.

DEEP BRAIN STIMULATION (DBS)

DBS of the subthalamic nucleus or globus pallidus has been FDA-approved and used in over 25,000 patients with movement disorders. The use of DBS in MDD is only a recent undertaking, with only 11 patients thus far being implanted and studied in the United States. The data on follow-up is also limited to three- to six-month maximum follow-up times. Two key anatomical targets have been studied for DBS in MDD: the ventral internal capsule (anterior limb)/ventral striatum (VC/VS) and the subgenual cingulate gyrus (Brodmann area 25). Each target was studied separately and their subsequent results are discussed below.

The surgical implantation procedure for DBS involves bilaterally implanting two custom-made quadripolar stimulating leads stereotactically under MRI guidance bilaterally. Placement is then verified by stereotactic CT. Either during the same surgical procedure or at a later date, an implantable pulse generator is implanted in the subcutaneous tissues of the chest wall, with extension wires tunneled down subcutaneously to connect the electrodes to the generator.

For those implanted in the VC/VS, the leads are targeted to remain within the anterior capsule in the coronal plane, with the distal tips extending into ventral striatum. For those implanted in Cg25, the ventral contact is centered in Cg25.

The implantation is performed under a local anesthetic to evaluate stimulation thresholds for efficacy or adverse effects. After implantation, voltage is progressively increased at each of the electrode contacts until the patient reports feelings of well-being. These range from "sudden calmness or lightness," "disappearance of the void," sudden brightening of the room, or a sharpening of visual details and intensification of colors. These changes are reproducible and reversible depending on the patient, level of stimulation, and location of the contacts (152). All patients following exposure to more than a certain voltage threshold (in one study more than 7.0 V) (152), developed stimulation dose–dependent adverse effects including light-headedness and psychomotor slowing. This also has been the experience of this author.

The antidepressant effects of DBS of the VC/VS in patients with severe OCD have been well described (142). The VC/VS contains neuronal connections implicated in MDD, and overlaps targets of ablative procedures for highly refractory MDD. Specifically, it overlaps that of the subcaudate tractotomy lesions discussed above, which have been used in more than a thousand patients with highly refractory depression. Patients in this initial use of DBS had severe and disabling MDD, refractory to multiple adequate trials of antidepressants from at least three different chemical classes, medication combinations, psychotherapy, and to BL ECT. It had been hypothesized and now substantiated with good evidence that VC/VS DBS can benefit patients with treatment-intractable depression. The following discussion is based on results from a study by Greenberg et al. (153).

Five patients were studied and followed up for three months. Presurgical psychotropic medications were generally continued throughout the DBS trials, though systematic efforts were made to gradually reduce doses of benzodiazepines and other sedating agents as clinical progress allowed. Categorical response was defined as 50% reduction in baseline total score on the HRSD and MADRS scales.

After the three-month single-blind phase, three of the five patients (60%) met the HRSD criterion for response. Four of five patients met the response threshold of a 50% decrease from baseline. Ratings on the MADRS suicidality item (No. 10) decreased for all four patients who had scores > 0 (indicating suicidal thinking) at baseline. Ratings on the Social and Occupational Functioning Assessment Scale improved from serious functional impairment at baseline to a score corresponding to moderate impairment at three months with most of the gain during the first month of DBS. Self-ratings of depressive symptoms, as measured by the Inventory of Depressive Symptoms-Self-Rated, also dropped during the three-month trial reflecting a mean, 56% decrease from baseline.

DBS-associated adverse effects were jaw tightness, paresthesias around the chest pulse generator, insomnia, and various undesirable mood states (agitation, anxiety, disinhibition, and hypomania) acutely associated with some DBS parameters in several patients. In all cases, these mood states reversed with DBS adjustment, mainly pulse width reduction from 210 to 60–150 μsec.

Of note is the fact that the first three patients had experienced stimulator battery depletion during chronic stimulation, accompanied by acute symptom worsening and return of their baseline depressive symptoms. In all cases, symptoms improved rapidly within one week when DBS resumed.

Depending on the rating scale used, three or four of five patients responded with a 50% reduction in depression severity after three months of DBS. Moreover, patients' social and occupational functioning improved.

Notably, all five patients had failed to benefit substantially from psychotherapy, multiple antidepressant trials, combination pharmacotherapy treatments, and ECT. That depression worsened in all three patients experiencing battery depletion, and improved again when DBS resumed provides further support that the stimulation itself produced the clinical improvements that were observed. The main stimulation-induced adverse effect was hypomania, which rapidly reversed when DBS parameters were changed.

Functional neuroimaging studies have demonstrated consistent involvement of Cg25 in acute sadness as well as in antidepressant treatment effects, suggesting a critical role for this region in modulating negative mood states (152,154,155). A decrease in Cg25 activity is reported with clinical response to antidepressant treatments including SSRI medications, ECT, TMS, and ablative surgery (154,156–160).

Connections from Cg25 to the brainstem, hypothalamus, and insula have been implicated in the disturbances of circadian regulation associated with depression (libido, sleep, and appetite) (161–165). Reciprocal pathways linking Cg25 to orbitofrontal, medial prefrontal, and various parts of the anterior and posterior cingulate cortices form the neuroanatomic substrates by which primary autonomic and homeostatic processes influence various aspects of learning, memory, motivation, and reward-core behaviors altered in depressed patients (161,166–168).

The use of chronic DBS to modulate Cg25 gray matter and interconnected frontal and subcortical regions was studied in six patients and was found to produce significant clinical benefits in patients with TRD (152). Categorical response in this study was also defined as 50% reduction in baseline total score on the HRSD. Remission was defined as an absolute HRSD-17 score of <8. By two months, five of six patients met the defined response threshold. At the six-month study endpoint, the antidepressant response was maintained in four out of six patients (66%). Of note is the fact that three of the subjects achieved remission or near remission of the illness. Comparable improvements were also seen in other rating scales; HDRS-24, MADRS, and Clinical Global Impression. The mean stimulation parameters used in this group at six months were 4.0 V, 60-µsec pulse width, at a frequency of 130 Hz.

The Mayberg study also correlated PET evidence of cerebral blood flow (CBF) changes in specific areas of brain with chronic stimulation. In fact, the identified CBF pattern change associated with DBS-induced antidepressant effects is comparable to other therapies for depression in those patients who respond to standard treatments. The pattern of reduced activity in the Cg25 and hypothalamus, together with prefrontal and brainstem increases during DBS are identical to changes reported with antidepressant response to medication (159). PET studies revealed decreases in CBF in medial frontal and orbital frontal cortex and CBF increases in dorsal cingulated cortex. These changes are similar to the pattern observed with cognitive behavioral therapy.

In summary, the initial findings that severe and extremely refractory depression improved after DBS are encouraging. More definitive controlled data are needed. Newer neurostimulators have enhanced battery life, minimizing risk of therapy interruption. Given the severity of illness in this subject population, and the potential for DBS-induced hypomania, future studies should be conducted cautiously, by specialized psychiatric/neurosurgery teams monitoring patients closely. Further development of this interdisciplinary treatment approach holds promise in meeting a critical need for otherwise untreatable major depression.

VNS

The FDA approved intermittent electrical stimulation of cranial vagus nerve X via a surgically implanted, programmable prosthesis for medically refractory partial-onset seizures in 1997. Four years later, and without the benefit of controlled data to establish its efficacy, the VNS Therapy™ System for delivery of cervical VNS was also approved as a treatment for medication-resistant or intolerant depression or BP disorder in Europe and Canada. Since that time, VNS has come to be regarded as one of the most promising new forms of therapeutic brain stimulation, a fact that reflects a tremendous need for better, long-term treatment of disabling depression, as well as great expectations for the application of new technologies in treating mental illness. In fact, the U.S. FDA issued full approval for treatment-resistant MDD, or TRD, in July, 2005, based on both open and case-controlled cohort data.

Anatomy of the Vagus Nerve

The vagus (Latin for "wandering") nerve is best known for its parasympathetic efferent functions, such as autonomic control and regulation of heart rate and gastric motility. It is a mixed nerve that is composed of sensory and motor fibers. Approximately 80% of the left vagus is composed of sensory afferent fibers, carrying information to the brain from head, neck, thorax, and abdomen (169). Through sensory afferent connections in the nucleus tractus solitarius (NTS), the vagus has extensive projections to brain regions that are thought to modulate activity in the limbic system and higher cortex (164,170,171). Pathways connecting the NTS with the parabrachial nucleus and the locus ceruleus carry afferent vagal input to norepinephrine-containing neurons that reach the amygdala, hypothalamus, insula, thalamus, orbitofrontal cortex, and other limbic structures (172).

Information on the VNS and Its Safety in Epilepsy Trials

The VNS therapy system includes a pocket watch–sized generator that is implanted subcutaneously into the left chest wall in a fashion similar to placement of a cardiac pacemaker (173). Via a separate neck incision, bipolar electrode coils are wrapped around the left vagus nerve near the carotid artery. The leads from these coils are subsequently tunneled under the skin for connection with the programmable generator. A telemetric wand connected to a portable computer is held to the chest (over the patient's clothing) to assess and control the stimulation parameters in a noninvasive office procedure.

The first human implants for a pilot study of cervical VNS were performed in 1988, in patients with medication-resistant epilepsy who were not candidates for neurosurgery (174). Collective data from these epilepsy trials showed that after two years of continuous VNS, categorical response rate (defined as 50% or greater reduction in seizure frequency) reached 43% and was maintained after three years (175). More importantly, the epilepsy studies demonstrated that cervical VNS was well tolerated, with adverse events rarely leading to discontinuation of VNS therapy (153). Pooled data from epilepsy clinical studies ($n = 454$) show minimal surgical complications associated with implantation: infection without explantation of the device (1.8%), infection with subsequent explantation (1.1%), hoarseness or temporary vocal cord paralysis (0.7%), and hypesthesia or lower left facial paresis (0.7%) (176). In the vast majority of cases, side effects related to the intermittent stimulation itself (i.e., voice alteration or hoarseness, cough, paresthesia, dysphagia, and dyspepsia) were judged to be mild or moderate, and decreased over time with continued VNS at the same stimulation level. Stimulation-related adverse events could be diminished by reprogramming the device to deliver a lower level of output current or a diminished pulse-width. Alternatively, a patient could completely abort a stimulation-induced adverse event by holding or taping a small magnet over the pulse generator. High continuation rates (72% at three years), lack of compliance issues or drug-interactions, and favorable practice and reimbursement economics have all contributed to the success of VNS in the treatment of patients with severe epilepsy. At the time of this publication, over 35,000 epilepsy patients worldwide have received cervical VNS (Cyberonics, Inc., data on file), and the treatment has been judged by the American Academy of Neurology's Technology and Therapeutics Committee as having "sufficient evidence ... to rank VNS for epilepsy as effective and safe, based on a preponderance of Class I evidence." (177).

The Rationale for VNS as a Potential Treatment for Depression

During the early epilepsy trials of VNS, patients frequently stayed in the same Gainesville, Florida hotel during follow-up visits. An astute observation made by a hotel clerk and reported to VNS investigator, B.J. Wilder, was that the VNS patients "seemed to be in better spirits as time passed." Anecdotal reports of mood improvements, apparently unrelated to reduction in seizure frequency, further inspired the VNS investigators to systematically assess mood and anxiety symptoms (178,179). Both retrospective data analysis and prospective assessments during epilepsy trials suggested that VNS was associated with reduction in depressive symptoms, even in the absence of improvement in seizures (180–182). In addition, the ever-growing number of modern anticonvulsant agents that have demonstrated efficacy in the treatment of mood disorder patients (e.g., carbamazepine, valproic acid, and lamotrigine) supported the possibility of using VNS in the treatment of depression. The similarities between VNS and ECT, which is considered the most effective antidepressant treatment, provided additional support to the hypothesis that VNS may be a useful depression treatment. Finally, a study of lumbar CSF components in epilepsy patients sampled before and after three months of VNS showed significant increases in CSF concentrations of gamma-aminobutyric acid (GABA) and trend-level decreases in glutamate (183). This study also found trends toward VNS-induced increases in levels of HVA, the major dopamine metabolite, and 5-hydroxyindoleacetic acid, the major serotonin metabolite. As the vagus nerve projects to mood regulation regions of the brain, the above-listed evidence provided a rationale for studying VNS in depression.

Open-Label Study of VNS for TRD

The efficacy and safety of VNS for nonpsychotic, chronic, or recurrent TRD was first studied in an open-label fashion in 30 patients at four U.S. academic sites (184). Patients enrolled in the study had either BP ($n = 9$) or UP ($n = 21$) forms of depressive affective illness and had failed trials for at least two classes of medications during the current depressive episode. The study design called for all subjects to undergo a two-week, single-blind recovery period after surgery. After recovery, the patients began a two-week period where the VNS was activated and the output current was progressively increased to the maximum tolerated level. After these first four weeks, the output level of the stimulator was fixed and stimulation continued for an additional eight weeks. Additionally, all patients in the trials were continued on their pre-VNS, stable psychotropic medication regimens for the entire course of the trial.

For the purpose of this study, the authors defined a "responder" as a patient who had a 50% or greater reduction in baseline on the HRSD. Study results showed that 12 of the 30 (40%) patients met the criteria after 12 weeks of VNS treatment. Substantial functional improvement was also seen with average scores on the Global Assessment of Function increasing from 40.6 to 61.9 in the acute study period of 12 weeks.

A second cohort of 30 patients with TRD, meeting similar inclusion and exclusion criteria, was added to the open-label study. A slightly less impressive response rate was seen in this group, with only 6 of 29 (20.7%) patients completing the study meeting the criteria for a "responder." The overall acute response rate was 18 of 59 (30.5%) for both groups in the trial, with 9 of the 59 patients (15%) meeting criteria for full remission of the depressive episode. Quality-of-life assessments suggested VNS was associated with improvements in vitality, social function, and mental health domains, even among patients who were considered VNS acute phase nonresponders (185). These results are particularly impressive given the study population, as the average participant had unsuccessfully tried over 16 interventions, both medication and nonmedication, prior to the trial.

When further analyzing the data, no dose–response relationship was detected with final output current. In addition, neuropsychological tests indicated neurocognitive improvements after VNS relative to baseline, especially in those who experienced decreased depressive symptoms (185,186). Finally, after placing the data in a regression model, the only identifiable predictor of response was degree of treatment resistance, as measured by the number of failed antidepressant trials. In general, more severely refractory patients experienced poorer responses to the 10-week VNS therapy.

In terms of safety, much like the epilepsy trials, VNS was also well tolerated with no patients discontinuing the study due to an adverse event. Most side effects were mild and were reported only during stimulation. The most common adverse events reported were hoarseness, coughing, shortness of breath during exercise, headache, and neck pain.

While the short-term results of the study were encouraging, the long-term pilot data generated even more enthusiasm for VNS in TRD. After one year of VNS, 10/11 (91%) acute responders from the first group of 30 had maintained their response, and 3 of the 17 (18%) of the initial nonresponders had achieved a reduction of depressive symptoms sufficient enough to meet "responder" criteria (187). When the entire sample ($n = 60$) participating in the study was followed to the one-year mark, response rate was 45% and remission rate was 27%. For those who had reached the two-year mark, there continued to be evidence of sustained or even enhanced response to VNS in 13/24 (54%) responders (188). It is worth noting that changes in dose or type of psychotropic medication and VNS stimulation parameters were not controlled after exit from the initial 12-week acute phase study, introducing the possibility that the observed improvements were not entirely attributable to the VNS. Nevertheless, the association of adjunct VNS with sustained depressive symptom reduction and improved functional status after two years is suggestive of antidepressant efficacy.

Placebo-Controlled Study of VNS for Depression

Given the positive results noted in the original open-label study, a push was made to investigate the efficacy of the VNS in the treatment of depression through a double-blind, sham-controlled study. This study was designed in a similar fashion to the original study, with the important exception that patients were randomized in a double-blind fashion to either active VNS or a sham VNS (device not turned on) condition. After completing the 12-week–long acute study, patients assigned to the sham arm of the study who still were depressed crossed over to the active stimulation arm, and long-term data was collected on all patients in the study. In addition, the investigators revised the study exclusion criteria to exclude those with the highest levels of treatment resistance (six or more failed trials in the depressive episode), because they appeared to have the worst predictive response rate in the previous open-label study.

Two hundred and twenty-one patients received VNS through this double-blind study. As in the previous study, acute safety and tolerability of VNS was demonstrated with 115/117 (98%) patients in the active treatment group tolerating the procedure. Placebo (sham) response rate was low at 10%, but only 15% of participants responded to acute, active VNS, which failed to statistically confirm the short-term antidepressant efficacy of the VNS therapy (189). Interestingly, patient self-reports on IDS were statistically significant.

When speculating on reasons for the difference between the placebo-controlled and open-label study, many have focused on possible inadequate low dosing of the VNS in the controlled study. A preliminary comparison of the output current delivered in the placebo-controlled depression study with that used in the initial open-label depression study, as well as the epilepsy studies suggests that stimulation set at 1.0 mA or higher is associated with higher rates of clinical response. Stimulation parameters were set at lower settings in the placebo-controlled study, compared to those used in the initial open-label depression studies and the epilepsy trials.

In light of the apparent gradual accumulation of more VNS responders over time in the open-label study, there has been considerable interest in the clinical course and the longer term outcomes experienced by the MDD patients who continue to receive VNS after finishing the acute phase trial. In a preliminary analysis, it was found that at 12 months, 30% of patients were "responders" and 17% were in remission ($n = 180$), and at 24 months, 33% were "responders" and 17% were in remission ($n = 157$) (190). In addition, long-term response rates from this second study showed that VNS has a sustained effect with 70% of those classified as "responders" at three months continuing to be classified as "responders" at two years. This data suggests that the response to VNS might simply take longer to exert an effect. It should be noted, however, that as in the open-label study, long-term data are not collected under controlled conditions, and it is therefore possible that changes in VNS parameters or antidepressant therapies could account for the change.

Finally, to better delineate the long-term efficacy of VNS, a prospective comparison cohort group of 125 patients was formed (191) with the same enrollment criteria as the randomized control trial. The second group was strictly observational in nature and did not receive any specific treatment other than community standard of care. In essence, this new group allowed the comparison between "standard of care" treatment and "standard of care" treatment plus VNS in a long-term setting. Using the same "responder" criteria of the HRSD from the first study, it was found that at 12 months, only 17% of the "standard of care" group responded as compared to the 30% in the VNS group. Furthermore, it was found that the remission rate was 7% in the "standard of care" group as compared to 17% in the VNS group (190). It is felt that this long-term and comparative data achieved the above-cited recent FDA approval.

VNS Mechanisms of Action Research in Depression

One of the most quickly advancing areas in VNS research is the ever-expanding neurobiology research on the direct action VNS has on brain regions and neurotransmitter systems implicated in mood disorders.

A SPECT imaging study conducted in six MDD patients receiving VNS in the open-label study found that at baseline, compared to normal controls, patients had reduced rCBF to left dorsolateral prefrontal, antero-lateral temporal, and perisylvian temporal structures, including posterior insula (180). After 10 weeks of VNS, these depressed patients showed increased rCBF in the superior frontal gyrus, right mesial (posterior hippo-campus), and lateral temporal cortex. The 10-week trial of VNS appeared to lead to resolution of classic rCBF abnormalities in depressed patients, espe-cially among those showing a favorable clinical response.

A PET study performed on seven patients with TRD after 10 weeks of VNS therapy found that, compared with baseline, metabolic activity was sig-nificantly higher in the BL orbitofrontal gyrus, left amygdala and parahippo-campal gyrus, BL thalamus, left insula, and right cingulate gyrus. Areas of decreased activity included the BL cerebellum and right fusiform gyrus. This data represents a combination of the effects of acute VNS stimulation and chronic effects of VNS on blood flow over 10 weeks of therapy (192).

A method for synchronized blood oxygenation level-dependent (BOLD) fMRI was developed to detect signals from the implanted device and link it to fMRI image acquisition (193). In depressed patients, BOLD fMRI response to VNS was shown in areas regulated by the vagus nerve: orbitofrontal and parieto-occipital cortex bilaterally, left temporal cortex, hypothalamus, and left amygdala. This newly developed fMRI technique was also used to examine whether BOLD signal changes depend on the frequency of VNS (194). Results confirmed that acute immediate regional brain activity changes vary with the frequency or total dose of stimulation. Additionally, results suggested that VNS exerts a dose-dependent modula-tory effect on other brain activities.

In the placebo-controlled study, lumbar CSF samples were collected in 18 patients, both before and after VNS therapy (195). Consistent with the

CSF findings reported for a group of seizure patients receiving three months of VNS, the CSF concentration of HVA, the major dopamine metabolite, showed a 21% increase in the depressed group when compared to the placebo group. However, unlike the CSF results obtained during the epilepsy trials, no changes in CSF GABA were detected. While categorical clinical response rates were low, the data suggested that an increase in CSF level of norepinephrine during VNS was correlated with better clinical outcome. This correlation with norepinephrine levels is of interest because of known anatomical connections and animal studies demonstrating that VNS exerts effects on higher brain regions via actions at the locus ceruleus, the major noradrenergic nucleus in the brain.

Sleep EEG studies have also measured apparent VNS-induced improvement in indices of sleep macro- and microarchitecture in patients with TRD (196). After 10 weeks of VNS, amplitude of sleep EEG rhythms was restored to near normal levels, and patients manifested significantly less awake time and "light sleep" time, and significantly more stage four (deep sleep).

Practical Considerations in the Use of VNS for Psychiatric Disorders

Surgical implantation of the VNS therapy system is considered a procedure of low technical complexity for a surgeon with experience in the head and neck area. The surgery typically takes between 30 minutes and one hour in the operating room, and is usually performed on an outpatient or day-surgery basis, without subsequent admission to the hospital for routine post-surgical recovery or monitoring. General anesthesia is used in the majority of cases, but regional and local anesthesia have been used in some centers. A device "programmer" who is knowledgeable with the operation of the VNS therapy system must be present, but not sterile, in the operating room to perform lead testing before surgical incisions are closed. A 4- to 5-cm incision is made in the neck for placement of the two stimulating electrodes, which coil around the vagus nerve. A second incision, similar in size, is made in the external chest wall (or alternatively in the axillary region for a superior cosmetic result) for insertion of the pacemaker-like pulse generator in the neck. A tunneling tool subcutaneously passes the electrodes to the site for connection with the pulse generator. The battery life of the currently available pulse generator model is approximately 8 to 12 years. Once the battery expires, a single surgical incision in the chest wall is needed for a replacement.

Because of the potential for heating of the electrical leads, whole-body MRI is contraindicated in patients who have the VNS pulse generator implanted. Special "send–receive coils" have been used to concentrate magnetic fields away from the neck area when MRI of the brain is necessary. Patients with the VNS therapy system are asked to carry identification cards and are educated about the risks of being in close proximity to strong magnetic fields. Diathermy, used in physical therapy, is also contraindicated.

The cost of the VNS therapy system and surgical implantation for cervical VNS is approximately $20,000, making it roughly comparable to the cost of a course of ECT for depression in an inpatient setting. If the generator battery life is an estimated 10 years, VNS costs can be calculated to approximately $2000 per year. Early success in establishing adequate terms of coverage and reimbursement by third-party payers has contributed to the wide-scale availability of VNS for patients with epilepsy in the United States.

Data regarding the optimal stimulation parameters for antidepressant effects are extremely limited. While it is tempting to imagine that VNS may someday replace psychotropic medications and the many undesirable side effects that accompany them, it is important to bear in mind that in the majority of cases to date, VNS has been investigated as an adjunct therapy rather than as a monotherapy. Patients' expectations for dramatic symptom recovery or even cure from severe psychiatric illness may be fueled by the introduction of new technology and the highly interventional nature of the device implantation. Management of such expectations should be undertaken with great care, particularly in depressed patients who are at a heightened risk of acting impulsively and self-destructively on feelings of disappointment and hopelessness.

CONCLUSIONS

ECT is the most effective acute form of antidepressant therapy available. It has been proven to be effective in between 85% and 90% of cases of major depression when compared with antidepressant medications, which are effective in 60% to 65% of cases (197,198). Long-term ECT data are much less robust. Thus, understanding the mechanism of ECT might be a major clue to understanding the etiology of depression. ECT treatment requires the induction of a series of convulsions, usually induced three times a week by the application of either BL or UL electrical shocks. The response is usually seen after four to eight treatments and usually results in reduction in the symptoms of depression with the fourth to sixth treatment. Thus, repeated convulsions are necessary for the therapeutic effect (199), and the drop in symptoms can occur in one to two weeks.

Routine clinical use of rTMS in psychiatric disorders is far from certain at the present time, but that may change as the results of larger well-controlled trials become available. None of the key effects has been rigorously replicated, and most of the positive findings are based on small samples in short duration trials. Depression is the condition with the most consistent evidence, but there are discrepancies among the initial studies in the magnitude and nature of effects. In addition to the usual concerns about sample comparability and the reliability of assessment, the therapeutic application of rTMS has particular methodological issues involving sham application and the parameters used.

In any case, the initial studies suggest that rTMS can exert a variety of both short- and long-term behavioral effects. On the optimistic side, they raise the possibility that focal modulation of cortical excitability can have therapeutic properties in psychiatric disorders and that TMS may prove informative about the anatomy and physiology of the neural systems involved in achieving therapeutic effects. At the clinical level, because its adverse effect profile is so benign, rTMS may ultimately offer a less invasive alternative to already established somatic interventions for severe or treatment-resistant illnesses.

In two cases, researchers report on the efficacy and the cognitive side effects of a treatment course of MST. The patients, suffering from a treatment-resistant episode of major depression, reached remission after treatment of depressive symptoms. The treatment was well tolerated and no side effects were reported, especially no subjective cognitive impairments. The cognitive measures assessed in the two studies indicate less severe objective cognitive side effects than those reported after ECT treatment. Verbal and nonverbal learning tasks improved significantly from baseline compared with that on completion of the MST trial. They demonstrate that magnetic seizure induction under general anesthesia is feasible in the treatment of psychiatric disorders. Recent brain imaging studies suggest that manipulations of ECT electrode placement and electrical dosage that are associated with greater efficacy produce more robust functional changes in prefrontal cortex. The enhanced control over both dosage and focality of stimulation that may be achieved with MST offers the capacity to restrict seizure induction to specific cortical areas, such as prefrontal cortex regions, and perhaps improve the efficacy and/or reduce the adverse effects of traditional convulsive treatment. Considerable evidence indicates that depending on the frequency of the magnetic pulses, rTMS may enhance inhibition or excitation in targeted brain regions. This leads to the possibility of selecting specific sites for seizure initiation and other sites as targets of inhibition. This approach offers the possibility of maximizing efficacy while halting seizure spread to further limit adverse effects. Additional studies are certainly needed to confirm the findings of these case reports. If they confirm that MST has significant antidepressant effects while maintaining a benign cognitive side-effect profile, the method could be seen as another major advance in the treatment of refractory major depression possibly complementing or even replacing ECT.

These new data are emerging at a time when there is renewed interest in the entire area of device-based approaches to major depression. ECT, TMS, MST, VNS, and DBS, while all are greatly different in their method of entry into the brain, as well as their invasiveness, nevertheless share in common the use of electrical stimulation of neurons as a route to therapeutic changes. By modulating disease-system pathways through the use of parameter changes (frequency, intensity, pulse width, and total dose), we will better understand the physiology and pathophysiology of the brain.

REFERENCES

1. Lisanby SH, Maddox JH, Prudic J, Devanand DP, Sackeim HA. The effects of electroconvulsive therapy on memory of autobiographical and public events. Arch Gen Psychiat 2000; 57:581–590.
2. Prudic J, Peyser S, Sackeim HA. Subjective memory complaints: a review of patient self-assessment of memory after electroconvulsive therapy. J ECT 2000; 16:121–132.
3. American Psychiatric Association. The Practice of ECT: Recommendations for Treatment, Training and Privileging. 2d ed. Washington, DC: American Psychiatric Press, 2001.
4. Sackeim HA. The cognitive effects of electroconvulsive therapy. In: Moos WH, Gamzu ER, Thal LJ, eds. Cognitive Disorders: Pathophysiology and Treatment. New York: Marcel Dekker, 1992:183–228.
5. Lerer B, Shapira B, Calev A, et al. Antidepressant and cognitive effects of twice- versus three-times-weekly ECT. Am J Psychiat 1995; 152:564–570.
6. McElhiney MC, Moody BJ, Steif L, et al. Autobiographical memory and mood: effects of electroconvulsive therapy. Neuropsychology 1995; 9:501–517.
7. Sackeim HA, Prudic J, Devanand DP, et al. Effects of stimulus intensity and electrode placement on the efficacy and cognitive effects of electroconvulsive therapy. N Engl J Med 1993; 328:839–846.
8. Sackeim HA, Prudic J, Devanand DP, et al. A prospective, randomized, double-blind comparison of bilateral and right unilateral electroconvulsive therapy at different stimulus intensities. Arch Gen Psychiat 2000; 57:425–434.
9. Bailine SH, Rifkin A, Kayne E, et al. Comparison of bifrontal and bitemporal ECT for major depression. Am J Psychiat 2000; 157:121–123.
10. Delva NJ, Brunet D, Hawken ER, Kesteven RM, Lawson JS, Waldron JJ. Electrical dose and seizure threshold: relations to clinical outcome and cognitive effects in bifrontal, bitemporal, and right unilateral ECT. J ECT 2000; 16:361–369.
11. McCall WV, Reboussin DM, Weiner RD, Sackeim HA. Titrated moderately suprathreshold versus fixed high-dose right unilateral electroconvulsive therapy: acute antidepressant and cognitive effects. Arch Gen Psychiat 2000; 57:438–444.
12. Abrams R, Swartz CM, Vedak C. Antidepressant effects of high-dose right unilateral electroconvulsive therapy. Arch Gen Psychiat 1991; 48:746–748.
13. Nobler MS, Sackeim HA, Prohovnik I, et al. Regional cerebral blood flow in mood disorders, III. Treatment and clinical response. Arch Gen Psychiat 1994; 51:884–897.
14. Sackeim HA, Decina P, Prohovnik I, Portnoy S, Kanzler M, Malitz S. Dosage, seizure threshold, and the antidepressant efficacy of electroconvulsive therapy. Ann NY Acad Sci 1986; 462:398–410.

15. Sackeim HA, Portnoy S, Neeley P, Steif BL, Decina P, Malitz S. Cognitive consequences of low-dosage electroconvulsive therapy. Ann NY Acad Sci 1986; 462:326–340.

16. Sackeim HA, Luber B, Katzman GP, et al. The effects of electroconvulsive therapy on quantitative electroencephalograms. Relationship to clinical outcome. Arch Gen Psychiatry 1996; 53:814–824.

17. Sackeim HA, Luber B, Moeller JR, Prudic J, Devanand DP, Nobler MS. Electrophysiological correlates of the adverse cognitive effects of electroconvulsive therapy. J ECT 2000; 16:110–120.

18. Prudic J, Olfson M, Marcus SC, Fuller RB, Sackeim HS. Effectiveness of electroconvulsive therapy in community settings. Biol Psychiat 2004; 55: 301–312.

19. Sackeim HA, Decina P, Kanzler M, Kerr B, Malitz S. Effects of electrode placement on the efficacy of titrated, low-dose ECT. Am J Psychiat 1987; 144:1449–1455.

20. Ng C, Schweitzer I, Alexopoulos, P, et al. Efficacy and cognitive effects of right unilateral electroconvulsive therapy. J ECT 2000; 16:370–379.

21. Awata S, Konno M, Kawashima R, et al. Changes in regional cerebral blood flow abnormalities in late-life depression following response to electroconvulsive therapy. Psychiat Clin Neurosci 2002; 56:31–40.

22. Blumenfeld H, McNally KA, Ostroff RB, Zubal IG. Targeted prefrontal cortical activation with bifrontal ECT. Psychiat Res 2003; 123:165–170.

23. Henry ME, Schmidt ME, Matochik JA, Stoddard EP, Potter WZ. The effects of ECT on brain glucose: a pilot FDG PET study. J ECT 2001; 17:33–40.

24. Nobler MS, Oquendo MA, Kegeles LS, Campbell C, Sackeim HA, Mann JJ. Decreased regional brain metabolism after ECT. Am J Psychiat 2001; 158: 305–308.

25. Perera TD, Luber B, Nobler MS, Prudic J, Anderson C, Sackeim HA. Seizure expression during electroconvulsive therapy: relationships with clinical outcome and cognitive side effects. Neuropsychopharmacology 2004; 29:813–825.

26. Luber B, Nobler MS, Moeller JR, et al. Quantitative EEG during seizures induced by electroconvulsive therapy: relations to treatment modality and clinical features. II. Topographic analyses. J ECT 2000; 16:229–243.

27. Geddes LA, Baker LE. The specific resistance of biological material—a compendium of data for the biomedical engineer and physiologist. Med Biol Eng 1967; 5:271–293.

28. Rush S, Driscoll D. Current distribution in the brain from surface electrodes. Anesthesie Analgesie 1968; 47:717–723.

29. Driscoll DA. An Investigation of a Theoretical Model of the Human Head with Application to Current Flow Calculations and EEG Interpretation. PhD thesis, University of Vermont, 1970.

30. Smitt JW, Wegener CF. On electric convulsive therapy with particular regard to a parietal application of electrodes, controlled by intracerebral voltage measurements. Acta Psychiatr Neurol 1944; 19:529–549.

31. Law SK. Thickness and resistivity variations over the upper surface of the human skull. Brain Topogr 1993; 6:99–109.

32. Hayes KJ. The current path in ECS. Arch Neurol Psychiat 1950; 63:102–109.

33. Weaver L, Williams R, Rush S. Current density in bilateral and unilateral ECT. Biol Psychiat 1976; 11:303–312.
34. Sackeim HA. Magnetic stimulation therapy and ECT. Convuls Ther 1994; 10:255–258.
35. Barker AT, Jalinous R, Freeston IL. Non-invasive magnetic stimulation of human motor cortex. Lancet 1985; 1:1106–1107.
36. Pascual-Leone A, Houser CM, Reese K, et al. Safety of rapid-rate transcranial magnetic stimulation in normal volunteers. Electroencephalogr Clin Neurophysiol 1993; 89:120–130.
37. Maccabee PJ, Eberle L, Amassian VE, Cracco RQ, Rudell A, Jayachandra M. Spatial distribution of the electric field induced in volume by round and figure '8' magnetic coils: relevance to activation of sensory nerve fibers. Electroencephalogr Clin Neurophysiol 1990; 76:131–141.
38. Maccabee PJ, Amassian VE, Eberle LP, et al. Measurement of the electric field induced in inhomogeneous volume conductors by magnetic coils: application to human spinal neurogeometry. Electroencephalogr Clin Neurophysiol 1991; 81:224–237.
39. BrasilNeto JP, Cohen LG, Panizza M, Nilsson J, Roth BJ, Hallett M. Optimal focal transcranial magnetic activation of the human motor cortex: effects of coil orientation, shape of the induced current pulse, and stimulus intensity. J Clin Neurophysiol 1992; 9:132–136.
40. Mills KR, Boniface SJ, Schubert M. Magnetic brain stimulation with a double coil: the importance of coil orientation. Electroencephalogr Clin Neurophysiol 1992; 85:17–21.
41. Epstein CM. Localizing the site of magnetic brain stimulation in humans. Neurology 1990; 40:666–670.
42. Lisanby SH, Luber BL, Schroeder C, et al. rTMS in primates: intracerebral measurement of rTMS and ECS induced voltage in vivo. Electroencephalogr Clin Neurophysiol 1998; 107:79P.
43. Lisanby SH, Luber B, Schroeder C, et al. Intracerebral measurement of rTMS and ECS induced voltage in vivo. Biol Psychiat 1998; 43:100S.
44. Lisanby SH, Moscrip T, Morales O, Luber BL, Schroederv C, Sackeim HA. Neurophysiological characterization of magnetic seizure therapy (MST) in nonhuman primates. Suppl Clin Neurophysiol 2003; 56:81–99.
45. Lisanby SH, Sackeim HA. Transcranial magnetic stimulation and electroconvulsive therapy: similarities and differences. In: Pascual-Leone A, Davey N, Rothwell J, Wassermann E, Puri BK, eds. Handbook of Transcranial Magnetic Stimulation. London: Arnold Publishers, 2002:376–395.
46. George MS, Lisanby SH, Sackeim HA. Transcranial magnetic stimulation: applications in neuropsychiatry. Arch Gen Psychiat 1999; 56:300–311.
47. Lisanby SH, Sackeim HA. TMS in major depression. In: George MS, Belmaker RH, eds. Transcranial Magnetic Stimulation (TMS): Applications in Neuropsychiatry. Washington, DC: American Psychiatric Press, 2000:185–200.
48. Wassermann EM, Lisanby SH. Therapeutic application of repetitive transcranial magnetic stimulation: a review. Clin Neurophysiol 2001; 112: 1367–1377.

49. Burt T, Lisanby SH, Sackeim HA. Neuropsychiatric applications of transcranial magnetic stimulation: a meta analysis. Int J Neuropsychopharmacol 2002; 5:73–103.

50. Mantovani A, Lisanby SH. Applications of transcranial magnetic stimulation to therapy in psychiatry. Psychiatric Times 2004; 21:56–72.

51. Gottesfeld BH, Lesse SM, Herskovitz H. Studies in subconvulsive electric shock therapy effect of varied electrode applications. J Nerv Ment Dis 1944; 99:56–64.

52. Hargrove EA, Bennett AE, Ford FR. The value of subconvulsive electrostimulation in the treatment of some emotional disorders. Am J Psychiat 1953; 109:612–616.

53. Ulett G, Smith K, Gleser G. Evaluation of convulsive and subconvulsive shock therapies utilizing a control group. Am J Psychiat 1956; 112:795–802.

54. George MS, Wassermann EM. Rapid-rate transcranial magnetic stimulation and ECT. Convuls Ther 1994; 10:251–254.

55. Sackeim HA, Devanand DP, Nobler MS. Electroconvulsive therapy. In: Bloom F, Kupfer D, eds. Psychopharmacology: The Fourth Generation of Progress. New York: Raven, 1995:1123–1142.

56. Nobler MS, Sackeim HA. Electroconvulsive therapy: clinical and biological aspects. In: Goodnick PJ, ed. Predictors of Response in Mood Disorders. Washington, DC: American Psychiatric Press, 1996:177–198.

57. Black DW, Winokur G, Nasrallah A. Illness duration and acute response in major depression. Convuls Ther 1989; 5:338–343.

58. Prudic J, Haskett RF, Mulsant B, et al. Resistance to antidepressant medications and short-term clinical response to ECT. Am J Psychiat 1996; 153:985–992.

59. Buchan H, Johnstone E, McPherson K, Palmer RL, Crow TJ, Brandon S. Who benefits from electroconvulsive therapy? Combined results of the Leicester and Northwick Park trials. Br J Psychiat 1992; 160:355–359.

60. Sobin C, Prudic J, Devanand DP, Nobler MS, Sackeim HA. Who responds to electroconvulsive therapy? A comparison of effective and ineffective forms of treatment. Br J Psychiat 1996; 169:322–328.

61. Daly JJ, Prudic J, Devanand DP, et al. ECT in bipolar and unipolar depression: differences in speed of response. Bipolar Disord 2001; 3:95–104.

62. Ottosson JO. Is unilateral nondominant ECT as efficient as bilateral ECT? a new look at the evidence. Convuls Ther 1991; 7:190–200.

63. Post RM, Putnam F, Uhde TW, Weiss SR. Electroconvulsive therapy as an anticonvulsant. Implications for its mechanism of action in affective illness. Ann NY Acad Sci 1986; 462:376–388.

64. Sackeim HA. The anticonvulsant hypothesis of the mechanisms of action of ECT: current status. J ECT 1999; 15:5–26.

65. Weiner RD, Fink M, Hammersley D, Moench L, Sackeim HA, Small I. American Psychiatric Association. In: The Practice of ECT: Recommendations for Treatment, Training and Privileging. Washington, DC: American Psychiatric Press, 1990.

66. Weiner RD, Rogers HJ, Davidson JR, Squire LR. Effects of stimulus parameters on cognitive side effects. Ann NY Acad Sci 1986; 462:315–325.

67. Strömgren LS. Is bilateral ECT ever indicated? Acta Psychiatr Scand 1984; 69:484–490.

68. d'Elia G, Raotma H. Is unilateral ECT less effective than bilateral ECT? Br J Psychiat 1975; 126:83–89.

69. Abrams R. Is unilateral electroconvulsive therapy really the treatment of choice in endogenous depression? Ann NY Acad Sci 1986; 462:50–55.

70. Sackeim HA, Devanand DP, Prudic J. Stimulus intensity, seizure threshold, and seizure duration: impact on the efficacy and safety of electroconvulsive therapy. Psychiatr Clin North Am 1991; 14:803–843.

71. Farah A, McCall WV. Electroconvulsive therapy stimulus dosing: a survey of contemporary practices. Convuls Ther 1993; 9:90–94.

72. Prudic J, Olfson M, Sackeim HA. Electro-convulsive therapy practices in the community. Psychol Med 2001; 31:929–934.

73. Letemendia FJ, Delva NJ, Rodenburg M, et al. Therapeutic advantage of bifrontal electrode placement in ECT. Psychol Med 1993; 23:349–360.

74. Krystal AD, Coffey CE, Weiner RD, Holsinger T. Changes in seizure threshold over the course of electroconvulsive therapy affect therapeutic response and are detected by ictal EEG ratings. J Neuropsychiat Clin Neurosci 1998; 10:178–186.

75. Karlinsky H, Shulman KI. The clinical use of electroconvulsive therapy in old age. J Am Geriatr Soc 1984; 32:183–186.

76. Spiker DG, Stein J, Rich CL. Delusional depression and electroconvulsive therapy: one year later. Convuls Ther 1984; 1:167–172.

77. Aronson TA, Shukla S, Hoff A. Continuation therapy after ECT for delusional depression: a naturalistic study of prophylactic treatments and relapse. Convuls Ther 1987; 3:251–259.

78. Sackeim HA, Prudic J, Devanand DP, Decina P, Kerr B, Malitz S. The impact of medication resistance and continuation pharmacotherapy on relapse following response to electroconvulsive therapy in major depression. J Clin Psychopharmacol 1990; 10:96–104.

79. Malcolm K, Dean J, Rowlands P, Peet M. Antidepressant drug treatment in relation to the use of ECT. J Psychopharmacol 1991; 5:255–258.

80. Grunhaus L, Shipley JE, Eiser A, et al. Shortened REM latency post-ECT is associated with rapid recurrence of depressive symptomatology. Biol Psychiat 1994; 36:214–222.

81. Lemstra A, Leentjens AF, van en Broek WW. Temporary results only in electroconvulsive therapy in therapy-resistant depression: retrospective study. Ned Tijdschr Geneeskd 1996; 140:260–264.

82. O'Leary DA, Lee AS. Seven-year prognosis in depression: mortality and readmission risk in the Nottingham ECT cohort. Br J Psychiat 1996; 169:423–429.

83. Flint AJ, Rifat SL. Two-year outcome of psychotic depression in late life. Am J Psychiat 1998; 155:178–183.

84. Prudic J, Sackeim HA, Devanand DP. Medication resistance and clinical response to electroconvulsive therapy. Psychiat Res 1990; 31:287–296.

85. Shapira B, Gorfine M, Lerer B. A prospective study of lithium continuation therapy in depressed patients who have responded to electroconvulsive therapy. Convuls Ther 1995; 11:80–85.

86. Sackeim HA, Prudic J, Devanand DP, et al. A prospective, randomized, double-blind comparison of bilateral and right unilateral electroconvulsive therapy at different stimulus intensities. Arch Gen Psychiatry 2000; 57: 425–434.

87. Boylan LS, Haskett RF, Mulsant BF, et al. Determinants of seizure threshold in ECT: benzodiazepine use, anesthetic dosage, and other factors. J ECT 2000; 16:3–18.

88. Husain MM, Rush AJ, Fink M, et al. Speed of response and remission in major depressive disorder with acute electroconvulsive therapy (ECT): a Consortium for Research in ECT (CORE) report. J Clin Psychiat 2004; 65:485–491.

89. Trivedi MH, Rush AJ, Pan JY, Carmody TJ. Which depressed patients respond to nefazodone and when? J Clin Psychiatry 2001; 62:158–163.

90. Nierenberg AA, Farabaugh AH, Alpert JE, et al. Timing of onset of antidepressant response with fluoxetine treatment. Am J Psychiat 2000; 157:1423–1428.

91. Koran LM, Gelenberg AJ, Kornstein SG, et al. Sertraline versus imipramine to prevent relapse in chronic depression. J Affect Disord 2001; 65:27–36.

92. Thase ME, Rush AJ, Howland RH, et al. Double-blind switch study of imipramine or sertraline treatment of antidepressant-resistant chronic depression. Arch Gen Psychiat 2002; 59:233–239.

93. Rodger CR, Scott AI, Whalley LJ. Is there a delay in the onset of the antidepressant effect of electroconvulsive therapy? Br J Psychiat 1994; 164:106–109.

94. Segman RH, Shapira B, Gorfine M, Lerer B. Onset and time course of antidepressant action: psychopharmacological implications of a controlled trial of electroconvulsive therapy. Psychopharmacology (Berl) 1995; 119: 440–448.

95. Petrides G, Fink M, Husain MM, et al. ECT remission rates in psychotic versus nonpsychotic depressed patients: a report from CORE. J ECT 2001; 17:244–253.

96. O'Connor MK, Knapp R, Husain M, et al. The influence of age on the response of major depression to electroconvulsive therapy: a C.O.R.E. Report. Am J Geriatr Psychiat 2001; 9:382–390.

97. The U.K. ECT Review Group. Efficacy and safety of electroconvulsive therapy in depressive disorders: a systematic review and meta-analysis. Lancet 2003; 361:799–808.

98. Kho KH, van Vreeswijk MF, Simpson S, Zwinderman AH. A meta-analysis of electroconvulsive therapy efficacy in depression. J ECT 2003; 19:139–147.

99. Pagnin D, de ueiroz V, Pini S, Cassano GB. Efficacy of ECT in depression: a meta-analytic review. J ECT 2004; 20:13–20.

100. Pascual-Leone A, Rubio B, Pallardo F, Catala MD. Beneficial effects of rapid-rate transcranial magnetic stimulation of the left dorsolateral prefrontal cortex in drug resistant depression. Lancet 1996; 248:233–237.

101. Triggs WJ, McCoy KJ, Greer R, et al. Effects of left frontal transcranial magnetic stimulation on depressed mood, cognition, and corticomotor threshold. Biol Psychiat 1999; 45:1440–1446.

102. George MS, Wassermann EM, Kimbrell TA, et al. Mood improvements following daily left prefrontal repetitive transcranial magnetic stimulation in patients with depression: a placebo-controlled crossover trial. Am J Psychiat 1997; 154:1752–1756.

103. Herwig U, Lampe Y, Juengling FD, et al. Add-on rTMS for treatment of depression: a pilot study using stereotaxic coil-navigation according to PET data. J Psychiatr Res 2003; 37:267–275.
104. Pridmore S, Rybak M, Turnier-Shea P, Reid P, Bruno R, Couper D. A naturalistic study of response in melancholia to transcranial magnetic stimulation (TMS). Ger J Psychiat 1999; 2:13–21.
105. Gershon AA, Dannon PN, Grunhaus L. Transcranial magnetic stimulation in the treatment of depression. Am J Psychiat 2003; 160:835–845.
106. Klein E, Kreinin I, Chistyakov A, et al. Therapeutic efficacy of right prefrontal slow repetitive transcranial magnetic stimulation in major depression: a double-blind controlled study. Arch Gen Psychiat 1999; 56:315–320.
107. Kauffmann CD, Cheema MA, Miller BE. Slow right prefrontal transcranial magnetic stimulation as a treatment for medication-resistant depression: a double-blind, placebo-controlled study. Depress Anxiety 2004; 19:59–62.
108. Kimbrell TA, Little JT, Dunn RT, et al. Frequency dependence of antidepressant response to left prefrontal repetitive transcranial magnetic stimulation (rTMS) as a function of baseline cerebral glucose metabolism. Biol Psychiat 1999; 46:1603–1613.
109. Padberg F, Zwanzger P, Thoma H, et al. Repetitive transcranial magnetic stimulation (rTMS) in pharmacotherapy- refractory major depression: comparative study of fast, slow and sham rTMS. Psychiat Res 1999; 88:163–171.
110. George MS, Nahas Z, Molloy M, et al. A controlled trial of daily left prefrontal cortex TMS for treating depression. Biol Psychiat 2000; 48:962–970.
111. Fitzgerald PB, Brown TL, Marston NA, Daskalakis ZJ, De astella A, Kulkarni J. Transcranial magnetic stimulation in the treatment of depression: a double-blind, placebo-controlled trial. Arch Gen Psychiat 2003; 60:1002–1008.
112. Grunhaus L, Dannon PN, Schreiber S, et al. Repetitive transcranial magnetic stimulation is as effective as electroconvulsive therapy in the treatment of non-delusional major depressive disorder: an open study. Biol Psychiat 2000; 47: 314–324.
113. Dannon PN, Dolberg OT, Schreiber S, Grunhaus L. Three and six-month outcome following courses of either ECT or rTMS in a population of severely depressed individuals—preliminary report. Biol Psychiat 2002; 51:687–690.
114. Janicak PG, Dowd SM, Martis B, et al. Repetitive transcranial magnetic stimulation versus electroconvulsive therapy for major depression: preliminary results of a randomised trial. Biol Psychiat 2002; 51:659–667.
115. Holtzheimer PE 3rd, Russo J, Avery DH. A meta-analysis of repetitive transcranial magnetic stimulation in the treatment of depression. Psychopharmacol Bull 2001; 35:149–169.
116. Martin JL, Barbanoj MJ, Schlaepfer TE, et al. Transcranial magnetic stimulation for treating depression. Cochrane Database System Rev 2002; 2:CD003493.
117. Martin JL, Barbanoj MJ, Schlaepfer TE, Thompson E, Perez V, Kulisevsky J. Repetitive transcranial magnetic stimulation for the treatment of depression. Systematic review and meta-analysis. Br J Psychiat 2003; 182:480–491.
118. Wassermann EM, Cohen LG, Flitman SS, Chen R, Hallett M. Seizures in healthy people with repeated 'safe' trains of transcranial magnetic stimuli. Lancet 1996; 347:825–826.

119. Conca A, Konig P, Hausmann A. Transcranial magnetic stimulation induces 'pseudoabsence seizure'. Acta Psychiatr Scand 2000; 101:246–248.

120. Hufnagel A, Elger CE, Durwen HF, Boker DK, Entzian W. Activation of the epileptic focus by transcranial magnetic stimulation of the human brain. Ann Neurol 1990; 27:49–60.

121. Tassinari CA, Michelucci R, Forti A, et al. Transcranial magnetic stimulation in epileptic patients: usefulness and safety. Neurology 1990; 40:1132–1133.

122. Dhuna A, Gates J, Pascual-Leone A. Transcranial magnetic stimulation in patients with epilepsy. Neurology 1991; 41:1067–1071.

123. Hufnagel A, Elger CE. Induction of seizures by transcranial magnetic stimulation in epileptic patients. J Neurol 1991; 238:109–110.

124. Claussen J, Witte OW, Schlaug G, Seitz RJ, Holthausen H, Benecke R. Epileptic seizures triggered directly by focal transcranial magnetic stimulation. Electroencephalogr Clin Neurophysiol 1995; 94:19–25.

125. Wassermann EM. Risk and safety of repetitive transcranial magnetic stimulation: report and suggested guidelines from the International Workshop on the Safety of Repetitive Transcranial Magnetic Stimulation, June 5–7, 1996. Electroencephalogr Clin Neurophysiol 1998; 108:1–16.

126. Lisanby SH, Luber B, Finck AD, Schroeder C, Sackeim HA. Deliberate seizure induction with repetitive transcranial magnetic stimulation. Arch Gen Psychiat 2001; 58:199–200.

127. Lisanby SH, Schlaepfer TE, Fisch HU, Sackeim HA. Magnetic seizure induction for the treatment of major depression. Arch Gen Psychiat 2001; 58:303–305.

128. Kosel M, Frick C, Lisanby SH, Fisch HU, Schlaepfer TE. Magnetic seizure therapy improves mood in refractory major depression. Neuropsychopharmacology 2003; 28:2045–2048.

129. Lisanby SH, Luber B, Schlaepfer TE, Sackeim HA. Safety and feasibility of magnetic seizure therapy (MST) in major depression: randomized within-subject comparison with electroconvulsive therapy. Neuropsychopharmacology 2003; 28:1852–1865.

130. Murray CJ, Lopez AD. Evidence-based health policy—lessons from the Global Burden of Disease Study. Science 1996; 274(5288):740–743.

131. Depression Guideline Panel. Clinical Practice Guideline, Number 5. Depression in Primary Care: Vol. 2. Treatment of Major Depression. AHCPR Publication No. 93–0551, Rockville, MD: U.S. Department of Health and Human Services, Public Health Service, Agency for Healthcare Policy and Research, 1993.

132. Fava M. Diagnosis and definition of treatment-resistant depression. Biol Psychiat 2003; 53(8):649–659.

133. Fava M, Davidson KG. Definition and epidemiology of treatment-resistant depression. Psychiatr Clin North Am 1996; 19(2):179–200.

134. Rush AJ, Ryan ND. Current and emerging therapeutics for depression. In: Davis KL, Charney DS, Coyle JT, Nemeroff CB, eds. Neuropsychopharmacology: The Fifth Generation of Progress. American College of Neuropsychopharmacology, 2002:1081–1095.

135. Simon GE, Lin EH, Katon W, et al. Outcomes of "inadequate" antidepressant treatment. J Gen Intern Med 1995; 10(12):663–670.

136. Greenberg B, Carpenter L, Friehs G, et al. Neurosurgery for Intractable Obsessive-Compulsive Disorder and Depression: Critical Issues Neurosurgery Clinics of North America, 2003.

137. Malizia AL. The place of stereotactic tractotomy in the management of severe psychiatric disorder. In: Katona C, Montgomery S, Sensky T, eds. Psychiatry in Europe: Directions and Developments. London: Gaskell, 1994:85–94.

138. Spiegel EA, Wycis HT, Freed MD, Orchinik MA. The central mechanism of the emotions. Am J Psychiat 1951; 121:426–432.

139. Sachdev P, Sachdev J. Sixty years of psychosurgery: its present status and its future [see comments]. Aust NZ J Psychiat 1997; 31(4):457–464.

140. MacLean PD. The Triune Brain in Evolution: Role in Paleocerebral Functions. New York: Plenum Press, 1990:580–635.

141. MacLean PD, Kral VA. A Triune Concept of the Brain and Behaviour. Toronto: University of Toronto Press, 1973.

142. Marino R, Cosgrove GR. Neurosurgical treatment of neuropsychiatric illness. Psychiatr Clin North Am 1997; 20:933–934.

143. Papez JW. A proposed mechanism of emotion. 1937 1995; 7:103–112.

144. Mindus P. Capsulotomy in Anxiety Disorders: A Multidisciplinary Study [Thesis]. Stockholm, Karolinska Institute, 1991.

145. Goktepe EO, Young LB, Bridges PK. A further review of the results of sterotactic subcaudate tractotomy. Br J Psychiat 1975; 126:270–280.

146. Strom-Olsen R, Carlisle S. Bi-frontal stereotactic tractotomy. A follow-up study of its effects on 210 patients. Br J Psychiat 1971; 118(543):141–154.

147. Hodgkiss AD, Malizia AL, Bartlett JR, Bridges PK. Outcome after the psychosurgical operation of stereotactic subcaudate tractotomy, 1979–1991. J Neuropsychiat Clin Neurosci 1995; 7(2):230–234.

148. Bridges PK, Bartlett JR, Hale AS, Poynton AM, Malizia AL, Hodgkiss AD. Psychosurgery: stereotactic subcaudate tractomy. An indispensable treatment (discussion). Br J Psychiat 1994; 165(5):599–611; 612–593.

149. Whitty CM, Duffield JE, Tow PM. Anterior cingulotomy in the treatment of mental disease. Lancet 1952; 1:475–481.

150. Kullberg G. Differences in effects of capsulotomy and cingulotomy. In: Sweet WH, Obrador WS, Martín-Rodríguez JG, eds. Neurosurgical Treatment in Psychiatry, Pain and Epilepsy. Baltimore: University Park Press, 1977:301–208.

151. Ballantine HT, Jr. Neurosurgery for behavioral disorders. In: Rengachary S, ed. Neurosurgery. Elsevier/North Holland Biomedical Press, 1985:2527–2537.

152. Mayberg HS, Lozano AM, Voon V, et al. Deep brain stimulation for treatment-resistant depression. Neuron 2005; 45:651–660.

153. Greenberg B, Carpernter L, Friehs G, et al. Deep brain stimulation for intractable major depression. In press.

154. Mayberg HS, Brannan SK, Mahurin RK, et al. Regional metabolic effects of fluoxetine in major depression: serial changes and relationship to clinical response. Biol Psychiat 2000; 48:830–843.

155. Seminowicz DA, Mayberg HS, McIntosh AR, et al. Limbic-frontal circuitry in major depression: a path modeling metanalysis. Neuroimage 2004; 22: 409–418.

156. Dougherty DD, Weiss AP, Cosgrove R, et al. Cerebral metabolic correlates as potential predictors of response to cingulotomy for major depression. J Neurosurg 2003; 99:1010–1017.
157. Goldapple K, Segal Z, Garson C, et al. Modulation of cortical-limbic pathways in major depression: treatment specific effects of cognitive behavioral therapy. Arch Gen Psychiat 2004; 61:34–41.
158. Malizia A. Frontal lobes and neurosurgery for psychiatric disorders. J Psychopharmacol 1997; 11:179–187.
159. Mottaghy FM, Keller CE, Gangitano M, et al. Correlation of cerebral blood flow and treatment effects of repetitive transcranial magnetic stimulation in depressed patients. Psychiat Res 2002; 115:1–14.
160. Nobler MS, Oquendo MA, Kegeles LS, et al. Decreased regional brain metabolism after ECT. Am J Psychiat 2001; 158:305–308.
161. Barbas H, Saha S, Rempel-Clower, N, Ghashghaei T. Serial pathways from primate prefrontal cortex to autonomic areas may influence emotional expression. BMC Neurosci 2003; 4:25.
162. Freedman LJ, Insel TR, Smith Y. Subcortical projections of area 25 (subgenual cortex) of the macaque monkey. J Comp Neurol 2000; 421:172–188.
163. Jurgens U, Muller-Preuss P. Convergent projections of different limbic vocalization areas in the squirrel monkey. Exp Brain Res 1977; 29:75–83.
164. Maclean PD. The Triune Brain in Evolution: Role in Paleocerebral Function. New York, NY: Plenum press, 1990.
165. Ongur D, An X, Price JL. Prefrontal cortical projections to the hypothalamus in Macaque Monkeys. J Comp Neurol 1998; 401:480–505.
166. Carmichael ST, Price JL. Connectional networks within the orbital and medial prefrontal cortex of macaque monkeys. J Comp Neurol 1996; 371:179–207.
167. Haber SN. The primate basal ganglia: parallel and integrative networks. J Chem Neuroanat 2003; 26:317–330.
168. Vogt BA, Pandya DN. Cingulate cortex of the rhesus monkey II: cortical afferents. J Comp Neurol 1987; 262:271–289.
169. Foley JO, Dubois F. Quantitative studies of the vagus nerve in the cat, I: the ratio of sensory and motor studies. J Comp Neurol 1937; 67:49–67.
170. Bailey P, Bremer F. A sensory cortical representation of the vagus nerve. J Neurophysiol 1938:405–412.
171. Dell P, Olson R. Projections 'secondaries' mesencephaliques diencephaliques et amygdaliennes des afferences viscerales vagales. C R Soc Biol 1951; 145:1088–1091.
172. Van Bockstaele EJ, Peoples J, Valentino RJ. Anatomic basis for differential regulation of the rostrolateral peri-locus coeruleus region by limbic afferents. Biol Psych 1999; 6:1352–1363.
173. Amar AP, Heck CN, Levy ML, et al. An institutional experience with cervical vagus nerve trunk stimulation for medically refractory epilepsy: rationale, technique and outcome. Neurosurgery 1998; 43:1265–1280.
174. Penry JK, Dean JC. Prevention of intractable partial seizures by intermittent vagal stimulation in humans: preliminary results. Epilepsia 1990; 31(suppl 2):S40–S43.
175. Morris GL, Mueller WM, E01-E05 VNSSG: Long-term treatment with vagus nerve stimulation in patients with refractory epilepsy. Neurology 1999; 53: 1731–1735.

176. Bruce DA. Surgical complications. Epilepsia 1998; 39(suppl 6):92–93.
177. Fisher RS, Handforth A. Reassessment: vagus nerve stimulation for epilepsy: a report of the therapeutics and technology assessment subcommittee for the american academy of neurology. Neurology 1999; 53:666–669.
178. Ben-Menacham E, Manon-Espaillat R, Ristanovic R, et al. Vagus nerve stimulation for treatment of partial seizures, I: a controlled study of effect on seizures. Epilepsia 1994; 35:616–626.
179. Handforth A, DeGiorgio CM, Schachter SC, et al. Vagus nerve stimulation for treatment of partial-onset seizures: a randomized active-control trial. Neurology 1998; 51:48–55.
180. Devous MD, Husain M, Harris TS, et al. The effects of VNS on regional cerebral blood flow in depressed subjects. Biol Psychiat 2002; 1525.
181. Harden CL, Pulver MC, Nikolov B, et al. Effect of vagus nerve stimulation on mood in adult epilepsy patients [abstr]. Neurology 1999; 52(suppl): A238–P03122.
182. Scherrmann J, Hoppe C, Kral T, et al. Vagus nerve stimulation: clinical experience in a large patient series. J Clin Neurophysiol 2001; 18:408–414.
183. Ben-Menacham E, Hamberger A, Hedner T, et al. Effects of vagus nerve stimulation on amino acids and other metabolites in the CSF of patients with partial seizures. Epilepsy Res 1995; 20:221–227.
184. Rush AJ, George MS, Sackeim HA, et al. Vagus Nerve Stimulation (VNS) for treatment resistant depression: a multicenter study. Biol Psych 2000; 47: 276–286.
185. Sackeim HA, Rush AJ, George MS, et al. Vagus nerve stimulation (VNS) for treatment resistant depression: efficacy, side effects, and predictors of outcome. Neuropsychopharmacology 2001; 25:713–728.
186. Sackheim HA, Keilp JG, Rush AJ, et al. The effects of vagus nerve stimulation on cognitive performance in patients with treatment resistant depression. Neuropsychiatry Neuropsychol Behav Neurol 2001; 14:53–62.
187. Marangell LB, Rush AJ, George MS, et al. Vagus nerve stimulation (VNS) for major depressive episodes: One year outcomes. Biol Psychiat 2002; 51:280–287.
188. Martinez JM, MS G, AJ R, et al. Vagus nerve stimulation shows benefits in treatment resistant depression for up to two years. APA 2002 Annual Meeting New Research Program [abstr NR21]. Philadelphia, PA, 2.
189. Rush AJ, Marangell LB, Sackeim HA, et al. Vagus nerve stimulation for treatment-resistant depression: a randomized, controlled acute phase trial. Biol Psych 2005; 58(5):347–354.
190. Rush AJ, Sackeim HA, Marangell LB, et al. Effects of 12 months of vagus nerve stimulation in treatment-resistant depression: a naturalistic study. Biol Psych 2005; 58(5):355–363.
191. George MS, Rush AJ, Marangell LB, et al. A one-year comparison of vagus nerve stimulation with treatment as usual for treatment-resistant depression. Biol Psych 2005; 58(5):364–373.
192. Chae J-H, Nahas Z, Lomarev M, et al. A review of functional neuroimaging studies of vagus nerve stimulation (VNS). J Psych Res 2003; 37:443–455.

193. Bohning DE, Lomarev MP, Denslow S, et al. Feasibility of vagus nerve stimulation-synchronized blood oxygenation level-dependent functional MRI. Invest Radiol 2001; 36:470–479.

194. Nahas Z, Lomarev MP, Denslow S, et al. Synchronized BOLD fMRI. Society of Biological Psychiatry 57th Annual Scientific Meeting and Convention Abstracts. Philadelphia, PA.

195. Carpenter LL, Moreno F, Kling M, et al. Effect of vagus nerve stimulation on cerebrospinal fluid monoamine metabolites, norepinephrine, and gamma-aminobutyric acid concentrations in depressed patients. Biol Psychiat 2004; 56: 418–426.

196. Armitage R, Husain R, Hoffman R, et al. The effects of vagus nerve stimulation on sleep in depression: a preliminary report. J Psychosom Res 1998; 54: 475–482.

197. Nobler MS, Sackheim HA. Electroconvulsive therapy. In: Henn FA, Sartorius N, Helmchen H, Lauter H, eds. Contemporary Psychiatry. Vol. 3. Berlin: Springer, 2001:425–433.

198. Shergill SS, Katona CLE. Pharmacotherapy of affective disorders. In: Henn, Sartorius, Helmchen, Lauter, eds. Contemporary Psychiatry. Vol. 3. Berlin: Springer, 2001:317–336.

199. Franco-Bronson K. The management of treatment-resistant depression in the medically ill. Psychiat Clin N Am 1996; 19:329–350.

200. Snaith RP, Price DJ, Wright JF. Psychiatrists' attitudes to psychosurgery. Proposals for the organization of a psychosurgical service in Yorkshire. Br J Psychiat 1984; 144:293–297.

201. Bingley T, Leksell L, Meyerson BA, et al. Long term results of stereotactic capsulotomy in chronic obsessive-compulsive neurosis. In: Sweet WH, Obrador Alcalde S, Martín-Rodríguez JG, eds. Neurosurgical Treatment in Psychiatry, Pain, and Epilepsy [Proceedings of the Fourth World Congress of Psychiatric Surgery, Sep. 7–10, 1975, Madrid, Spain]. Baltimore: University Park Press, 1977:287.

202. Rauch SL, Greenberg BD, Cosgrove GR. Neurosurgical treatments and deep brain stimulation. In: Sadock VA, ed. Kaplan & Sadock's Comprehensive Textbook of Psychiatry/VIII 32 1/19/05. Philadelphia: Lippincott Williams & Wilkins. In press.

203. Breit S, Schulz JB, Benabid AL. Deep brain stimulation. Cell Tissue Res 2004:19.

204. Greenberg BD, Price LH, Rauch SL, et al. Neurosurgery for intractable obsessive-compulsive disorder and depression: critical issues. Neurosurg Clin N Am 2003; 14(2):199–212.

205. Elger G, Hoppe C, Falkai P, Rush AJ, Elger CE. Vagus nerve stimulation is associated with mood improvements in epilepsy patients. Epilepsy Res 2000; 42:203–210.

206. Schachter SC, Saper CB. Vagus nerve stimulation (progress in epilepsy researsch). Epilepsia 1998; 39:677–686.

207. Fulton.

208. Ballantine.

11

Medication and Psychotherapy Options and Strategies: The Future

Timothy J. Petersen and George I. Papakostas
*Massachusetts General Hospital/Harvard Medical School,
Boston, Massachusetts, U.S.A.*

Thomas L. Schwartz
*Department of Psychiatry, SUNY Upstate Medical University,
Syracuse, New York, U.S.A.*

INTRODUCTION

Despite the significant advances that have been made during the last several decades, much remains to be learned about pharmacotherapy and talk therapy treatments for major depressive disorder (MDD). We stand at a point of potentially massive change in our understanding of what are the most effective tools in our psychotherapeutic and pharmacotherapeutic armamentarium, and what are the most effective ways to utilize these tools. Several domains that represent the most promising and compelling areas of MDD-focused research are highlighted in the following section.

COMBINING PSYCHOTHERAPY AND ANTIDEPRESSANT MEDICATIONS: SEQUENTIAL APPLICATION

As described in the previous chapter there is mixed evidence as to whether antidepressant and psychotherapy combination treatment during the acute illness phase actually offers greater efficacy than either modality alone.

Factors that account for the mixed nature of this evidence include the patient characteristics of the given study sample, dosing of both antidepressant and psychotherapy treatments, study therapist experience level, and research site (e.g., primary vs. specialty care). Several studies published during the last 10 years suggest that using antidepressant medication during the acute phase of treatment, followed by the introduction of evidence-based psychotherapy, may result in a better long-term illness course when compared with the traditional acute phase antidepressant or psychotherapy combination treatment. This sequential strategy also potentially offers the therapist more focused treatment targets, in part because the patient has already experienced relief from acute phase symptoms. Whether this strategy will prove to be more effective than more traditional strategies is unknown. Studies with large sample sizes, well-characterized patients, and easily replicable therapies are needed to draw firm conclusions.

Stemming from the investigation of a sequential treatment approach is an exciting development pertaining to modification of the traditional cognitive-behavioral therapy (CBT) treatment model. In particular, the work of G.A. Fava, in developing well-being therapy, shows great promise in both being a better fit for the clinical presentation of patients' post acute phase treatment and potentially quite effective in reducing risk for relapse and recurrence. Again, larger sample sizes and broader research settings are needed to extend this line of research.

CONCEPTUAL SHIFT FROM COGNITIVE CONTENT TO COGNITIVE PROCESS

One of the fundamental tenets of the mechanisms by which cognitive-based psychotherapies work is that a depressed person experiences thoughts that contain depressive themes. These thoughts are a primary focus of such treatments, and successful modification of content is supposed to lead to affective change. However, in recent years, two new psychotherapies have been pioneered, both of which challenge the notion that thought content change is necessary for depressive symptoms to improve. The first new therapy is mindfulness-based cognitive therapy (MBCT), a group psychotherapy developed by Segal and Teasdale. Significantly informed by the work of Jon Kabat Zinn, MBCT posits that the way in which patients relate to negative thoughts, rather than alteration of content, is key to effectively treating depressive symptoms. In this treatment, patients are taught to decenter themselves from their negative thoughts and regard thoughts as cognitive events rather than necessary truths. The very limited number of empirical studies that have been conducted suggest that this treatment may be effective in improving long-term illness course, but the jury is still out as a more definitive trial has just gotten underway. The second such treatment is acceptance and commitment therapy (ACT), developed by Steven Hayes and colleagues (1). This treatment emphasizes the reduction of avoidant behavior by increasing a patient's awareness of thoughts, feelings, memories, and physical sensations that have been feared and avoided. Patients learn to recontextualize and accept internal events, develop greater clarity about personal values, and commit to needed behavior change. ACT is a clearly different method than MBCT, but still retains the shift from a focus on thought content alteration to an emphasis on the degree of importance that a patient places on his or her internal state.

These two new schools of therapy represent a distinct paradigm shift in the field and potentially could revolutionize the assumptions upon which evidence-based psychotherapy for depression are based. Practitioners and consumers alike should pay close attention to results of ongoing, larger clinical trials involving these two forms of psychotherapy.

DISMANTLING AND INTEGRATING TREATMENTS

Neil Jacobson and colleagues, in their groundbreaking study that compared the efficacy of the components of CBT versus the entire CBT-manualized treatment package, found that the entire package did not offer any incremental benefit. This was a novel idea, and certainly counter to the original treatment methods as described by Beck and colleagues. It could be that the behavioral activation component of CBT is just as effective as delivering the entire treatment package, but more research is needed to confirm this. Similarly, treatment that only includes the cognitive components of CBT is worth future study as well. Distilling treatments into their most and least effective components is a worthy endeavor, and could decrease the costs of treatments and change the way in which practitioners are trained.

As we know from Garfield and Bergin's seminal text, most psychologists in practice identify themselves as practicing "eclectic" therapy. Thus, it is the minority of psychologists on the front line that adhere to only one school of thought and practice. In parallel with efforts to dismantle known psychotherapeutic treatments, other recent developments have blended conceptualization and methods of existing psychotherapies. Perhaps the best example is McCullough's recent development of the cognitive behavioral analysis system of psychotherapy (CBASP), which represents a creative mix of cognitive, interpersonal, developmental, and psychodynamic techniques. Although designed specifically to address the needs of chronically depressed patients, the integration of techniques drawn from different schools into a formal system of psychotherapy is another promising avenue for further research. A larger-scale CBASP study is currently underway and results will help shape future practice in this domain.

INTERPERSONAL PSYCHOTHERAPY

Interpersonal psychotherapy (IPT) is less widely practiced than CBT for a variety of reasons. One reason may be that IPT has a less "cookbook" feel to it than CBT, and because of this, potentially less immediate appeal to practitioners seeking out specialized or advanced training. A second reason may be that IPT has historically been closely connected to biological psychiatry in that depression is viewed, in collaboration with the patient, as a medical illness. It is possible that some psychologists have reacted to this by more closely aligning themselves with CBT and other schools of psychotherapy. Despite this, it is important for efforts to be made to further test IPT as a treatment to help prevent relapse and recurrence, and also to determine what are the "active ingredients" of IPT. For this reason, it would be helpful to conduct dismantling studies with IPT. Long-term IPT studies have been promising and IPT utilizing fewer visits are showing good effectiveness as well.

SPECIALIZED POPULATIONS

With greater recognition of the prevalence of depression across a spectrum of medical disorders, the demand to understand how to appropriately modify evidence-based treatments has grown. Efforts have been made to customize CBT and IPT to fit the needs of specialized populations such as HIV-positive patients, postpartum women, elderly patients, Parkinson's patients, and multiple sclerosis patients. However, much work remains to be done in understanding the unique needs of patient groups that vary along the lines of age, medical status, ethnicity, etc.

DISSEMINATION OF EVIDENCE-BASED TREATMENTS

A great challenge facing all health care fields is translating research findings to frontline clinical practice. For example, it is not uncommon for a rural psychologist to have limited access to postgraduate training to keep up to date with current best practices. For many such practitioners, work demands and logistical constraints make it impossible to attend conferences that are typical venues for dissemination of the latest research findings and novel clinical developments. The Association for the Advancement of Behavior and Cognitive Therapies (AABCT), which many regard as the premier organization for practitioners of evidence-based psychotherapeutic treatments for depression, recently reported that most attendees at its annual meeting describe their primary affiliation as an academic research setting. Clearly those most in need of access to research findings and continuing education are not attending this annual meeting in great numbers. Organizations such as AABCT should make outreach efforts to increase attendance of these practitioners and thereby increase dissemination of this knowledge base.

Another important area to consider is decreasing waiting time between submission of a scientific paper for review and publication. It is not unheard of for the time between submission and print to well exceed one year. To the extent possible, journals with high citation impact should seek ways to streamline this process so that members of the profession have access to important research findings in as timely a manner as possible.

A final area to consider is expansion of the training requirements of all clinical mental health training programs to include greater emphasis on attainment of competence in evidence-based psychotherapeutic treatments for MDD. The obvious starting point for this expansion is the increased effort put in by the American Psychiatric Association and the American Association of Directors of Psychiatric Residency Training to make their accreditation process more stringent.

PSYCHODYNAMIC TREATMENT MODELS: WHAT'S NEXT?

Despite a high degree of intuitive appeal and clinical efficacy in some patients, psychodynamic therapies have lost significant favor as a primary modality for treatment of MDD. In some senses, these therapies have suffered due to their proponents' lack of attention to the completion of rigorous, large-scale studies to establish efficacy. Part of the problem lies in just how to manualize such a treatment and then how to measure therapist competence and adherence. A considerable amount of research work is underway to investigate the therapy process variables that may account for the efficacy of such interventions. This is an intellectually compelling question, but seems to be a secondary research question to be answered. Efforts would be better placed in establishing a network to conduct large-scale trials using a treatment manual that captures what is being delivered in real-world practice settings. In this way, how psychodynamic psychotherapy fits into our menu of treatments for depression will begin to be elucidated.

BALANCING EFFECTIVENESS AND EFFICACY RESEARCH

Critics of the traditional randomized controlled trial design (efficacy research) point out that patient samples used for such studies are not generalizable. To an extent this is true, but to really advance the field, a balance needs to be achieved between the limitations of both efficacy trial designs and the newer effectiveness trial model. The advantage of the effectiveness design is that few exclusion criteria are utilized and that the study takes place in the real-world venues (e.g., primary care settings). Because of this, patient samples derived from effectiveness research are more representative of the general population of interest (e.g., depressed outpatients). However, along with these advantages comes a decrease in our ability to determine what was responsible for symptom change. Use of a hybrid design, retaining the strengths of both models, is a step in the right direction.

IMPROVING DETECTION OF MDD

Almost every trained clinician can quote the nine symptoms of MDD. However, the diagnosis may be missed given the variability and fluctuation of symptoms as noted in previous chapters. The use of both clinician- and patient-rated scales should continue to be studied because it may allow better detection and more aggressive treatment to full remission of symptoms. Rating scales may also be employed to detect comorbidity, which is often a key component to resistant MDD. Particularly in the face of busy clinical practices, direct patient entry of scales and information into practice software or web-based applications may allow for real-time data collection, scoring, and documentation. These services exist regionally and often can be modified as per clinician preferences. Our practice utilizes ClinicTracker software by J.A.G. Products, LLC that allows us to streamline data collection for both clinical trials and regular clinic visits. This is a paperless system where patients interact with a laptop computer just prior to their visits. Other ideas include the use of a central website and web-based electronic medical record. These often employ data fields that may be used to track patient outcomes. Also, a web-based system may allow patients to log on from home and complete scales, in case patients felt they were in an impending relapse. Poor scores could be flagged and clinicians alerted. Again, the goal of any of these techniques is to drive more aggressive MDD treatment.

USE OF TARGET SYMPTOM PROBLEM LISTS AND PHARMACODYNAMIC THEORY

This theory is mostly due to the work of Stephen M. Stahl, who has spent much time and work pioneering the idea that the key symptoms, which overlap in several categorical mental disorders, i.e., inability to focus in MDD, generalized anxiety, and attention deficit disorder, may have a unifying pathological set of dysfunctional neurocircuits. If one cannot focus, then the noradrenergic system may be functioning poorly and that facilitating norepinephrine activity may alleviate the key symptom of inattention in any of these disorders. In fact, noradrenergic medications are approved by the Food and Drug Administration (FDA) to treat these categorical illnesses. This would support the theory of rational polypharmacy or pharmacodynamic theory where a psychopharmacologist might not only pick medication based on categorical FDA approvals but also based upon the pharmacodynamic profile of the individual agent that is purported to fix the underlying circuit which will ultimately promote resolution of a particular MDD symptom. This type of advanced pharmacotherapy could promote better symptom resolution and the same practices may allow clinicians to combine medications for better tolerability.

MANUALIZATION OF PSYCHOPHARMACOPSYCHOTHERAPY

In the current outpatient treatment milieu where the splitting of psychophar-macotherapy and psychotherapy is commonplace, many psychopharmacolo-gists use FDA approvals and symptom-based approaches to treat MDD patients. Given the high noncompliance rates with psychotropics and office visits, it would make intuitive sense to see if the true combination of pharma-cotherapy and psychotherapy in a single sitting is truly effective in the management of the MDD patient. Dewan and colleagues have studied and suggested that combined medication and psychotherapy techniques in single office visits may be a more cost-effective way of treating MDD patient; but there is little outcome-based evidence to support this new versus split prac-tice. It would make intuitive sense to manualize a form of psychotherapy (supportive–directive) that can be easily and efficiently applied in a typical medication management session, and then study these outcomes to determine if there is reasonable efficacy and improvement in compliance.

TECHNOLOGY

As discussed in previous chapters, the advent of neuroimaging and neuroge-netics is both fascinating and confusing. Both the employed techniques and the data collected are in their infancy and are often conflicting in nature. However, great strides in the use of these techniques occur frequently. The ability to predict treatment response and choose the right modality first should be pivotal in treating the MDD patient. Similar to the pharmaco-dynamic theory used to support rational polypharmacy to alleviate particu-lar externally valid, phenotypic MDD symptoms, simple imaging or genetic testing may be able to tell us more quickly which internal neural systems are malfunctioning. Based on this data our initial treatment could be the ultimate treatment. This could alleviate many weeks of continued patient suffering because multiple, "best guess" drug trials will not be needed.

PHARMACOTHERAPY

Since the serendipitous discovery of the monoamine oxidase inhibitors in the 1950s and the tricyclic antidepressants in the 1960s, several specific pharma-cotherapies have been developed for the treatment of MDD (XGIP, MF chapter). Despite these advances, a significant proportion of patients who are treated for MDD remain symptomatic.

Clearly, greater research efforts are needed to further refine the treat-ment of MDD. Such efforts can be directed in one of three major areas: (i) the development of novel pharmacotherapies, (ii) the refining of existing pharmacotherapies and pharmacotherapeutic strategies, and (iii) the identifi-cation of biologic as well as clinical factors that may help to define a subgroup of MDD patients who are particularly responsive to certain treatments.

The Development of Novel Pharmacotherapies

So far, all pharmacotherapies approved for the treatment of MDD in the United States exclusively focus on the direct manipulation of the monoaminergic neurotransmitter systems, most of which possess either serotonergic or noradrenergic, or combined serotonergic and noradrenergic activity. Over the course of the past ten years, there have been several agents with nonmonoaminergic (direct) mechanisms of action that have also been as potentially promising in the development of novel treatments for MDD. Such agents have included neurokinin-1–receptor antagonists, *N*-methyl-D-aspartate–receptor antagonists, corticotrophin-receptor antagonists, corticosteroid-receptor antagonists, and phosphodiesterase inhibitors, as well as natural remedies including hypericum perforatum, chromium picolinate, and l-acetylcarnitine. Unfortunately, to date, such leads have failed to result in the development and approval of novel antidepressant treatments. As a result, almost all contemporary pharmacotherapies available for the treatment of MDD continue to be based, more or less, on the same mechanism of action as those agents we first stumbled upon in the middle of the past century. Clearly, greater priority and emphasis needs to be placed on enhancing our ability to identify agents early on in preclinical phases of development, which have the potential of being developed as safer and more effective treatments for MDD than those presently available. Identifying and refining biological correlates of clinical improvement in MDD, such as those discussed in previous chapters, can greatly accelerate this process.

Refining Existing Pharmacotherapies and Pharmacotherapeutic Strategies

Here too, there have been several interesting leads as discussed previously. A number of studies, for example, suggest better outcome during the short-term treatment of MDD for patients treated with a combination of two antidepressant agents such as 5-hydroxytryptamine 2 antagonists or α-2 antagonists (i.e., mirtazapine or mianserin) or the tricyclic antidepressant desipramine with the selective serotonin reuptake inhibitors (SSRIs), or a combination of standard antidepressants with other agents including the benzodiazepines, *S*-adenosyl-l-methionine, folate, zinc, the calcium channel blocker nimodipine (for vascular depression), or the steroid synthesis inhibitor metyrapone. However, experience from double-blind, placebo-controlled trials is limited, with the majority of double-blind studies focusing on older agents with differing effectiveness, including lithium, triiodothyronine, and pindolol. For instance, a number of promising adjunctive pharmacotherapeutic strategies including modafinil, the atypical antipsychotic agents, and dopaminergic agents such as bupropion, pramipexole, or ropinirole, and the psychostimulants have yet to be subject to controlled investigation while other leads have yet to be replicated. Clearly, focusing our clinical practice on choosing a "good enough" initial treatment strategy for the majority of MDD patients, and then elaborating on refining treatment approaches for non- or incomplete responders may unnecessarily prolong the treatment of many MDD patients. More studies are needed to examine whether we can achieve better outcomes from the onset of treatment by combining one or several of the multitude of agents currently available.

The Identification of Factors to Define a Particularly Responsive MDD Subgroup

A number of studies have focused on several biologic markers including genetic factors, neuroimaging factors, and neurophysiologic factors that predict a greater likelihood of poorer response to standard antidepressant treatment (mostly the SSRIs). Similarly, an increasing number of reports suggest that certain symptoms or symptom clusters including anxiety (1), insomnia (2), sleepiness or fatigue (3), and painful symptoms of depression (4) may be more responsive to treatment with certain agents. However, to date, prospective, double-blind, randomized studies focusing on whether the presence of these biologic markers or symptom clusters at baseline in MDD patients confers an increased likelihood of achieving remission of the disorder during treatment with one versus another pharmacotherapeutic agent have yet to be published. Here too, there is an opportunity to further refine the standard of care in MDD by combining existing treatments with predictors of outcome. Therefore, such studies should also become a priority.

CONCLUSIONS

Over the last several decades, great strides have been made in our understanding of which psychotherapies are most effective for treating depression. We now have two primary evidence-based psychotherapies (CBT and IPT) that are increasingly being practiced by mental health professionals throughout the world. Despite this progress, a multitude of questions remains unanswered. These include how to best apply these treatments, whether some of the more recently developed treatments that represent significant paradigm shifts will prove efficacious in larger studies, how to best adapt our treatments to patients with significant comorbidities, what aspects of depression are important to consider in selecting treatments, and how evidence-based treatments can best be disseminated to front line treatment settings. Answers to these questions will help shape the field for the coming decades.

In parallel, we have many of the same questions and issues in regard to pharmacotherapy. There appears to be a pipeline dedicated to facilitating monoamine transmission and very few treatments that are "out of the box." With available resources, we must get better at providing safer, more aggressive treatment for the MDD patient. This should include early and better detection of depression with rating scales and improved training, use of imaging and genetics, and finally rational polypharmacy to promote better effectiveness and tolerability.

BIBLIOGRAPHY

Brannan SK, Mallinckrodt CH, Brown EB, Wohlreich MM, Watkin JG, Schatzberg AF. Duloxetine 60 mg once-daily in the treatment of painful physical symptoms in patients with major depressive disorder. J Psychiat Res 2005; 39(1):43–53.

Fava M, Entsuah R, Rummala R. Venlafaxine versus SSRIs and placebo in the treatment of anxious depression. 158th Annual Meeting of the American Psychiatric Association, Atlanta, Georgia, 2004.

Hayes SC, Strosahl KD, Wilson KG. Acceptance and commitment therapy: an experiential approach to behavior change (paperback), Guilford Press, 1999.

Papakostas GI, Donahue RM, Nierenberg AA, Nutt DJ, Fava M. Resolution of sleepiness and fatigue in the treatment of major depressive disorder: a comparison of bupropion and the selective serotonin reuptake inhibitors. 45th Annual Meeting of the American College of Neuropsychopharmacology, Waikokoa, Hawaii, 2005.

Papakostas GI, Fava M. Monoamine-based pharmacotherapy. In: Licinio J, ed. Biology of Depression: From Novel Insights to Therapeutic Strategies. 1st ed. Weinheim: Wiley-VCH Verlag, 2005:87–140.

Winokur A, Baker RA, Simmons JH, Jansen WT, Jan Schutte A. Comparative sleep improving effects of mirtazapine versus SSRIs: a meta-analysis of individual patient data. 8th World Congress of Biological Psychiatry, Vienna, Austria, 2005.

Index